Bargaining for Life

D0171314

University of Pennsylvania Press
Studies in Health, Illness, and Caregiving in America
Joan E. Lynaugh, General Editor

A complete listing of the volumes in this series appears in the back of this book.

Bargaining for Life

A Social History of Tuberculosis, 1876–1938

Barbara Bates

University of Pennsylvania Press
Philadelphia

Library of Congress Cataloging-in-Publication Data
Bates, Barbara, 1928–
    Bargaining for life : a social history of tuberculosis, 1876–1938
    Barbara Bates.
        p.   cm. — (Studies in health, illness, and caregiving in America)
    Includes bibliographical references and index.
    ISBN 0-8122-3120-1 (cloth). — ISBN 0-8122-1367-X (pbk.)
    1. Tuberculosis—Pennsylvania—History.   I. Title.   II. Series.
    [DNLM: 1. Tuberculosis—history—United States.   WF 11 AA1 B3b]
RC309.P4B38   1992
614.5′42′09748—dc20
DNLM/DLC
for Library of Congress   91-40040
                                                                    CIP

To

MARY BACHMAN CLARK

whose life and stories
introduced me
to a wider world

Contents

Part III. Adjustments and Compromise, 1914–1938

Part IV. A Retrospective View

Illustrations

GRAPHS

TABLE

Acknowledgments

Writing history incurs many debts and I acknowledge them happily. Several people shared with me their personal knowledge and photographs or suggested additional sources: Mary S. Bracken, Bruce Darney, Clayton Fox, Edward M. Keck, Mr. and Mrs. Albert Maier, Maxim and Jean Maranuk, Kathryn Riordan, and Walter Ziegler.

Fellow students and colleagues gave me valuable references and other useful leads: Lillian Brunner, Gail Farr, Bruce Lewenstein, Edward Morman, and others whom I may have inadvertently overlooked.

Then there are those who staffed the libraries and archives and who suggested, found, carried, and retrieved (often over and over again) the indispensable volumes. I especially appreciate the help of Jean Carr at the College of Physicians of Philadelphia, Dr. Anthony Zito and Sr. Anne Crowley at Catholic University, Norma Harberger at Episcopal Community Services, and David Weinberg at the Center for the Study of the History of Nursing, University of Pennsylvania.

Special thanks go to the people who read the manuscript, criticized it, made suggestions, and gave encouragement. Those who read one or two chapters in their early versions include Lee Cassanelli, Vanessa Gamble, Gloria Hagopian, Janet Meininger, Katherine Ott, Carroll Smith-Rosenberg, Rosemary Stevens, and Meryn Stuart. Most gracious of all were those who read the entire book in one of its several "almost final" forms: Janet Golden, Mathy Mezey, Nancy Tomes, Charles Rosenberg, and Joan Lynaugh. It was Charles Rosenberg who first told me of the Flick papers, thus changing the course of my life. I would also like to thank him for his subsequent guidance, his generosity, and his example. Joan Lynaugh made an additional contribution. Occasionally, over more than a decade, she persuaded me to think about something else.

Mary Norris skillfully edited a late version of the text, and Barbara Jones, the copyeditor for the University of Pennsylvania Press, contributed further to the final manuscript. Yvonne Keck Holman, Alternative Productions, created the graphs and map.

Introduction

Throughout the nineteenth century, tuberculosis (or consumption as it was then called) was the most common cause of death in the United States, as in much of western Europe. Year after year, the disease sapped the strength of its victims and took its deadly toll of lives. Although individual men and women tried to escape its effects and were helped in their efforts by caretakers, there was no public outcry, no social campaign to fight the disease. Consumption developed gradually and mysteriously; it seemed beyond the reach of human control.

In the last decades of the nineteenth century, however, there emerged a new optimism about the disease and more aggressive attempts to deal with it. In 1882, Robert Koch discovered the tubercle bacillus, the bacterial cause of tuberculosis, and in 1885 Edward L. Trudeau, encouraged by the results of institutional treatment in Europe, opened the first successful sanatorium in the United States. As physicians and social leaders gradually recognized that consumption was infectious and not necessarily hopeless, they began to promulgate new laws, educational programs, and institutions with which to combat it. Two exhilarating convictions became the driving force for sanatoriums and hospitals. First, the disease was preventable. By controlling the patients' behavior and by separating the afflicted from their families and from the rest of society, the spread of tuberculous infection could be stopped. Second, consumption was curable, at least if detected soon enough. If patients could be persuaded to live properly—an intermediate objective that also made institutionalization desirable—they could regain their health and once again become productive members of their communities.

Historians of this subject have traditionally focused on either the medical knowledge of tuberculosis, as it developed over the centuries, or on the social movement to control the disease. The protagonists in these histories are usually physicians or social reformers who led the campaign against tuberculosis. When patients appear in these stories at all, their role is typically passive: as beneficiaries of advancing knowledge and an expanding system of care or, more recently, as victims of popular fear and institutional segregation. This view is partly due to traditional assumptions about historical forces and leadership and partly due to the scarcity of primary sources with which to examine the experiences and motivations of the patients, their families, and others who helped to take care of the sick. As a result, only part of the story has been told.

A previously unexplored collection of letters, preserved by Dr. Lawrence F. Flick and his family, helps to correct this deficiency. It widens the historical view to include not just tuberculosis as a disease but also the chronically ill people afflicted by it, not just the social campaign against tuberculosis but also the interactions of patients and their caretakers, and not just the leaders of the movement but also the families, friends, clergymen, superintendents of institutions, nurses, and a variety of physicians— all with their own reasons to participate in the care of the tuberculous. In this broader view, the patients, together with their families and other advocates, emerge as fascinating and varied men and women and as protagonists in their own right, bargaining with their caretakers, helping to shape and expand the institutions, and affecting the outcomes of the tuberculosis campaign.

All these men and women are in the foreground of this study. In the background are the rise of scientific medicine, the growth of health-related institutions and voluntary organizations, the development of trained nursing, the conservative concerns about coddling the poor and creating dependency, the growing calls upon governments to provide medical care, and a highly competitive society in which opportunity was stratified by class, race, and gender. By examining this microcosm, I believe, we can see the interplay among individual experience, family relationships, professional behaviors and interests, scientific knowledge, values, politics, and social structure.

My study began in the late 1970s with four naively simple questions. What was it like to have tuberculosis? Who took care of the patients? What characterized the relationships among the patients, their families, and their other caretakers? How did the answers to these questions change during the nineteenth and twentieth centuries? As the work progressed, other questions emerged. What induced men and women to undertake the hazardous and discouraging job of caring for consumptives? What implicit bargains were involved in the work? How did institutions mediate these relationships? How did medical knowledge, cultural values, and local politics affect health-related policies and the caretaking process? How did the structure of society, including class, gender, and race, influence them? How and why did caretakers and officials of state and local governments favor the care of curable patients over the care of the chronically and hopelessly ill? What were the results of the antituberculosis campaign and how did they differ from those intended by its leaders? I hope that the answers to these questions shed some light on how society has dealt—and may still deal— with the problems of chronic illness and prolonged dependency.

The sixty-two years encompassed by this study witnessed profound changes. Consumption, which in the nineteenth century had been attributed to a constitutional weakness and unhealthful habits or surroundings, became a communicable disease caused by a specific microorganism. Diagnostic methods improved. Treatment changed from the mere amelioration of symptoms, adjustment of bodily processes, and choice of a new environment to a hygienic regimen of fresh air, nutritious food, and supervised rest and exercise. In the 1920s and 1930s, surgical treatment seemed to offer additional hope. Care of the sick shifted in part from homes to institutions and from families or friends to physicians and nurses. The cost of care, once the burden of families and perhaps of a local almshouse, was lightened by charity and, increasingly, by government.

The men and women who created and built the new institutions linked them to one or more societal missions—overarching goals that served to justify the work and attract support for it. These missions included the salvation of souls, the prevention of disease, the cure of the sick, and the eradication of tuberculosis through research.

Within the institutions, patients and caretakers sought their own rewards. Patients wanted to live longer, to get personal care, treatment, and basic subsistence, and at times to protect their families from infection or to escape conditions at home. They paid in various ways, including gratitude, obedience, relinquishment of personal pleasures and freedom, loneliness, and money. When they lacked money, they sometimes paid with their labor and ultimately, if their families agreed in advance to an autopsy, with their bodies. Caretakers earned training, knowledge, clinical experience, advancement in their careers, a gratifying sense of service to others or to God, and a modest amount of money.

Vast expenditures and effort went into building the new system of care for the tuberculous, but there were flaws in the plan. Physicians and nurses overestimated their ability to educate patients and thus make them noninfectious to others. Physicians could not usually identify and select for treatment the patients with truly early disease—those most likely to re-

cover. For various reasons, men and women often delayed institutionalization until they had advanced or even hopeless disease. For these people, as
for many others, physicians had no cure. Although the tuberculosis movement had promoted sanatoriums with curative goals, most of the patients
there were chronically ill and dependent. Tuberculous men and women
hoped to recover, but they also used the institutions to meet their basic
needs. Many physicians and other leaders had long been reluctant to encourage dependency, but they helped to create a system that accepted it.
Institutional life was usually not attractive enough, however, to retain
patients throughout their terminal illness. Most tuberculous patients continued to die at home, thus exposing others to infection at a particularly
dangerous stage of the disease.

This study focuses primarily on Philadelphia and eastern Pennsylvania,
where Dr. Flick and his colleagues worked. Flick was arguably the most
innovative of all the leaders in the nation's campaign against tuberculosis.
Along with two New Yorkers—Edward L. Trudeau, founder of the Adirondack Cottage Sanitarium, and Hermann M. Biggs, a public health
official—he is typically cited as one of the three U.S. physicians who had
the greatest impact on the movement. He founded the Pennsylvania Society for the Prevention of Tuberculosis, the first voluntary organization of
its kind; he started and directed Pennsylvania's first successful sanatorium;
he planned and directed a research institute for the study, prevention, and
treatment of tuberculosis; he developed two nursing schools for consumptive women; and he treated a large number of private patients. He dealt
with the rich and the poor, with the powerful and the helpless, with the sick
and their families, and with diverse men and women who had interests in
the welfare of individual patients and in the developing system of care.
With no discernible effort to distort or conceal, he also saved his correspondence with these people; he felt confident that the record would speak for
itself.

The nature of this correspondence both limits and enlarges the gener-
alizability of a study that uses it. The history is chiefly Northeastern and
based in an urban area; its flavor would be different if it focused on
Colorado Springs or another such mountainous area that catered to consumptives. Only a major city could have supported the variety of approaches to the care of tuberculous patients that Philadelphians developed.
The research institute that Flick founded in 1903 was unique, and Pennsylvania's expansive state system of care made it somewhat atypical among its
counterparts in the United States. Nevertheless, most of the ideas, goals,

and methods described in this story resembled those in other regions where tuberculosis was a major problem. The unusual multiplicity of Flick's activities widens the historic view and, most important, the variety of men and women whose lives are illuminated by the correspondence deepens our understanding.

The care of chronically ill consumptives developed in ways that differed from the hospital care of acutely ill or injured people. Tuberculosis institutions began later, they were less likely to be urban, and technical advances in medicine and surgery had much less impact. Sanatoriums had more in common with nineteenth-century health resorts and hydropathic institutions than with modern hospitals. Both the segregation of patients and the therapeutic regimen in sanatoriums echoed the moral therapy of nineteenth-century insane asylums. Two additional features that distinguished the care of the tuberculous were the fear of infection and the chronicity of the illness. The impact on family and social relations was accordingly magnified.

The bracketing dates of this study have meaning. In 1876 the Philadelphia Protestant Episcopal City Mission founded the first organization in the region that devoted its efforts specifically to consumptives; in 1938 Flick died. By the time of Flick's death, all the major new methods of fighting the disease were firmly in place and mortality rates had diminished remarkably. Effective chemotherapy, however, was still a decade or more away.

Throughout the book, I have used actual rather than fictitious names for two reasons. First, there is no clear dividing line between caretakers, whose names are traditionally used by historians, and the sick, whose names are often concealed. Many of the persons who appear in this narrative, including Flick, played both roles; they were caretakers but also had tuberculosis. Second, the sick men and women themselves influenced the system of care and its results. Although history has often ignored this influence, I do not want to compound this omission by keeping the patients anonymous. By not citing their places of residence in many instances and by omitting names in a few cases, I have tried to avoid giving any possible offense.

Part I of the book, "Tuberculosis and the Beginnings of Change, 1876–1903," focuses mainly on the last quarter of the nineteenth century. Chapter 1 introduces Flick and describes his initial attempts to prevent the spread of the infection. It also discusses the late-nineteenth-century understanding of the disease. Chapter 2 deals with the treatment of tuberculosis, both from a medical viewpoint and through the experiences of Flick's private patients.

Chapters 3 and 4 focus on poor consumptives and on two organizations that tried to help them: the Philadelphia Protestant Episcopal City Mission and the Free Hospital for Poor Consumptives. Chapter 5 describes the planning and the start of the first sanatorium in Pennsylvania, the Free Hospital's White Haven Sanatorium.

The early twentieth century witnessed major and pervasive changes in the care of consumptives. These are the subject of Part II, "New Systems of Care, 1903–1917." Between the turn of the century and the nation's entry into the First World War, the tuberculosis campaign gathered momentum. Voluntary organizations, philanthropists, entrepreneurs, and governments all involved themselves in building new institutions for the treatment of tuberculous patients. Chapters 6 and 7 focus on the Henry Phipps Institute—an unusual organization that combined research with patient care. For a little more than a decade, the hope of conquering the disease through scientific investigation justified the care of sick and dying patients, but this hope could not be realized. Chapters 8 and 9 trace the development of the White Haven Sanatorium. Chapter 9 also includes the state health department's competing system of care and the ideological conflict between the voluntary and the governmental efforts. Chapter 10 deals with the private sanatoriums.

Nurses and pupil nurses played an essential role in all these settings. They and the training schools for consumptive women that Flick initiated at the Phipps Institute and at White Haven are described in Chapters 6 and 9, and nurses who became proprietors of private sanatoriums appear in Chapter 10. Chapter 11 concentrates on the training of nurses and on their work in private duty or in institutions. Chapter 13 describes the Visiting Nurse Society of Philadelphia and the efforts of one of its nurses to take care of tuberculous patients, prevent the spread of disease, and preserve the integrity of families at the same time.

Chapter 12 details the experiences of one private patient and his caretakers. Chapter 14 examines the methods of persuasion used to influence patients' behavior and the circumstances that also affected their choices of treatment. It closes by reviewing the factors that underlay the growth of tuberculosis institutions and by introducing some of the doubts as to their effectiveness.

Part III, "Adjustments and Compromise," deals with the period from about 1914 to 1938. After a period of rapid change, the tuberculosis movement began to lose momentum. Chapter 15 describes the economic constraints on the system, partial retrenchments, the search for new and more successful treatments, and the efforts of institutions to survive under straitened economic conditions. Chapter 16 focuses on the experience of black people and on two belated and segregated methods of providing care for the group who had the highest tuberculosis death rates in the region.

Part IV provides "A Retrospective View." Chapter 17 examines the decline of tuberculosis and its possible causes. Chapter 18 reviews the changes that occurred between 1876 and 1938 and draws some parallels with the care of the chronically ill today.

Readers may wish to know the "truth" about tuberculosis: what causes it, how it is transmitted, and why only some people contract it and die of it. Physicians now understand tuberculosis as a specific infectious disease caused by a rod-shaped germ, the tubercle bacillus. Although a related organism infects cows and may on occasion cause human disease, most people contract their infections from other human beings who have active pulmonary tuberculosis. When diseased persons cough, or even when they talk or sneeze, they may spray clouds of bacilli-laden droplets into the surrounding air. Most of these droplets cause no harm; even when they are inhaled by another person, their relatively large size prevents them from reaching the tiny air sacs of the lungs. Instead, they settle out in higher portions of the respiratory tract, where the body's defenses eliminate the bacilli. Other droplets sink to the floor or ground, where the germs may linger but seldom, if ever, endanger anyone. As some of the droplets fall through the air, however, their moisture evaporates rapidly, leaving light, dry residues called droplet nuclei. These minute particles waft about in the air and are small enough to penetrate into the air sacs of a new host, carrying the seed of infection with them.[1]

Droplet nuclei that reach these air sacs probably each contain only one to three tubercle bacilli. Special defensive cells in the lungs ingest the bacilli and usually destroy them. Instead, however, bacilli may multiply and kill the cell in which they lie. By a complex series of reactions, the body then mobilizes further cellular defenses, and a small area of inflammation—a tubercle—develops at the site of invasion. This pulmonary tubercle, along with a similar one in a lymph node that drains the involved portion of lung, constitutes the initial infection. During the first few weeks of this process, when bodily defenses are relatively weak, bacilli often travel fairly freely through the circulatory system and establish small foci of infection elsewhere in the body. Most people, however, never have a discernible illness. That infection has occurred is detected by a skin reaction to a tuberculin test.[2]

Although infection is usually a silent process, the body changes in two important and contrasting ways. First, it develops acquired resistance, an accelerated capacity to defend itself against future invasions of tubercle bacilli. Reinfection may occur but becomes less likely. Second, the body now harbors viable bacilli within the lungs or elsewhere, possibly for decades. Should resistance falter, these bacilli may escape the scar tissue in which the body has encapsulated them and spread the infection to adjacent or other tissues, most commonly in the lungs. A person then has the disease called tuberculosis.[3]

Factors causing infection and factors promoting tuberculous disease are different. A first infection depends on proximity to someone with active tuberculosis, but brief encounters are rarely enough. Prolonged and close exposure to a person whose sputum carries a large number of bacilli is usually required. Such a person probably has advanced disease of the lungs but does not necessarily feel ill. A poorly ventilated environment, where droplet nuclei recirculate without being exposed to the lethal effects of sunlight, further enhances the risk.[4]

The chances that tuberculous infection will proceed to disease depend on several factors, most notably age and the recency of infection. A person's resistance is especially poor at three times in life: the first three years, the period between puberty and the approximate age of twenty-five, and old age. During the first of these periods, children are also more likely to develop disease in areas outside their lungs. They may then die of tuberculous meningitis (an inflammation of the lining of the brain) or of miliary tuberculosis, a generalized form of the disease. At any age, tuberculosis is most likely to develop during the first year or two after infection. The risk falls gradually after that, but may never disappear.[5] Large variations in resistance have yet to be explained. Differences in inherited resistance, in psychosocial and economic factors, in nutrition, and in the magnitude and frequency of exposure to tubercle bacilli have all been postulated. In most settings, however, such factors are coexistent, hard to measure, and impossible to separate. Interpreting trends in the past is accordingly difficult.

Briefly stated, these are the facts about tuberculosis as physicians currently understand them. Most of this book, in contrast, deals with a different kind of reality: the human experience of tuberculosis as a chronic illness, the responses to it, and the efforts of caretakers to cope with that illness while also trying to fight the disease.

Part I

Tuberculosis and the
Beginnings of Change,
1876–1903

1. Doctor Flick and Tuberculosis

For Lawrence Francis Flick in the 1930s, the section near home in Philadelphia was rich with bittersweet memories; he had lived there on Pine
Street, near 8th Street, for almost half a century. A few blocks north and
west of his house lay the Jefferson Medical College, which he had entered in
1877. When his classmates had passed him up bodily over the benches in a
college ritual, one of them had noticed "a decided infirmity" in the seat of
his trousers—evidence of the poverty with which Flick had started his
medical career. Several blocks east of the college he had boarded with the
Stone family, in whose house he had met his future wife. Their marriage
had taken place at nearby St. Mary's Church, five and one-half blocks from
the couple's present dwelling.[1]

One block east of their home and then a block south to Lombard
Street was the Henry Phipps Institute, which he had helped to establish in
1903. He disapproved of the work there now. After the University of
Pennsylvania had replaced him as the director in 1910, the Institute had
abandoned its hospital, and now, as he saw it, the physicians were wasting
much of their time on nontuberculous patients. The White Haven Sanatorium, in contrast, was still performing creditably, just as it had since 1901,
when he had opened it. This institution—founded for poor people—lay
miles away in the Pennsylvania mountains, but the nurses there still sent
him flowers on special occasions. He had established their training school
and another like it at the Phipps Institute. The private sanatoriums in the
town of White Haven were starting to close in the 1930s; running one was a
difficult business. Flick had tried it himself in 1913, right near his home on
Pine Street, but had given it up after a year. He still maintained his office,
however, and he was still pursuing his life's goal—preventing tuberculosis.
His latest project involved the Frederick Douglass Memorial Hospital,
where he was trying to organize a special ward for black patients with
tuberculosis.

Flick himself had had the disease as a young man. Since 1928 the aged
physician had again been plagued by recurrent illness—infections, pains in

his chest, and high levels of blood sugar for which he took insulin. He had "twice looked into the valley of death," as he expressed it to friends in the 1930s, and sensed a sword hanging over his head "which may drop at any time."[2]

Although an invalid during his last ten years of life, Flick was neither idle nor isolated. He and his beloved wife had successfully raised seven children, and two daughters still lived with them at home. All three women devoted much of their lives to his needs. The daughters helped in his office, and after his wife died suddenly in 1934 they took over the household and cared for their father. "The loss of wife and mother was a great blow to us," Flick wrote to a brother eighteen months later, "but we still look upon her as part of our family, and of our home. She is entombed right outside of our Church where I am near her body every day when I make my visit to the Blessed Sacrament." It was the same church in which they had been married, had had their children baptized, and had "knelt side by side in receiving the Holy Sacrament for nearly fifty years." Each day that his health permitted during this final decade, Flick went to his office to see a few patients. He continued to support his family, and people continued to want his medical advice.[3]

Few of his patients would have suspected that Flick had not wanted to practice medicine. He had studied it in hope of regaining his health, but his interests had always been broader. As a boy he had wanted to study law. As a young physician he had tried his hand in politics but had lost a bid for the state legislature in 1888, his only attempt at public office. He had had a flair for journalism, had written for newspapers as a young man, and later had almost succeeded in starting a Roman Catholic newspaper. He read extensively, favoring Goethe, Schiller, Newman, and Shakespeare. He liked history, had written some himself, and had helped to establish two Roman Catholic historical societies. None of his efforts to escape the practice of medicine had succeeded. As he explained to Sister M. Cosmos in 1937, "Our dear Lord always brought me back and kept me straight in line. Now at the end of my career I realize the wisdom of His direction and I thank Him for it."[4]

In the 1930s, Flick was reviewing his life and sharing some recollections. For much of his career he had led what he called a crusade against tuberculosis. As a young man, after his health had improved, he had consecrated his life " 'to the welfare of those afflicted with the disease and to the protection of those who had not yet contracted it.'" The work was his "thank-you to God." He had labored remarkably hard, had sacrificed time and income, had found pleasure in his achievements, but also had suffered defeats and humiliations. Before he died, he wanted to set the record straight by publishing the truth about the crusade.[5]

It was not an easy task to publish anything in the middle of the Great Depression. No editor wanted his materials, and Flick had to print them privately, burdensome as he found the costs to his dwindling resources. The long illness in 1928 had depleted his capital, and what securities he still possessed had dropped in value. He owned three buildings close together on Pine Street, in one of which he lived and worked, but few people could afford to rent the rooms now and his income was small. Dr. Joseph Walsh, an old friend and colleague, twice offered to help him financially, but twice Flick declined. The aged physician himself paid for the printing of a pamphlet on the tuberculosis crusade in 1932, printed a second in 1935, and in 1937, with a loan of eight hundred dollars from his son John, paid for the publication of his last book, *Tuberculosis*. He was then eighty. In these three works, together with a "Short Life Story" published by the Philadelphia County Medical Society in 1933, he summarized his contributions and his criticisms of other efforts.[6]

The campaign against tuberculosis, according to Flick, could be measured by its outcome, the dramatic fall in death rates after 1900. This decline, he asserted, was directly attributable to the isolation of advanced consumptives in hospitals and sanatoriums. Here he had led the way. If his opponents had not deviated from this purpose, he believed, the disease would already have disappeared. As he saw it, the Pennsylvania Society for the Prevention of Tuberculosis, which he had founded in 1892, had diverted its funds away from the all-important segregation and care of the tuberculous poor and had wasted its Christmas Seal income on building its own salaried organization. Its educational efforts, in Flick's opinion, had been worthless. The state, in spite of its vast expenditures on tuberculosis, had also done little to protect the public. It too had failed to concentrate its efforts on what Flick believed to be the most dangerous source of infection—men and women with advanced or terminal disease.[7]

During the 1930s Flick occasionally considered writing his reminiscences, but doubted his strength for the work. He thought that his son Lawrence, a newspaper editor, or his daughter Ella, a writer with historical interests, might some day record the history of the crusade. In any case, he had the story "securely stored away" in his library. During the 1880s he had started to save some letters that he received, and in 1900 he had begun to save them all. Late in 1903, he had also begun to keep copies of all the letters that he wrote. Through this correspondence and related materials, he hoped that the truth would be finally told, his leading role confirmed, and his policies vindicated. This collection has lain largely untouched for fifty years; the following pages could not have been written without it.[8]

Flick's Background and Early Years

The society in which Flick conducted his crusade against tuberculosis was far removed from that of his forebears and childhood. Both of his parents had immigrated to western Pennsylvania in the early 1830s—his father, John, then eighteen, from Alsace, France, and his mother, Elizabeth Sharbaugh, from Bavaria. Both families spoke German and both were attracted to the growing Roman Catholic settlement in the Allegheny mountains near what is now Carrolltown, in Cambria County. John and Elizabeth were married in 1840. Lawrence was born in their new farmhouse on August 10, 1856, the ninth of their twelve children and the second of five sons.[9]

Delicate health and a fondness for study earned young Lawrence a privileged place in the hard-working family. His stern and exacting father excused him from the more arduous chores on the farm, leaving him time to spend with his beloved mother, a calm, dignified, affectionate woman "known for her quiet sense of humor" and "adored by her husband and children." At the age of six Lawrence began to attend the local schools, and at thirteen he left home for St. Vincent's College, a Benedictine school in Beatty, Pennsylvania. There he established himself as an excellent student in the classical program and made some lifelong friendships.[10]

Illness and loss soon disrupted the boy's life. Early in November 1869, just two months after he had left home, his mother died of typhoid fever. Life on the farm changed permanently. St. Vincent's became a second home for Lawrence and his younger brother Edward—the only members of the family to acquire an advanced education. Illness interrupted the boy's life again in February 1874, three months before he expected to receive his diploma. The Benedictine fathers, suspecting consumption, sent him home for a long rest.[11]

Uncertainty plagued young Flick for the next two and one-half years as he attempted to better his health and decide on his future. He set arduous schedules for himself, studied, wrote for newspapers, stumped for a temperance campaign, taught school, and even tried an outdoor job as a

trackman for the Lehigh Valley Railroad. Taking long rides on horseback (then frequently prescribed for consumptive patients), he also accompanied the local priest and the family physician, Dr. Michael Wesner, on their calls through the mountains. For a year Dr. Wesner took him into his office during part of every day, and Flick finally decided on a medical education. He had saved some money from teaching, borrowed more from his father, and in the fall of 1877 matriculated at Wesner's alma mater, Jefferson Medical College in Philadelphia.[12]

Despite straitened circumstances, Flick did well in the two-year program at Jefferson, graduating with a medal in surgery in March 1879, but he was still unwell and undecided about his career. Throughout medical school he had also attended law lectures, and during his second year he had entered the office of Benjamin Brewster as a law student. Even during his internship at Philadelphia Hospital he continued working in Brewster's office for one or two hours every day. Although he developed a febrile illness during the latter part of his internship, the young physician opened a private office for the practice of medicine in the summer of 1880, but by the following spring he felt too sick to continue. Two physicians finally diagnosed consumption and, offering the typical recommendation of the time, advised him to travel west.[13]

The prospect of leaving Philadelphia must have caused great distress. The serious, diffident student had gradually fallen in love with Ella J. Stone, the daughter of master locksmith Thomas S. Stone and his wife, Ellen, with whom he had boarded during medical school. For six months or so he searched for alternatives to going west. He visited Atlantic City and Cape May, both reputedly healthful; he spent some time on his father's farm; and he stayed for a while with an old friend, Father Michael Bergrath, pastor of St. Patrick's Church in White Haven, Pennsylvania—but all to no avail. Finally, in October 1881, he started west from Carrolltown, unsure of his future but placing his trust in God. He and Ella had promised themselves to each other, and she decided to wait for him, regardless how long he took to get well.[14]

The journey west proved lengthy, lonely, and discouraging. Flick found Colorado, his first destination, too cold for his liking and continued on to Santa Fe, Albuquerque, El Paso, Tucson, and Los Angeles. The climate of southern California seemed more agreeable, and he finally found work to support himself—nailing orange crates together and sorting and packing fruit. For a time he seemed to improve in both strength and weight—the result, he believed, of a better diet. Instead of the unpalatable and expensive hotel food that he had had to eat along the way, he had devised a cheap and agreeable substitute: six quarts of milk daily at only four cents a quart, and one main meal at midday. As the weather turned warm in the spring, Flick's condition worsened again, however, and he headed toward home. After a brief visit in Philadelphia, he reached his father's farm early in July 1882. There, and at White Haven again, his health began to improve as he followed a program of horseback-riding, light farmwork, reading, writing, and drinking milk. By the spring of 1883 he felt well enough to resume his practice, and in 1885 he and Ella were married. In 1887, after the birth of their second child, they moved from the Stone household into their own home at 736 Pine Street.[15]

Flick did not intend to specialize in tuberculosis; he dreaded the disease and would have preferred to avoid it. Tuberculous men and women, probably attracted to a physician who seemed to have cured himself, however, actively sought him out. He treated these patients by the methods that he had used successfully on himself. Encouraged by his results, he grew less fearful of the disease and more confident in his practice.[16]

Consumption in the Late Nineteenth Century

When Flick was starting to practice medicine in 1880, only a rare physician considered consumption infectious. The idea was not a new one, however; it had waxed and waned since the time of the ancient Greeks. In 1865 J. A. Villemin, a French physician, began to report data to show that the disease could be transferred from one animal species to another by inoculation. The germ theory, developed by Louis Pasteur and others, was gaining acceptance, and in 1882 Robert Koch's demonstration of the tubercle bacillus convinced at least some physicians that the ancient scourge, consumption, was communicable. Learned authorities, however, still disputed the growing evidence. While it was clear to any observer that smallpox spread fairly rapidly from one victim to another, tuberculosis could not be tracked so easily. This disease could develop years after infection, there was no way to identify it in its milder forms, and even advanced cases were sometimes overlooked. When physicians did make the diagnosis, they seldom found a source of infection. "It is with extreme rarity that a case of tuberculosis in a human being can be traced to another," wrote Dr. James Tyson, professor of clinical medicine at the University of Pennsylvania, in his 1896 textbook of medicine. "In a practice of thirty years, including large general hospital service, I can recall but a single instance of probable communication of the disease, and this was from a husband to the wife, who was his faithful nurse for years." When physicians observed families in which several members had died of the disease, they could just as easily have attributed the misfortune to heredity, to constitutional predisposition, to unfavorable climatic conditions, or to the damp soil on which they all lived together. If tuberculosis were infectious, they somtimes reasoned, everyone in the patient's household should be diseased.[17]

Diagnosing tuberculosis was far from easy. Early symptoms, if present at all, were often subtle: "a short and insidious cough, with a feeling of lassitude, and a decline in general health," as Jacob Da Costa, one of Flick's personal physicians, described them in 1881. At times, there was "pain in the affected lung and a somewhat quickened circulation" or even a hemorrhage from the lungs. The symptoms might develop "after a severe bodily or mental fatigue" or be "traceable to some neglected cold." Many people, especially the poor, would not seek medical attention for such an array of symptoms. If they did, physicians could easily misinterpret the meaning of their complaints.[18]

Physicians whose diagnostic skills were relatively advanced examined a patient's chest with particular care. Flattening of the chest wall with diminished expansion on breathing might raise suspicion of underlying disease. If the upper portion of the chest sounded dull to their tapping fingers, they could infer that tuberculous tissue had replaced the normally resonant, air-filled lungs. Through a stethoscope they might hear altered breath sounds or the soft, ominous, crackling sounds, called rales, that they associated with inflammation. This cluster of signs characterized what late-nineteenth-century physicians labeled incipient or early tuberculosis. Present-day x-ray studies would almost certainly demonstrate that such a person's disease—if indeed tuberculous—had passed beyond the early stage.[19]

As the disease progressed, its manifestations became more obvious but could still mislead the average physician. Appetite diminished, debility worsened, breathlessness developed, and the cough became increasingly severe and productive of large amounts of phlegm. Fever was common, and exhausting night sweats added their miseries to the racking cough. On the other hand, the "deceptive blush" that fever imparted to the cheeks, the "increased lustre of the eye," the "singular hopefulness" of the patient, and the temporary improvements could all engender false optimism in both the physician and the patient's family. They also confounded the doctors' efforts to judge the efficacy of treatments.[20]

Late in the illness, examination of the chest could document the spread of infection to other parts of the lungs. Hollow breath sounds and cavernous voice sounds heard through a stethoscope indicated the development of large cavities—holes within the lungs remaining after inflamed tissue broke down into dead, bacilli-laden material, which the patient then coughed out.[21] By this time, every portion of the body might give evidence of advanced disease: the hollow eyes and gaunt face; the sticklike limbs from which the muscles seemed to have melted away; the sharp, bony outlines and knobby joints; the prominent ribs and hip bones; the withered breasts and sunken abdomen—in sum, the picture of shriveled and wasted flesh that had given tuberculosis its two ancient names, phthisis (from the Greek *phthiein*, to waste away) and consumption.

Flick and the Early Campaign Against Consumption

Flick was not the first physician in Philadelphia to argue that consumption was contagious, but he did so relatively early and very persistently. In a series of papers starting in 1888, the young physician, barely established in practice, repeatedly tried to convince his colleagues to support this idea and the consequent measures that society should take to reduce the danger of infection. Phthisis, he declared, was indisputably contagious. Although a person might inherit a certain predisposition to the disease, the infection itself was not hereditary. People who had phthisis in their families no longer needed to worry about themselves or merely accept their fates; they could actively prevent the disease by avoiding contagion and by living in healthful ways. The poor, he admitted, had "neither the power nor the knowledge to escape its clutches" but were "like dumb cattle . . . driven by their necessities into the very face of death." Here was a job for government, for sanitary science placed in the service of the state.[22]

For government to do its job, Flick argued, it had to know where the danger lay. Consumption, therefore, had to be put on the list of reportable diseases, along with smallpox and diphtheria. Boards of health could then make sure that every consumptive's house, especially the room used for sleep, was properly disinfected. Through these boards, government should also educate the people as to the infectiousness of sputum and the proper methods of protecting themselves. Consumptives should not be allowed to work in situations in which they might contaminate the clothing, food, or drink of others. "To obviate hardships in such cases," Flick suggested in

1888, "the government should make provision out of the public treasury for the maintenance of such people," perhaps by granting pensions or offering an asylum.[23]

In 1890 Flick proposed a more modest and more medical solution for the consumptive poor—special hospitals devoted to the disease. Arguing that such hospitals had reduced the death rates from consumption in England and Wales after 1848, he supported them on grounds of both humanitarianism and self-protection. It is "no longer a question of helping your neighbor alone," he asserted. "It is a question of helping yourself—of protecting yourself and your family . . . against a most loathsome disease, which is almost certainly fatal." The consumptive "wants hospital treatment," he added. "His poverty, his helplessness, his utter despair of recovery . . . and his serious interference with the efforts of his poor relatives to support themselves and him, make him want it. He has wanted it for years."[24]

It was a radical message for a young physician to take before a conservative medical establishment. Not only was Flick challenging some cherished beliefs about the cause of consumption, he was also advocating a fairly new approach to public health through governmental action. Since the mid-nineteenth century, increasing numbers of municipal governments had organized permanent boards of health to combat the filth and disease of their expanding cities, and similar boards at the state level followed thereafter—in Pennsylvania, in 1885. Flick had made useful contacts with board officials at both levels of government. Although these boards paid little attention to consumption during the nineteenth century, they provided models for combating infectious diseases and organizational structures from which to launch future campaigns against tuberculosis. They also seemed to threaten the authority of practicing physicians, as did some of Flick's recommendations.[25]

Flick's background and personality did not make him a likely figure to change the dominant ideas of his fellow physicians, nor did they readily qualify him for a place in the city's medical leadership—an elite group drawn primarily from old, successful Philadelphia families, most of whom were Protestant. A Roman Catholic, immigrant farmer's son from western Pennsylvania who had married a locksmith's daughter would naturally find it hard to compete socially, even though both families had succeeded financially. Although Flick's wife was light-hearted and sociable, Flick himself lacked some of the social graces and confidence that might have smoothed his way upward. He was a handsome man in the late 1880s and

1890s. His face and trunk had filled out since his illness, he wore a neatly trimmed beard, and in informal moments his face lit up with a warm smile. In public appearances, however, he was not a very good speaker; his voice was weak, tired easily, and sometimes broke with emotion. Blunt in his opinions, self-righteous, and even abrasive in conflict, he alienated some of the men who might have helped him. Sensitive to snubs and injustice, he sometimes fought back, sometimes withdrew into the security of his family and his religion. He avoided most social engagements unless they were directly connected with his work. He stayed away from the theater, liked no sports or games, and had no hobbies of the lighter sort. A loving husband and father, he felt most comfortable at home. He also liked to take long walks by himself, especially in the poorer parts of the city; he found them, he said, more interesting.[26]

Professionally, Flick's qualifications were good but not superior. Lack of a high-school or college diploma did not prevent admission to medical school during this period, but a physician destined for leadership would probably have had one. Flick's medical education at Jefferson and his internship at Philadelphia Hospital were both to his advantage, but neither institution was the city's most prestigious and he had not gone further. He had assisted no senior physician who might have acted as his mentor, he had not studied in Europe, and he had held no positions on hospital staffs or dispensaries—all typical stepping-stones in a distinguished career. His tendencies to write for newspapers and to air disparaging opinions, moreover, had alienated some leading physicians. As an intern, outraged by the conditions and politics at the Philadelphia Hospital, he had written a pseudonymous series of critical letters to the city's newspapers. It was not a way to make medical friends or connections. Nevertheless, Flick was studious, knowledgeable, hard-working, morally upstanding, and ambitious. In 1880 he became a member of the Philadelphia County Medical Society; in 1888 he was elected to the College of Physicians of Philadelphia, an elite medical society; and in 1890 he was elected to a second prestigious group, the Pathological Society of Philadelphia. His opinions deserved to be heard even if his colleagues disagreed with him.[27]

Physicians in the county medical society and at the College of Physicians greeted Flick's ideas on contagion with skepticism and hostility. Despite the experiments with tubercle bacilli reported by Koch and others, many of these physicians found other ways to interpret the data. While an animal inoculated with the bacilli might get tuberculosis, some acknowledged, this observation failed to prove transmission of the germs from person to person under natural circumstances. If bacilli were everywhere, as the laboratory men were reporting, why did relatively few people become diseased? Additional factors must be important: heredity, nutrition, bodily resistance, damp soil, or infected milk and meat. Disinfection, moreover, was impracticable, unenforceable, and likely to divert efforts from more important measures such as improving sanitation.[28]

Reporting of cases to the board of health proved equally controversial. Flick and some like-minded colleagues managed to persuade the county medical society to approve the measure, but other medical groups, most notably the College of Physicians, opposed it. In a special meeting in January 1894, members of the College expressed their concerns over two principal issues. First, reporting would simply add hardship to the lives of the unfortunate patients, they asserted, "stamping them as the outcasts of society," treating them as dangerous "criminals guilty of consumption," and pursuing them from house to house like marked men. Second, reporting infringed on the rights and responsibilities of private physicians. "Is not the intelligent physician the proper health officer?" asked Jacob Da Costa. "Is not what he says sufficient?" The city's board of health, he pointed out, already had the right to put an unsanitary house into better order, "but let it leave the care of the individual where it belongs—to the conscientious physician." The College voted against the measure, and case-reporting in Philadelphia was delayed until 1904.[29]

Flick's proposal for a tuberculosis hospital, in contrast, met with little objection; those who discussed this paper supported the idea almost unanimously. They did so, however, for strikingly different reasons: because it would restrict the spread of consumption, or create public uneasiness over contagion, or improve the patients' nutrition, or provide for special nursing or the necessary kinds of exercise. Starting a hospital appealed both to doctors who believed in contagion and to those who did not, just as Flick had intended. Laurence Turnbull, the only practitioner to express a mild dissent, thought that a hospital for consumptives would be too depressing, the coughing there too disturbing to the other patients, and the air heavily contaminated and therefore dangerous. Consumptives "do not require a hospital so much as a home," he asserted, "with good food, medicine, and a little money." When this was impossible, special homes such as the two managed by the Philadelphia Protestant Episcopal City Mission were suitable substitutes.[30]

A home for consumptives, however, with its implications of incurability and custodianship, had relatively little appeal to an increasingly confident and aggressive segment of the medical profession that preferred to treat patients, not simply take care of them. Flick, agitating for a hospital in a style that was becoming characteristic, distributed a thousand reprints of his paper "where they would do the most good," and within a few months "several earnest physicians," Flick among them, joined forces to create the Rush Hospital for Consumption and Allied Diseases. They thought that "the treatment of consumptives could be improved," as one of its staff members later observed, "by a more thorough study of its nature, conditions and causes, and by therapeutic efforts along new lines." Rush Hospital incorporated in September 1890, opened a dispensary in 1891, and accepted its first hospital patient in 1892. Flick, however, soon found himself in conflict with other members of the board who did not believe in the contagiousness of the disease, and, either by his own volition or at their request, he resigned in 1893.[31]

The Pennsylvania Society for the Prevention of Tuberculosis

Meanwhile, Flick had been developing his own society—one that would promulgate the concept that tuberculosis was contagious and teach the public how to prevent the disease. On April 22, 1892, about twenty-five interested men and women, most of them laypersons, met in his office and decided to organize. On May 6 the group elected its officers, with Flick as the president, and agreed upon its objectives: to prevent tuberculosis by promoting the doctrine of contagiousness, by instructing the public, by supplying the consumptive poor with protective materials and teaching them how to use them, by furnishing the consumptive poor with hospital treatment, by cooperating with boards of health in preventive measures, and by advocating appropriate laws. In 1895 the group incorporated as the Pennsylvania Society for the Prevention of Tuberculosis—the first organization of its kind in the country.[32]

　　The new voluntary society, scraping along on a skimpy budget, produced and distributed thousands of copies of tracts—educational leaflets that carried its messages not only to Philadelphians but to people throughout the country who requested them. Three persistent themes repeated themselves through the leaflets: tuberculosis was contagious; the germs could enter the body through the stomach, the lungs, or an open wound; and the disease could be prevented if only consumptives themselves and those around them would take the necessary precautions.[33]

Patients and their families could prevent the spread of infection without depriving themselves of comfort or companionship, Flick asserted in these tracts, but they had to alter their way of life. Not only must consumptives control and disinfect their sputum but they should also have their own separate dishes and eating utensils. These should be boiled after each use, and all their linens and bedclothes should be boiled before being laundered. Consumptives must not kiss on the mouth, should preferably not shake hands, and must keep their living rooms and bedrooms clean and frequently aired.[34]

The public at large, moreover, should take its own measures for self-protection. Do not buy food from consumptives, the leaflets urged; wash your hands after any contact with them and before eating. Avoid inhaling dust in a consumptive's room or anywhere on the premises unless you are sure that the patient is very careful to disinfect all sputum. Never put coins or other small objects into your mouth: "They may have been used by a consumptive just before falling into your hands. . . . *Never allow* clothing or furniture that has been used by a consumptive or that has been kept in a house occupied by a consumptive to come into your house or room until it has been thoroughly disinfected." Before changing residence, the counsel continued, inquire about whether the house has been occupied by a consumptive; if so, be sure that it has been thoroughly disinfected before you move. Some of this advice, such as that involving cleanliness and disinfection, long antedated the germ theory and had been widely promoted to prevent a variety of other diseases thought to result from filth. The more-specifically targeted sputum precautions reflected the newer bacteriological insights. Whatever their origins, most of the recommendations were to continue largely unchanged for roughly half a century. Whether they would reassure the sick or the public, as Flick anticipated, remained to be seen.[35]

The movement that Flick was starting in Philadelphia and others were starting elsewhere, most notably in New York City, embodied a changing attitude toward consumption and its victims. The disease was no longer a private affair; it touched on the public's welfare and health. Apathy, sympathy, and even charity toward the afflicted no longer sufficed as responses. Because consumptives were dangerous to others, they needed to learn and adopt specific behaviors, and the healthy too needed to take precautions lest they become infected themselves. The required educational efforts exceeded the capacities of private physicians and demanded the participation of informed laypersons and public health officials. The helpless poor needed a particular kind of attention, preferably in special hospitals. Such institutions would combine the humanitarian impulse with the public's enlightened self-interest and the aspirations of medicine. It was a grand vision illuminated by bacteriological science and social reform.

It was also a vision far removed from the traditional ways in which doctors treated their private patients late in the nineteenth century. When consumptive patients sought Flick's advice in the 1890s, most of his recommendations were based on older ideas that he and his patients shared.

2. The Quest and the Treatment

Bacteriological insights into the cause of consumption were almost irrelevant to its treatment in the late nineteenth century. Although some physicians adopted new rationales for their old therapies, most of their recommendations had long been familiar to physicians and patients alike. Health, they believed, depended in part on environment; if a person sickened in one setting, changing it seemed prudent or even mandatory. Health depended, too, on the way people lived, the food they ate, and the proper balance of rest and exercise. Physicians, including Flick, guided their patients in all such matters. They also used a variety of remedies to strengthen the body, regulate its functions, and ameliorate symptoms. Patients—vulnerable and dependent in their illness—asked for medical guidance even from hundreds of miles away. They wanted recommendations for travel, climate, food, and companions; they wanted their symptoms interpreted and treatments prescribed.

In the free-enterprise system of nineteenth-century America, a beneficial environment, health advice, and various remedies could all be purchased, and invalids shopped for what they could afford. Although physicians competed to provide these services, they were far from alone in the marketplace. As the nation expanded, railroad companies and other community interests promoted the healthfulness of newly accessible regions and enticed tuberculous men and women westward and southward in search of cure. Patent medicines—branded as quackery by medical leaders—vied with physicians and their prescriptions. Late in the century, tuberculosis sanatoriums entered the competition. While most of these claimed salutary locations, they also promised health-promoting daily regimens, nutritious diets, medical supervision, and a greater chance of cure.

Consumption and Climate

Rose Farren, a young consumptive from Philadelphia, spent the summer and fall of 1893 as might any person of means in a similar predicament—in search of recovery. In August she stayed with her father at the Pocono Mountain House, a summer resort in Pennsylvania; in September she went to Massachusetts; and by November she had returned to Philadelphia, where her father was considering the winter's itinerary. Flick, Rose's physician, was ill in November, and Mr. Farren turned to Dr. William Pepper for advice. "Most of the places you name are excellent," wrote Pepper to Flick on November 27, but "do you you think that a journey involving so many changes of residence is as good as a more prolonged stay in some spot which has shewn itself very suitable?" A skilled physician of the late nineteenth century had to match healthful localities not only to the particular malady but also to the patient's temperament and, in this case, to the temperaments of key family members. "Would Mr. Farren become impatient and restless if in one of these places all was going well, and it was better that they should continue [there] for some time[?]" Pepper asked. "I have no criticism of the itinerary," he noted tactfully, but, if Miss Farren showed that a moderate elevation suited her well, "I distinctly prefer that . . . they should stay on there and omit some of the distant and elevated points. You know his temperament so well that I defer entirely to your judgment."[1]

Beliefs that certain airs, soils, and waters affected health or produced illness had roots in ancient medicine, and many Americans found their faith confirmed by observation. As early as the mid-eighteenth century, colonists sought out the mineral springs of Virginia, for example, and as transportation improved in the nineteenth century the well-to-do flocked in increasing numbers to White Sulphur Springs, Saratoga Springs, and a number of other resorts that promised healing waters, pleasant scenery, entertainment, and an amiable or stimulating social life. While a trip to such establishments offered diversion and pleasure, it also promised a respite from the icy winters of the North, the steamy, fever-ridden summers of the South, and the crowded, dirty cities of the eastern seaboard. Moreover, the purging effects of the waters when taken internally or their effects when used as a bath were entirely congruent with nineteenth-century concepts of disease. They would restore the body's balance and bring relief from conditions as diverse as rheumatism, dyspepsia, nervous disorders, and phthisis.[2]

As the western territories were explored, tales of the pure, salubrious air filtered back through the malarial Mississippi River basin and on toward the East, and invalids, many of them consumptive, joined the lumbering wagon trains to search for health in the West. Although the Civil War interrupted this migration, it resumed after the war, and by the 1870s western businessmen, railroad companies, state officials, and physicians were actively promoting the curative properties of their regions. Consumptives followed the lures and streamed into Colorado, southern California, Texas, New Mexico, and Arizona—among them, in the early 1880s, the young Dr. Flick.[3]

The East had its own competitive boosters, and eastern resorts advertised regularly for a share in the invalid trade. Boasting of climate, scenery, or mineral springs, of their bright, airy rooms and excellent food, they promised good health, pleasure, entertainment, and the cure of diseases. The Hygeia Hotel in Old Point Comfort, Virginia, for example, labeled itself the "Unrivaled Health and Pleasure resort of the Atlantic Coast," while the Ocean View Hotel on Block Island, Rhode Island, aimed its appeal at "worn-out business men, overworked professional men," and "nervous and delicate women." Proprietors of a new pier in Atlantic City, New Jersey, advertised its health-giving ocean climate:

A well known fact without presumption,
Physicians say it cures consumption.[4]

Enthusiastic local physicians did indeed support such claims. In 1880 and again in 1884, Boardman Reed, an Atlantic City physician, reported to his medical colleagues on the favorable effects of the coastal resorts. "My observations have led me to the conclusion that, as a rule, consumptives in the early stages . . . do well at the sea-shore, at least in that locality," he wrote in 1884. "The great majority . . . have progressed favorably during their stay there. Quite a number of persons having a portion of one lung consolidated have become permanent residents of the place on account of the marked improvement." Similar medical testimonials lauded regions as different as Bethlehem, New Hampshire, and Aiken, South Carolina. In 1889 Dr. Bushrod W. James soberly recommended to consumptives the ocean climate of the East Coast; the mild, moist climate of Florida; the White, Green, Adirondack, Allegheny, and Rocky Mountains; the cold, dry winters of Minnesota; the warm, dry climate of the Southwest; and the pine forests of the Carolinas and Georgia. Each region had its own assets, and James expected physicians to individualize their climatic prescriptions.[5]

In 1884 a group of physicians, troubled by the conflicting or frankly uninformed climatic recommendations made by their medical colleagues, banded together to form the American Climatological Association. They wanted "to revive and further a knowledge of climatology" and to disseminate to the profession the "well-known and indispensable facts" concerning localities, the indications for selecting them, the ways of traveling to them, and the accommodations for living once invalids arrived. Too many Americans, a vocal element among these physicians emphasized, were spending their money in European spas and resorts. American health resorts and mineral waters equaled those in Europe, they argued, but were failing to compete because American medicine had not yet systematized and disseminated the relevant knowledge.[6]

The climatologists devoted much of their early attention to phthisis. Two observable facts supported the logic of this approach. First, some localities seemed free of the disease or at least had very low death rates among their native populations. Second, consumptives who went to such places appeared to improve. Medical scientists, the physicians reasoned, should describe the climatic variables that characterized the different localities, correlate them with the prevalence of disease and with the frequency of recoveries, and deduce from their observations which attributes of climate made the critical differences. In 1862 Henry I. Bowditch, a distinguished Boston physician, had published such a study of Massachusetts, concluding that damp soil bred consumption. Bowditch could not explain how a damp environment might produce such a dire effect, but he was sure that patients should try to escape it, much as they would flee from a region threatened by yellow fever.[7]

Members of the Climatological Association proceeded with further investigations. For various regions, they compiled measures of altitude, humidity, temperature, sunlight, dampness of the soil, ozone in the air, and emanations from pine and balsam forests. Some found fault with the crowding and foul air of the cities and the indoor, sedentary lives of those who dwelt there. The task was large, the volume of data impressive. A skeptic, however, might notice that many of the otherwise disparate conclusions shared one characteristic: physicians tended to discover health-giving attributes in their own locales.[8]

Flick was a member of the Association between 1889 and 1891, but his experiences in the West had made him doubt that the values of climate could outweigh the disadvantages of leaving home, at least for persons of average means. A warm climate encouraged an invalid to live outdoors, he acknowledged, and camping out in the territories had produced some "most remarkable cures." Because pure salt air improved the appetite, a sea voyage could be beneficial, and nonporous (and therefore damp) soil might indeed contribute to phthisis. Nevertheless, it "is much better that a consumptive have home comforts in the worst climate in the world," he argued, "than that he be compelled to undergo the tortures of boarding-house or fourth-class hotel at a health resort." The average consumptive "had better remain at home, unless his home is in a large city, and then he should go into the neighboring country. . . . Let him dress warm, take outdoor exercise whenever he can, eat plenty of light, nourishing food, take ample rest and sleep, and he will get along much better . . . than he would with small means in the most model consumption climate."[9]

The Therapeutic Regimen

Although most members of the American Climatological Association placed greater faith in climate than Flick did, few would have challenged his recommendations for fresh air, good food, and suitable combinations of rest and exercise. These constituted the hygienic regimen that increasing numbers of physicians were promoting as the most effective treatment for consumption. Among the elements of this regimen, Flick considered nutrition the most important. If the body was to fight disease and repair itself, it must be given enough of the right materials, he believed, and consumptives should force into their systems large amounts of easily digestible food. He instructed most of his patients in a daily menu that resembled the one he had found successful in his own case: one substantial meal, not less than three quarts of milk, and six raw eggs.[10]

With physiological reasoning typical of late-nineteenth-century health advice, Flick explained other parts of the regimen. Fresh air aided the body's nutrition by supplying oxygen, and outdoor activities stimulated the appetite. Rest conserved a person's energy. Exercise, therefore, should be restricted when patients had fever or were below weight and should be increased gradually as they recovered. Two less vigorous activities aided the circulation: regular sponge baths and rubbing the body with coarse towels.[11]

This program differed from the more drastic treatment of early-nineteenth-century medicine, which included repetitive bleeding and purging for consumption and other diseases. Reformers within and outside the profession had attacked such heroic measures as useless or even lethal, and for much of the century several competing sects of practitioners had challenged orthodox medicine. Physicians, beleaguered by critics and competitors, had gradually changed their methods and had even adopted some of the sectarian treatments. While they still cited Hippocrates or other ancient authorities to legitimate their therapeutic approaches, their sources of practice were more eclectic.[12]

There are few better examples of this eclecticism than the hygienic regimen promulgated for tuberculosis. In addition to Greek and Roman precedents, the regimen echoed the preachings of nineteenth-century health reformers who, especially since the 1830s, had zealously promoted the use of diet, fresh air, and exercise. These were the same ingredients that the nineteenth-century German sanatoriums were using to treat consumptives, with encouraging results. Hermann Brehmer had founded the first of these sanatoriums in 1859. Although Brehmer had based his therapeutic program on a medical theory, he had also been influenced by Vincent Priessnitz, a charismatic peasant healer who earlier in the century had popularized a series of water treatments known as hydropathy. These treatments, along with a dietary regimen and outdoor activities that Priessnitz also promoted, attracted hundreds of patients yearly, and hydropathic institutions spread across Europe.[13]

In the 1840s they appeared in the United States, and hydropathy became one of the several sects that competed with regular American medicine. Men and women of means, already accustomed to resorts, started to take the water-cure. Hydropathists adapted their treatments to the ideas of health reform, and orthodox physicians borrowed from both sets of practices. Although hydropathy lost much of its popularity after the Civil War, a few of its institutions persisted as hygienic sanitariums. Water treatments survived in regular medical practice under the name of hydrotherapy.[14]

The hygienic regimen for tuberculosis, often including water treatments, thus became an integral part of several traditions. It had roots in orthodox medicine, in sectarian practice, and in popular health reform. It found added support in the German successes in treating tuberculosis, but it was already familiar to many in the United States.

The regimen, as practiced by many physicians in the late nineteenth century, was not always benign, however, nor did it exclude drugs. Flick had special confidence in two of these—iodine and creosote. Of the various forms of iodine, he preferred iodoform, then europhen; he used them both as oily inunctions. He asked his patients to "rub from a teaspoonful to a tablespoonful into the armpits and into the inside of the thighs once or twice a day"—a procedure that took from half to a full hour. Along with the iodine, he often recommended gradually increasing doses of pure beechwood creosote in hot water, to be taken by mouth three times a day before meals. For "building-up purposes," Flick prescribed several tonics of the day, including strychnine, arsenic, phosphorus, and iron. Digitalis quieted a rapidly beating heart, he believed, while bicarbonate of soda, magnesia, and bismuth were useful for a "congested" stomach, pepsin and hydrochloric acid helped a "sluggish" stomach and liver, and pancreatin improved digestion.[15]

When tubercular deposits affected the lungs, Flick advised the counterirritant remedies familiar to most nineteenth-century patients—fly-blisters, plasters, and dry cupping. The action of a fly-blister depended on an extremely irritating extract prepared from a beetle (*Cantharis vesicatoria*, or Spanish fly). "I place an ordinary fly-blister over the affected lung, front or back, and allow it to remain in place about an hour," Flick explained in the *Medical News* in 1899. "I then have the plaster removed and the skin washed with warm water. In the course of a few hours a large vesicle [blister] will rise and as the epidermis has not been broken the serum is retained and in twenty-four hours is reabsorbed. During the process of reabsorption of the serum chills, malaise and some fever are liable to occur." When patients were "too timid" to apply a fly-blister, he substituted plasters made of other irritating substances such as croton oil or tartar emetic. In dry cupping, a partial vacuum was created in a bell-shaped glass either by using a small suction pump or by burning a few drops of alcohol or ether in the glass. The cup, placed on the patient's skin, sucked the tissues into it, thus creating the presumably therapeutic redness and congestion.[16]

Although physicians developed various and changing explanations of how these treatments helped consumptives, none of the measures were new. Perhaps the growing therapeutic confidence came not from the methods used but from the new, specific, and tangible targets against which they were directed. Consumption could no longer be ascribed to "an angry Providence," as Flick expressed it in 1896, but was caused by a "vexatious little organism" that people could now see through a microscope, study, and learn to destroy.[17] Even if bacteriology had not yet yielded a definitive cure, favorable reports from European sanatoriums that used the hygienic regimen gave physicians a reason to hope.

Search for the Proper Place

While Flick promoted a careful, complicated regimen of home treatment, he also recommended resorts to people of means such as the Farrens, and many of his patients sought this kind of advice. "I have a notion to go 'way up in the mountains' somewhere, next month for 2 weeks," wrote Joseph A. Michel in July 1894, "and as I know you are acquainted in Penna. could you prompt me some quiet resting place? I think it better for me than the seashore, and expect to get 'big and fat' as I go alone." July was a likely time for such questions as working consumptives planned their vacations. Elwell Stockdale, a salesman for a local paper company, mailed his inquiry on July 3, 1897. "I meant to ask you this morning about your opinion as to whether I had better spend my vacation at the Seashore or mountains," he wrote. "I had sort of decided to go to Atlantic City but it struck me the mountains might do me more good. Will you be so kind as to drop me word." By July 6 Stockdale had received Flick's answer and had decided to go to Mount Pocono.[18]

Other men and women planned trips of much greater duration and distance. With a diagnosis as serious as consumption, no brief vacation in a nearby resort sufficed for them; they thought they needed a longer, more radical change of environment even if it disrupted their lives. Mrs. Charles Rea, from York, Pennsylvania, for example, planned to leave immediately for Florida, where she would stay with her parents and depend on the curative qualities of the climate, together with rest, creosote, inhalations, iodoform, and strychnine.[19]

Some of Flick's patients found agreeable places in Pennsylvania where they could arrange for their prescribed regimens, obtain their medications, and enjoy the pleasures of resort life. In 1893 Mrs. Eleanor N. Gilbert, for example, found the Highland House in Wernersville much to her liking. The milk, butter, and cream were good, the eggs fresh, and the "lofty piazza (in effect private) on which I _live_, is itself a comfort that I might not find elsewhere." T. A. Gaffney, who spent July 1896 at Mt. Sunset Home in Wernersville, found the scenery "superb," the air "strong and bracing," and a little squab that the hotel had sent her "delicious." "We took a splendid drive yesterday," she wrote, "carriage, pair-horses, driver and three ladies."[20]

Farther away, Father Wertenbach formed a favorable first impression of the Piney Woods Inn, a large hotel in Southern Pines, North Carolina. "I am nicely situated," he reported cheerfully in January 1898. "The first thing I did was to arrange for the 3 qts of milk. The proprietor was astonished and seemed to doubt my capacity for that amount. I'll disabuse him of the impression after a few days trial." Out in the West, Dr. Jno. J. Gilbride finally found a ranch to his liking. On an exclusive diet of skimmed milk, he wrote in 1899, "I gain 7 pounds in 3 weeks. I began to gain the day I struck the town (6,000 ft altitude). . . . I am using the Europhen and oil. . . . I feel confident of complete recovery."[21]

If consumptives devoted themselves to pleasures less modest than diets of milk or taking a ride in a carriage, they neglected to write to Flick about them. Physicians decried the imprudence and dissipations of resort life: drinking, smoking, dancing, playing cards in closed and stuffy rooms, staying inside during the daytime, or overexerting outdoors. Transgressing the laws of nature was tantamount to transgressing the laws of God, Flick explained, using a combination of religious and physiological language common at the time. It brought "in its train a penalty which . . . may well be accepted as coming from God." Excessive indulgence of any kind scattered the vital forces, weakened the nervous system, and predisposed a person to consumption. "A single severe fatigue during the active stage of tuberculosis," he cautioned, "may be the turning-point from the road to recovery to the road to death. Many a consumptive has returned from a long walk or drive upon which he entered as a good case with the death-mark upon him."[22]

Whatever pleasures the invalids may have enjoyed, they often found life at resorts wearing indeed. Weakened by illness, often separated from family and friends, noticing new and worrisome symptoms for which they wanted yet dreaded an explanation, consumptives often felt lonely, vulnerable, frightened, and melancholy. Even the best resorts could disappoint them. While the climate of a place might be famous, the weather was frequently wretched. Stockdale found it "awful" in the Pennsylvania mountains; the nights were so damp he never ventured outside. It rained incessantly at Old Point Comfort, Virginia, and the days turned "ugly" and "disagreeable" at Southern Pines. Consumptives had difficulties, moreover, in securing the proper nourishments that would meet Flick's dietary requirements and also tempt a queasy appetite made worse by the side effects of creosote. Before her delicious squab, T. A. Gaffney had faced this problem:

> I try to find something to eat, but it is quite an effort at times. The [hotel] doctor said it would be impossible to get stale bread even for toast. They send me milk toast made of fresh bread night and morning. The last two mornings it was black as a coal. Of course I did not touch it. I begged a cracker off a doctor who sits at our table at dinner time. I took for dinner some soup a few beats [sic], a little beef, tea, milk and black raspberry pie. . . . If I don't get some good bread to eat I will die of starvation.[23]

Expenses of board and medications nagged some of the travelers, while the worries of home or business impinged unpleasantly on the lives of others. Gaffney's sister fell seriously ill at home, for example, and news from the office interrupted Edward S. Dunn's stay at Old Point Comfort. "I feel that it would be foolish to return [home] . . . and will postpone my time limit a few days," he explained to Flick, but "I fear it is impossible to steal another week from duty."[24]

Even worse, for some, were the miserable loneliness and the lack of care and attention so important to the sick. Gaffney, writing to Flick dutifully from the hotel piazza, reported that Miss Cope, who had accompanied her to Wernersville, "has gone walking with a party. I have to remain at home, it is rather lonely. If I don't get better in three weeks I am coming home." About a week later Miss Cope was replaced by a neighbor, Miss O'Neal, but the latter could stay for little more than two weeks. As her term neared its close, Gaffney appealed to Flick for another companion. "Miss O'Neal will leave next Monday. I can't be left alone, if the family know of no one, perhaps you do. I have to know before Saturday." Mathias Hau, whose health was "failing rapidly" in Southern Pines, ached with a similar feeling: "I intend to leave here in a few weeks for the North. What will you advise, to go to the Adirondack Mountains, or to go to a hospital and stay till the end comes. . . . Here I have no care and attention whatever, am alone at night, and in day time have only a colored cook in the house. Really, it was this lonelyness and want of care that may [made] me so wretched."[25]

For many consumptives, the want of care had medical as well as personal aspects. They felt sick, developed complications, and ran out of medications in places that had no druggists; they wanted symptoms explained and treatments advised. J. S. Campbell, for example, reported to Flick on the state of his tongue, cough, pulse, and temperature. "With frequent Flax Poultices" he had almost cleared up the pain in his chest, but he had only two powders left and wanted further instructions. "Am writing hurriedly in order to catch mail to send Special delivery," he wrote expectantly, "so I may receive answer this P.M." "What is your idea of me taking a warm bath, in a few days, after I get stronger[?]" asked William Beggs, who was starting off for Atlantic City. From Bethlehem, Pennsylvania, Joseph Michel reported that he had caught cold. "Can you help me, so far away[?]" From Cape May, New Jersey, another man revealed his need in the opening line of his letter: "I don't think I know exactly how I am till I have somebody to tell me."[26]

Alternative Treatments at Home

Even a week in the country lay far beyond the resources of most consumptives. The diagnosis, moreover, often brought little relief from life's usual responsibilities. Somehow patients adjusted their treatments to their daily schedules, but they were often unable to slacken their work. In August 1895, for example, George M. Chester wrote to Flick from Newark, New Jersey:

> I am alive but, I have been having it pretty rough for past year. . . . I felt pretty fair up to last spring April when . . . I moved back to Newark and into the Express biz again and all summer I have had from 12 to 17 hours a day to put in and I stood it fairly well, until about 2 weeks ago and I broke down again and for past week I have been having hemorrhages . . . and I am pretty well run down, although not near as bad as when you started in on me and Dr. I am working for $40⁰⁰ a month just think of it. I cannot live on that in the City let alone ever thinking of reducing my indebtedness to you—which I assure you I have not forgotten   Dr. I had to stop taking Creosote it upset my stomach so and I have tried it several times . . . now Dr. if I am not imposing on you, can you send me a prescription to stop hemorrhages and the linament again and whatever other treatment or orders you think necessary   I am inside at office work and I suppose that is no benefit to me, but I must work   I cannot see my family want—I trust you will pardon me for telling my troubles but it is a matter of life and death with me and has been for nearly 3 years   I trust . . . that I shall hear from you soon.

Flick, accustomed to treating his patients by mail, sent Chester some prescriptions, and almost a month later the patient reported that his hemorrhages had stopped and he felt better. "I did not loose [*sic*] much time, could not afford too," he wrote, "but I think your Letter acted as a tonic. . . . I am not well and I may never be but I am not throwing up the sponge."[27]

Not all consumptives turned to physicians for help and treatment. Some were too poor to pay a physician's fee, while others preferred or perhaps merely sampled the various remedies available. In advertisements virtually indistinguishable from news, the daily newspapers trumpeted cures for consumption. "NEW LIFE AND HOPE FOR CONSUMPTIVES" read the headline of a full-page, illustrated "article" in the Sunday *Philadelphia Inquirer* on March 5, 1899. "Dr. Slocum's Treatment Snatches Thousands from Death's Very Door. . . . You, too, can be cured if you will only begin in time. Don't delay." On another page of the same paper the Copeland Institute offered treatment by inhalations. "It reaches the deepest recesses of the lungs. . . . It heals the sore spots. It kills disease germs. It cures Bronchial

Catarrh and prevents Consumption. If taken in time it will cure Consumption in its early stages." No governmental regulations restricted claims such as these in the nineteenth century, nor were sellers required to reveal the ingredients of their remedies, which often included alcohol and morphine. Moreover, medical credentials at this time could be meaningless or frankly fraudulent. As a result, people had few, if any, reliable ways to judge the quality of their doctors or the worth of the treatments.[28]

Mrs. S. S. Erricson faced this problem in 1900. She had visited the "Koch Doctor," whose bespectacled and bearded likeness to Dr. Robert Koch added an air of scientific legitimacy to his advertisements in the local papers. Uncertain about the advice received, she wrote to the Philadelphia Board of Health, which in turn referred her to Flick. "I write you as advised. . . . I have been examined by the Koch Doctor. and informed that I have tubercular disease of the lungs but can be cured by them. I have also been told my trouble was catarrhal and bronchial inflammation by others. now as I am a poor woman with no friends or relatives in the city to advise . . . please tell me if they or any one can cure me. I dont think my case very far advanced."[29]

While Mrs. Erricson may have had early tuberculosis, if she had the disease at all, others were not so fortunate. For many consumptives, the struggle of living merged gradually into the stark realities of dying. Even then the quest continued. Physicians, doing the best they could, prescribed their various treatments; desperate patients placed their confidence in some of the remedies and rejected others. Dr. Elmer E. Keiser reported regularly on a man whom Flick had seen in consultation:

> Nov. 29. 1897 . . .
> I saw Mr. Miltenberger this morning . . . pulse still remains quite rapid 122. . . . Temperature was 100° F. Expectoration quite free . . . some night sweat. . . . less cough than formerly. . . . He is quite hopeful that the next few weeks will find him much improved. . . . I shall increase the strychnia as you have suggested.

> Dec. 8, 1897 . . .
> I have been following your instructions in regard to the dry cupping of Mr. Miltenberger every other day. . . .
> There are no signs of iodism [iodine toxicity] from the europhen. His appetite has improved but slightly and he finds it difficult to drink more than a quart of milk daily.

> Dec. 20. 1897 . . .
> Our patient is much the same. . . . I have endeavored to allay [the cough] with 1/4 gr[ain] doses of codeine in a teaspoon of Syr. Pinus Alba comp. every

two hours but without success. I have again suggested your seeing the patient
and the young man insists on waiting until after Christmas to see if there will
be no change. He now takes the Europhen inunctions twice daily, and increasing doses of strychnia, now 1/20 gr. t.d. [three times a day] and I apply the cups
(dry) every other day.

[Undated, circa Dec. 21, 1897]
Our patient has been pretty much the same . . . growing weaker. . . . He has
declined to have any more cupping because he thinks it does him no good, and
the family of course coincide with him. . . .

He feels very much discouraged in every way but fortunately he has great
faith in the inunctions which makes him at all tractable.

12.22.97 . . .
Mr. Miltenberger would like you to come out tomorrow evening. . . .
Trains leave Broad St. Sta at 5.02 and 5.19 P.M. also at 4.29 P.M. Kindly let
me know and I will meet you at the Tacony Station.[30]

Almost every year in the 1890s, more than twenty-five hundred people in
Philadelphia died of pulmonary tuberculosis. Little wonder that both consumptives and their physicians clutched at the chance of cure.

Rumor and Hope

In 1890 Robert Koch, who eight years earlier had identified the bacterial
cause of tuberculosis, announced that he had found an effective treatment.
The scientist had noted that a healthy guinea pig, when injected with a
culture of tubercle bacilli, showed no initial reaction but about two weeks
later developed a local nodule that then broke down into a persistent skin
ulcer. When a tuberculous guinea pig was inoculated, however, the skin
soon hardened at the site of injection, ulcerated, and healed. The animal's
prior infection had somehow protected it from a second exposure. Repeated injections of a substance derived from the bacilli, Koch reasoned,
would enable the body to slough away infected tissues and heal itself in a
comparable manner. From the fluid in which he had grown the bacilli,
Koch prepared a "lymph," or tuberculin as it was later called, tested it in
animals, and arranged for its trial in patients. Some of these subjects
improved dramatically, and Koch concluded that, for early cases at least, the
treatment was curative. Physicians and patients alike rushed hopefully to
Berlin to observe or participate in the new treatment. It gradually became
evident, however, that Koch's report had been premature. His tuberculin—
used in doses too large on patients too ill with extensive disease—was not

effective. Nevertheless, the hope lingered that some modification in the dose or preparation of tuberculin might prove beneficial. A few U.S. physicians, notably Edward L. Trudeau at Saranac Lake, New York, and Karl von Ruck in Asheville, North Carolina, as well as a number of European scientists, began the search. Soon they were making cautiously optimistic reports.[31]

Word of the new treatment swept like flame through communities of invalids. Miss Annie Fitzer heard of it in Tryon, North Carolina, a reputedly excellent place for consumptives. Hoarseness and cough had compelled her to give up teaching two years earlier, but she had improved at Southern Pines. Now she was living in Tryon, where a part-time teaching position allowed her "to get the climate" and she could spend her afternoons outdoors. "I am taking Tablets of Iron, Strychnine and Arsenic and drinking Porter," she informed Dr. Flick. "Am I . . . taking all that I should take . . . ?" Her principal question dealt with a new form of tuberculin. Her friends had seen wonderful improvement in a case of advanced consumption and were urging her to use it. Was it dangerous? she asked. "Would you advise me to use it? . . . I am sorely perplexed as to what is best to do, and I have a horror of Consumption, which I fear is on my track."[32]

From Idaho, Charles H. Pratt inquired on behalf of his daughter. He and his wife had relinquished their home in Minneapolis to take the young woman to Phoenix and Tucson, but she had not recovered. Along with Mrs. Pratt, she was now living in a tent at thirty-five hundred feet. "Is there any place in the world where the Koch method of treatment by inoculation is so successfully tried, as to to make it worthwhile to go there[?]" he asked. "Pardon this from a stranger." Flick suggested that Pratt write to von Ruck and Trudeau, but both these physicians were looking for early, not chronic, cases and it seems unlikely that either would have encouraged the trip.[33]

While news of tuberculin attracted attention, so did reports of another therapeutic innovation, the sanatorium (or sanitarium as it was spelled in the early years)—an organizational reformation of resort hotels and lodgings that was to challenge the resorts themselves. Here consumptives could presumably enjoy the advantages of a salubrious climate and count on the institution to provide the proper food, fresh air, activity, and rest that leading physicians considered so essential. Tuberculosis sanatoriums differed from health resorts in two significant ways: they specialized in the care of consumptives, and they promised closer supervision of the treatment.

Early sanatoriums in the United States were based in part on German models, particularly those established by Hermann Brehmer in 1859 and by

Peter Dettweiler in 1876. Brehmer's regimen reflected his medical and climatological beliefs: a proper location in the mountains, a liberal diet, wine, fresh air, and exercise, graded to prevent fatigue. In keeping with the Priessnitz influence, he also used a number of hydropathic treatments, including body rubs, sponge baths, showers, and his own special "forest douche"—a forceful stream of ice-cold water that fell on the patient from a height of five meters. Dettweiler, a previous patient and assistant of Brehmer, modified this program in his own sanatorium. He emphasized rest rather than exercise, and instituted the careful supervision that was to become popular among leading U.S. physicians.[34]

In 1882 Edward L. Trudeau, a consumptive physician from New York City, first learned of Brehmer's sanatorium and decided to follow his example. Trudeau had been diagnosed as having the disease ten years earlier and, like Flick, had followed the usual advice to leave his medical practice for a healthier environment. Travel, however, only seemed to make his condition worse. Anticipating his death, he decided to go to New York's Adirondack Mountains, not because he expected to benefit from the climate but because he loved the forest, its wildlife, and the good hunting that he had once enjoyed there. Gradually his health improved and, in a pattern typical of many tuberculous physicians and other healers before and after him, he decided to treat others with the methods that had worked in his own case. Brehmer's success gave him encouragement, and with the financial support of patients and friends he opened his small Adirondack Cottage Sanitarium at Saranac Lake in 1885. This was to become the best-known sanatorium in the United States.[35]

Despite faltering starts and some failures, other men and women established sanatoriums and attracted clienteles. Among the successful was Karl von Ruck, who opened the Winyah Sanitarium in Asheville, North Carolina, in 1888. Reports of the sanatoriums began to appear in the medical literature, and interested laypersons heard of the innovation. Patients, relatives, and friends began to write for Flick's opinions. Dr. Edward J. Nolan, for example, was urging his sister, Mrs. Eleanor Gilbert, to leave the Highland House at Wernersville and go instead to Asheville. He wanted Flick not only to give them advice but also to intercede with von Ruck on her behalf. Mathias Hau wrote for the address of the sanatorium in the Adirondacks that Flick had recommended. For the winter months, he noted, "it would be very good to have a similar institution in Southern Pines."[36]

For those Americans who wanted to enter sanatoriums late in the

nineteenth century, however, the nation's small number of fledgling institutions provided only a few opportunities. Some consumptives decided
to try their luck in Europe—among them Elwell Stockdale, who was doing
poorly despite his stay in the mountains. Dr. Edward O. Otis, a Boston
physician to whom Stockdale had written for advice, had recommended
Dettweiler's sanatorium at Falkenstein, near Frankfurt-am-Main, and
Stockdale arrived there late in November 1898. The young salesman, just
twenty-five years old and unable to speak German, was greeted with bad
news. "I find much to my surprise and sorrow that my right lung is also
affected," he wrote dejectedly to Flick. "I have always tried to console my
self with the fact that some people live a long long time on one lung and
that has always been my hope but I never heard of anyone living with no
lungs." Stockdale's characteristic faith and optimism, however, sustained
him. "You see there are so much for me to live for that it worries me—
Outside of my self which of course is something—there is my mother and
father to thing [sic] of and if I can't work why—well I simply must and I
cant help from feeling the Lord will see how important it is and let me get
well."[37]

He started promptly on the Dettweiler regimen:

> At 7[30] a man comes and wakes me up and rubs me hard with a coarse towel,
> this is to warm up the blood and prevent danger of taking cold in getting up.
>   1st breakfast at 8—all the milk and bread and butter I can eat and one cup
> of coffee. Then starts the cure which is merely sitting in a reclining chair
> (wrapped up warm) in an open pavilion . . . here we live our life and on which
> they wholly depend for the cure. at 10 we go in to sort of a 2nd breakfast
> consisting of milk and bread and butter. Then chairs till 1 which is dinner
> chairs till 7 which is supper chairs till 10 at night and to bed. at 4 and 9 milk is
> served to us at the chairs.[38]

Stockdale slowly made progress. For most of December his physicians
allowed him to stay in his chair only until 6 P.M., but by the end of the
month they promoted him to the later hour. Gradually, too, as the months
wore on, his morning rubs were changed—from a dry rub, to one with
alcohol and water, and finally to the ice-cold douche. Food and drink were
consistently plentiful, if expensive and not always to Stockdale's taste.
"Raw meats are the thing here," he explained; "it goes hard at first . . . but
you must get used to it and eat it all." Brandy, sherry, wine, and beer all cost
extra, adding to the daily charge of two dollars for food and one dollar for
sleeping. Dr. Otis, he complained, had not been told of these extras and,
furthermore, had underestimated the average stay. "It is all rot for your

friend Otis to say in that pamphlet that 3 months is the average stay," he wrote in April. Tell him "to burn up those pamphlets—or else change it to 6 to 8 months to be cured."[39]

In June 1899, Stockdale's physicians gave him a guardedly optimistic assessment but confirmed his fears about the need for prolonged treatment. His lung was better and they predicted healing by fall, but "it will be very weak and I must do 'cure' all winter till it gets thoroughly strong," he reported. "They say it will be suicide for me to come home for even if I did no work the temptations of friends etc and the lack of facilities to do cure would be such that they fear it would break open. They tell me I must go to Davos in the Alps for the winter and then I will be a complete cure and stronger than for years." Stockdale went to Davos, as advised, and probably stayed at one of the many hotels or lodgings that catered to invalids in that beautiful Alpine valley.[40]

The two kinds of environment that Stockdale saw in Europe symbolized past and future in the treatment of consumptives. "'Hilares mox sani,'" read an inscription in the largest hotel in Davos. The merry are soon well. In Brehmer's sanatorium hung a contrasting motto: "'Die Patienten kommen nicht um sich zu amüsiren sondern um geheilt zu werden' (Patients do not come here to amuse themselves, but to be cured)."[41] In the competition between resorts and sanatoriums, the latter would eventually prevail. Among the several reasons for their success were the organized services that spared their clienteles the worries of making their own arrangements and that also gave them a sense of support and hope.

Sanatoriums and hospitals were to grow in importance and numbers throughout the first half of the twentieth century. In 1895, Flick began to involve himself in this work as he turned his attention to a large and quite different group of consumptives—those who were also poor. The poor, of course, did not go to resorts or faraway sanatoriums; most could not even afford to pay a physician. In his practice, however, Flick had observed both their suffering and the dangers to which they exposed their families. At least two organizations in the city were already caring for poor consumptives— Philadelphia's municipal government and the Protestant Episcopal Church.

3. Helping Poor Consumptives

In August 1876, a missionary from the Philadelphia Protestant Episcopal City Mission found a young, consumptive Frenchman lying on the floor and covered by only a worn-out blanket. When the blanket was lifted, bones could be seen through holes in his skin. Some friends had managed to get the man admitted to a hospital, but because he was incurable the hospital had sent him home. Meanwhile, his landlord had arranged for the legal seizure of the sick man's possessions in lieu of some overdue rent. The man, his wife, and their three children were destitute.[1]

Philadelphia was a city of both hardship and opportunity in the late nineteenth century. In 1870, a population of roughly 674,000 made the city the second largest in the nation; by 1900, this number had risen to 1,293,000. Men and women had been crowding in from neighboring regions and also from Europe. Between 1870 and 1900, about a fourth of the city's populace had been born abroad. Among these, the Irish constituted the largest segment and the Germans the next. In the 1880s, increasing numbers of Russian Jews and Italians began to arrive. These and others spread out through the city, concentrating in sections where jobs were available. Most, though not all, of the men found work. As a railroad hub and an inland port on the Delaware River, Philadelphia was a center of commerce, with a diversified industry that included textiles, clothing, shoes, lumber, construction, and printing. Wages were often low, especially for unskilled labor, and relatively few workers could accumulate savings. Teen-aged children often contributed to a family's income by getting jobs, and some households took boarders. Economic security, however, was usually tenuous; cyclical depressions, seasonal layoffs, sickness, and accidents could quickly impoverish a family.[2]

Relief for the poor in Philadelphia, as elsewhere in the United States, was a local responsibility, and the municipal government fulfilled this duty in several ways. In 1870, the city's Guardians of the Poor provided "outdoor relief" to 36,522 needy persons by distributing groceries, fuel, medicines, and other incidentals at a cost of $61,805—$1.69 per person. The Guardians paid physicians to visit and treat some of the sick and apothecaries to fill the doctors' prescriptions. The Guardians also managed the Philadelphia Hospital and Almshouse, which in 1870 averaged 3,273 inmates: 842 in the hospital, 786 in the insane department, 165 in the children's asylum, and 1,480 in the "outwards"—areas intended for paupers presumably able to work.[3]

While a sense of social responsibility on the part of the city's leaders shaped the Almshouse, so did their desires to keep public expenditures low and dependency at a minimum. In terms of expense, the Almshouse seemed a success in 1873: the average cost was only $1.77 per inmate per week. In the opinion of Dr. Isaac Ray, who had recently served on the Board of Guardians, however, the institution needed reform: the hospital's wards were overcrowded, its floors and walls were deteriorating and dirty, and ostensibly-recovered patients provided most of the nursing care. In language that expressed both his concern and his social distance from the inmates, he described the Almshouse as "a continuous pile of buildings" that harbored "one seething mass of infirmity, disease, vice and insanity." In addition to the insane, the sick, orphans, and foundlings, this group included men and women who, through "misfortune, or sickness, or innate shiftlessness, or feebleness resulting from vicious indulgences, have become unable to support themselves."[4]

Ray's image of the Almshouse reiterated descriptions of the American city through much of the nineteenth century, as the worried middle and upper classes tried to cope with the social upheavals engendered by urbanization, industrialization, and immigration. According to typical judgments of the time, the moral defects of the poor helped to explain their condition, yet society should try to improve it. Throughout the century, various groups of private citizens had attempted to relieve the lot of the deserving poor by means that included religous instruction, work, schools, asylums, hospital care, and material aid. Those deemed undeserving because of attributes such as intemperance, laziness, or promiscuity were left to the Guardians and the Almshouse.[5]

On the medical wards of this institution, where tuberculous men and women mingled with other patients, phthisis caused 27 percent of the deaths in 1870—more than any other condition. In the insane department the figure was 36 percent. In neither the hospital nor the city at large, however, did consumption attract much attention. Unlike cholera or smallpox, it caused no sudden epidemics, no fears of contagion. Although 7 percent of the city's deaths from consumption in 1870 occurred at the Almshouse, most of the victims of the disease died at home.[6]

During the final quarter of the nineteenth century, attitudes began to change, and two church-related organizations inaugurated special programs to assist consumptives who were also poor. Each organization offered the aid in an effort to relieve human suffering, but each did so in a way that would serve additional purposes of its own. The Philadelphia Protestant Episcopal City Mission, which entered the work in 1876, had evangelical goals. In a moral struggle against crime, vice, and disorder, its clergymen linked temporal relief to spiritual instruction. They tried to lead their consumptive patients to Christ, thus, they believed, saving their patients' souls. As time went on, two more medical objectives emerged in the Mission's work: curing consumption and preventing its spread to others. It was in this later period, in 1895, that the Free Hospital for Poor Consumptives entered the field under Roman Catholic auspices. Under Flick's leadership, its goals were both medical and humane. The Free Hospital offered institutional care, thus segregating infectious patients and, by protecting the public, saving lives.

A Christian Response: The Philadelphia Protestant Episcopal City Mission

In 1870, the Right Reverend William B. Stevens, Bishop of Philadelphia, appealed for support of a new organization to bring "the remedial and elevating principles of our holy religion" to people who needed it. This organization, the Philadelphia Protestant Episcopal City Mission, was to include preaching, religious services in public institutions, and "visiting such poor and sick persons as have no recognized pastors, and giving them, as occasion may require, temporal as well as spiritual help and comfort." Reflecting contemporary hopes and anxieties common to Protestant clergy and zealous laypersons alike, Stevens believed that these efforts would serve to Christianize Philadelphia. They would help to prevent crime, make the useless useful, turn paupers into producers, and give homes to the outcast, thereby "introducing order, sobriety, and cleanliness." They would constitute "a means of doing our blessed Lord's work in a neglected field . . . thus seeking His glory, and the salvation of souls." The bishop had already appointed an experienced pastor, the Rev. Samuel Durborow, as superintendent of the City Mission, and both lay and clerical visitors assisted in the work.[7]

Needs of the sick poor soon commanded special attention from the superintendent and his assistants. The sick lacked food, among other necessities, and in the winter of 1875–76 the City Mission opened its first diet kitchen. Broth, custard, bread pudding, oranges, farina, wine, and other "delicate but nutritious food . . . without which medicines, medical skill, and even careful nursing would in many cases avail but little" were sent into the homes of those who needed them. When visitors found a family destitute, they also contributed bedding, clothes, coal, medicines, and small amounts of money.[8]

As the missionaries visited the sick, they became increasingly aware of the plight of poor consumptives. The "lingering nature" of their disease and the "extreme debility" with which it was associated seemed to entitle them to "compassionate regard." Early in 1876, the Board of Council for City Missions authorized the first step toward establishing an institution: the solicitation of a special fund to relieve such invalids. They thus inaugurated a new department within the Mission, the Home for Poor Consumptives. In 1877, when the Mission established a central office at 411 Spruce Street, it equipped several of the rooms upstairs as a temporary hospital where needy consumptives could be received. The bishop named the building the House of Mercy.[9]

Applicants to the Home for Poor Consumptives had to meet two criteria. First, like other recipients of charity in the nineteenth century, they had to be judged worthy—truly needy of help, not simply lazy or otherwise responsible for their own plight. Second, the medical condition of each applicant had to be certified by a respectable physician. Thus doubly legitimated, poor consumptives became proper subjects for relief. Most patients during the early years stayed in their own homes, where they received food, medicines, other necessities, and even a little whiskey (a commonly prescribed remedy). Physicians attended them as needed, and a missionary visited regularly. When the home surroundings proved too unwholesome or impoverished to permit adequate care, the Mission moved patients to suitable private homes and paid for their board and nursing. A few such patients—mainly if not entirely women—were admitted to the House of Mercy.[10]

Trying to help poor consumptives often distressed and exhausted the missionaries, but it also brought them emotional and spiritual satisfactions and a sense of accomplishing something worthwhile. During the winter of 1880–81, for example, the Rev. Dr. Thomas L. Franklin, who had assumed the spiritual charge of the Mission's consumptive patients, had an average of sixty-five of them under his care. They were scattered not only through the heavily populated parts of the city but also in outlying areas—far from the central office downtown. "The work of visitation during the past winter has been severe," reported Franklin,

> in bitter cold, in snow drifts, in slush, through narrow snow-and-ice-blockaded streets, by day and by night, at all hours, as late as three o'clock in the morning, wending my way home from ministering to the dying. Many days in the worst weather of the last hard winter, out in the streets all day, one day from eight o'clock in the morning until midnight, and then only entering my residence to be notified of a call to go to a dying man, and remaining with him until near daylight.
>
> This labor, I have reason to believe, has not been in vain. Many lives were rescued that would have been lost but for the sympathy and aid of the Mission, and in several instances I have been privileged to lead to the Cross souls that died in hope, and are doubtless now rejoicing in the joy of their salvation.[11]

Lay visitors—frequently women—assisted the clergymen and shared in their trials and rewards. "My pen fails me to depict the scenes of sufferings and distress which I have witnessed," wrote Mrs. Agar in 1879, yet there were satisfactions in giving both temporal and spiritual comfort. "An old lady, a consumptive and extremely destitute, with nothing to eat, and hardly any clothing, when told that the Mission would relieve her wants, put up her hands and exclaimed, 'I knew my Father in Heaven would not forget me, but would send Christian friends to help me!' A sick woman, in the last stages of consumption, asked me to read the Bible and pray with her, and when I had done so, drew me to her and kissed me, saying, with her eyes filled with tears, 'O God, bless you and those who sent you to comfort me!'"[12]

Spiritual attention was an important part of the care at the House of Mercy as well as in patients' homes. "Several of our family of consumptives have departed their life within the year," reported Miss Susan Nevins, who served as Matron there, "and we can say, without the slightest hesitation, that they all had the precious gospel of our blessed Lord and Saviour, Jesus Christ, plainly, kindly and earnestly presented to them in the daily religious service in common with the other patients, as well as in private at their bed-side."[13]

Relatively few of the Mission's patients, however, entered the House of Mercy—a fact that its limited space only partly explained. Despite the "wretched abodes" and "terrible sufferings" that troubled the visitors, most consumptives chose to remain at home. The Mission's annual report in 1878 noted with interest that, of all the persons under its care during the year, "not more than one in twenty desired removal from their homes." Most "were so reluctant to leave their families that, if forced to choose, they preferred to *suffer* at home, instead of enjoying every comfort that any institution could afford." This predilection of consumptives diminished in subsequent decades but never disappeared.[14]

An Institution Versus Care at Home

The Mission's leaders had originally intended to build an institution, and in 1881 a legacy of $190,000 increased the likelihood of a new Home. Dr. William M. Angney, physician in charge at the House of Mercy, strongly favored one, partly for its preventive benefits. In 1881, even before Koch's discovery of the tubercle bacillus, Angney was beginning to worry about the contagiousness of consumption. Many patients on the Home's list, he warned, lived in close, ill-ventilated quarters. More than once he had seen a consumptive father sleep in the same room with his wife and several small children. While he acknowledged the common prejudice against entering a hospital and the strength of family love—even among the poor—he felt the "urgent necessity" of erecting a new building. It should be out of the city where patients could escape the heat of the summer and enjoy the benefits of sunlight, fresh air, and exercise.[15]

Furthermore, Angney noted, some of the patients needed the discipline that only an institution could provide. In the fall of 1880, the Mission had opened a house for male consumptives at 111 Queen Street, but the patients had proved unruly. Most of the men lacked homes and family ties, he explained in 1882, and many had "led reckless lives." Because of their unacceptable behavior, the Mission had discontinued the service, leaving itself no means of caring for homeless men. Now the only alternative for these unfortunates was the Almshouse. The Mission, Angney urged, should build its own hospital.[16]

Moral, familial, and fiscal values, however, argued for the Mission's original methods. Although an institution provided a merciful shelter for those without resources or relatives, Superintendent Durborow acknowledged, kindness, the need to preserve families, and organizational economy favored their care at home. Showing no concern for contagiousness in the homes of the Mission's patients, he explained his position in the annual report of 1883. "[Suppose] the victim of this malady is a mother who has been left with a large family of children, some of whom perhaps are old enough to contribute by their small earnings to the scant support of the household. The mother's presence is necessary to preserve the home—to keep her children together, to maintain the strong tie of maternal affection . . . and to exercise, as her strength permits, a motherly influence over their conduct and lives." On the other hand, if the father and husband fell sick, he continued, all would depend "on the wife, who by taking in sewing or washing, or going out for day's work" could get together "a meagre subsistence." The sick husband could then look after the little ones in her absence. Two evils could thus be avoided: the common dread of being taken to a hospital, and the breakup of homes and families. Instead, sufferers could pass their last days among those they loved. Care at home also cost less and avoided the unsanitary crowding of a ward in a large hospital.[17]

A gift of a beautiful eleven-acre estate in 1885 helped to settle any disagreements about methods, and the board began to plan for its new Home in Chestnut Hill, just outside the city limits of northwestern Philadelphia. It would try to create a private, homelike atmosphere for consumptive patients, admit them without charge, and keep them indefinitely, even to the end of their days. The Home would continue its spiritual work, of course: regular religious services and solace to dying patients. It would "try to lead them to trust in the mercies of our adorable Redeemer, who alone could give them, if penitent and believing, an entrance into the everlasting rest."[18]

One question proved controversial: what class of consumptive patients to admit. Should the Home continue to take only advanced cases whose outlook seemed hopeless, or should it include patients in earlier stages of the disease? During a trip to England in 1877, Superintendent Durborow had first learned of the possible curative value of hospital care, at least for patients with incipient disease, and Dr. Angney was growing optimistic. As early as 1881, he thought he could claim the cure of Martha D., a seventeen-year-old girl who had been admitted to the House of Mercy almost a year and a half earlier. Subsequent patients gave further, if less dramatic, cause for optimism: some left the Home improved, and a few even returned to work.[19]

The board decided to try an experiment: it would admit some early cases to its new Home in Chestnut Hill and make provision there for curative treatment. This change in policy, the board believed, would actually benefit advanced cases by reducing their dread of the institution. Even if "Hope for all" could not be written over its portals, "Despair for all" would not appear there, frightening away prospective patients as if from the gate to Hell. To symbolize the change, the board cautiously named its new institution the Home for Consumptives: For Their Relief and Care.[20]

The Home at Chestnut Hill opened in the spring of 1886 with two substantial structures: a massive, ornate building that contained offices, reception rooms, a hall, and a chapel, and one brick-and-stone pavilion (or cottage) that housed the patients. Women patients were moved into this cottage from the House of Mercy, freeing the latter to admit men. During the year that ended in March 1887, the Mission cared for 210 patients: 18 percent of them in the new Home, 18 percent at the House of Mercy, and 64 percent in their own homes or in those of friends. The new facilities, which slowly expanded in capacity, began to change the location of care-giving. In 1900, the Mission reported 207 patients treated during the year: 55 percent at Chestnut Hill, 21 percent at the House of Mercy, and only 24 percent at home.[21]

Tensions persisted between medical and spiritual goals—between the prolongation and saving of lives that appealed to the physicians and the relief and comfort promoted by the clergy. Dr. Robert Bolling, the first physician to serve the Home at Chestnut Hill, wanted it to become a model hospital that would rank with the best in England and Berlin. To this end, he urged in 1887, the Home should equip itself with "all the modern appliances for the Pneumatic and Gaseous treatment[s]"—methods of administering germicides by inhalation or by enemas. Dr. Angney had just started to try the gaseous enemas at the House of Mercy. Bolling also recommended "improved microscopes for the study and differentiation of the cases" and platform scales for weighing the patients on admission and discharge. The Mission did not immediately accede to these requests, and in 1891 Bolling repeated them. European physicians were reporting success with such treatments, he noted, and one was charging gross neglect on the part of any physician who failed to use them.[22]

Bolling's recommendations partly reflected changes in medical thought and organization. Specific diagnosis was becoming more important in medical practice, microscopic examinations were therefore increasingly necessary, and effective treatments seemed almost at hand. In 1890, Flick's paper on special hospitals for tuberculosis was received well by his colleagues, and in 1891, the Rush Hospital for Consumption and Allied Diseases, which Flick had helped to establish, opened its dispensary. The hospital itself accepted its first patients the following year. Sanatoriums were also beginning to attract attention, and their medically supervised regimen offered promise.[23]

Therapeutic results at both Chestnut Hill and the House of Mercy, as if to confirm the growing optimism, seemed remarkably good for a disease long considered hopeless. Over the four years from 1887 through 1890, Bolling and Angney reported that roughly one-third to one-half of their patients improved. Superintendent Herman L. Duhring, who replaced Durborow in 1889, distrusted the doctors' claims. In 1890, at the height of the tensions between clergy and physicians, his report to the board praised the Mission's work with consumptives. Its homes had done "more than could any Hospital for that dreadfully common disease—about which physicians to this hour are only guessing. We speak carefully," he continued, "for nursing, not medicine, has to this day done the most for the Consumptive. True, remedies are pronounced successful, and we are told the disease can be cured, but deaths are as numerous as ever. Just as we were told last winter of a successful operation, but the patient died!"[24]

Home to Hospital

Even in the modest institution at Chestnut Hill, which sheltered about two dozen consumptives in the early 1890s, the physicians and the clergymen were playing their typical roles in the evolution of the American hospital. Medical authority, based on diagnosis, treatment, and the promise of bodily healing, was challenging more traditional Christian stewardship. Over the next few years, both groups accommodated, but physicians achieved the principal gains. While the clergymen still took an interest in chronically ill patients, they began to adopt the curative goals so dear to physicians. In 1892, the new bishop, the Rt. Rev. O. W. Whitaker, spoke favorably of the "careful study and skillful treatment" that were producing such good results at the new Home, and the Rev. Dr. Franklin praised the care and environment there. He found the conditions so superior to those in the patients' homes that he was starting to blame the patients for their own fates. If the Home "fails to cure, it is owing to the strange reluctance of the consumptive to enter it," he asserted, "and then the Home is blamed for not working a miracle. Let the consumptive seek it in the incipient stage of the disease."[25]

The clergy backed their praise of the Home with medical equipment that enabled the physicians to expand their diagnostic and therapeutic methods. According to the annual report in 1893, the Rev. Dr. Fulton donated the long-desired scales for the "systematic weighing of patients"— the very symbol of therapeutic optimism. The Home also acquired an excellent microscope for bacteriological work and all the instruments with which to treat the nose and throat. During the same year the physicians treated several patients with a new form of tuberculin, and reported "satisfactory results." In 1894 Dr. M. Hannah McKirachan, resident physician at Chestnut Hill, observed with pleasure that one patient had gained 24 1/2 pounds. Furthermore, Dr. Waldenburg's compressed air apparatus for inhalation treatments had arrived from Germany, and results with it seemed encouraging. Dr. McKirachan also noted the beginnings of a special department on the second floor of one of the cottages where Dr. Jacob Solis Cohen, a distinguished laryngologist, could try new treatments on a few of the "worst cases in the house." With its new scales, its new equipment, its newly appointed resident physicians, and its therapeutic research, the Home at Chestnut Hill was becoming a hospital.[26]

A change in the name of the institution confirmed this transformation. In the spring of 1894, five visiting physicians suggested the change in order to alter the kind of patient admitted. If the Home were called a "Hospital for the Relief and Cure of Chronic Chest Diseases or Lung Diseases," the doctors reasoned, it would more readily attract the early, more curable cases—those who still hoped they were not consumptive. At the same time, the name would not prevent the admission of patients with more advanced disease. Again a compromise was reached. In 1898, the annual report of the City Mission began to list the institution as the Hospital for Diseases of the Lungs at Chestnut Hill (Home for Female Consumptives).[27]

Several factors probably account for the changing attitudes of the clergy. First, they were surely aware of the growing optimism with which physicians were treating consumptives, not only in their own institution but also elsewhere. Second, the new environment at Chestnut Hill may well have raised their hopes and expectations. Insofar as the disease thrived in the dirty, crowded, impoverished conditions of the city, its victims could only benefit from the salubrious atmosphere of the new Home, its plentiful food, its cleanliness, and its careful supervision—all part of the hygienic regimen that leading physicians were recommending. Third, the apparently good results of the work must have begun to impress the clergy, just as they had the physicians. Between 1877 and 1890, the annual death rate fell from 53 percent of all patients treated to only 23 percent. The proportion of patients discharged as improved, moreover, rose from 1 percent in 1877, to 9 percent in 1882, and to 35 percent in 1890. Starting with the annual report in 1891, Mission leaders, thus emboldened, began to list and underline the percentages of patients discharged as improved during each year after 1890.[28]

Behind the Statistics: Crisis and Compromise

Neither treatment nor environment, however, explain the better results; the cure of advanced consumption was not that easy. As the Mission's published statistics were merely the first in the state to demonstrate, it was chiefly admission and discharge practices that determined an institution's results. During the 1880s, Mission leaders reduced the proportion of seriously ill patients, and the mortality rates and the rates of improvement responded accordingly.

The principal drop in the Mission's death rates occurred abruptly between the years ending in the spring of 1882 and the spring of 1883 (see Table 3-1). It coincided with a marked increase in the discharge rate, a decrease in the number of patients cared for during the year, and a fiscal crisis in the City Mission. The Mission's work with consumptives had expanded rapidly, reaching a peak of 182 patients and placing "a heavy drain" on the organization's resources. In October 1882, Mission leaders had found it necessary to close its four diet kitchens temporarily in order to reduce expenses. Statistics show that they also went further: they reduced the load of consumptive patients by terminating services, most of which during this period went to patients at home. The discharge rate increased drastically, from 12 percent of the patients reported in 1882 to 48 percent of the patients reported in 1883. The action affected many of the most advanced cases, whose deaths, therefore, never appeared in the Mission's records. While 45 more patients were discharged during the year ending in 1883 than during the year before, 37 fewer died in the Mission's care.[29]

These patterns persisted: a relatively high discharge rate and a lower mortality rate. By 1888, two years after the Home at Chestnut Hill had opened, two additional trends are discernible. First, the mortality rate fell even further. A change in patient selection almost certainly contributed to this apparent improvement. With its attractive new facility and its emerging optimism, the Home achieved what the physicians were urging—the admission of consumptives with somewhat less-advanced disease. In 1894, the matron at Chestnut Hill was able to report an exceptionally good year; on several occasions she had not had a single bed patient. A letter from one of the Mission workers, Miss A. F. Devereux, points to more stringent admitting policies as the cause of the matron's good fortune. "[I] beg to report a very sad case," she wrote to Flick in 1895; "[she] is too ill to be received at the [Chestnut] Hill and is in great need." Second, increasing proportions of patients were being removed from the Mission's care. As the

TABLE 3-1. Results, Patients of City Mission, Spring 1876–Spring 1890. Single-line boxes highlight the changes in 1883: proportionately more patients were discharged and fewer died. Double-line boxes show the increase in removals and the further decline in mortality after the Home at Chestnut Hill opened. Rounding error explains minor discrepancies in the percentages.[29]

Year ending spring	Total no. patients treated	Departed alive						Died		Remaining	
		Total		Discharged		Removed					
		No.	%	No.	%	No.	%	No.	%	No.	%
1877	103	20	19	—	—	—	—	55	53	28	27
		—	—	6	6	14	14				
1878	97	24	25	—	—	—	—	45	46	28	29
		—	—	5	5	19	20				
1879	71	17	24	—	—	—	—	27	38	27	38
		—	—	8	11	9	13				
1880	89	12	13	—	—	—	—	37	42	40	45
		—	—	12	13	0	0				
1881	146	14	10	—	—	—	—	69	47	63	43
		—	—	—	—	—	—				
1882	182	32	18	—	—	—	—	85	47	65	36
		—	—	21	12	11	6				
1883	137	68	50	—	—	—	—	48	35	21	15
		—	—	66	48	2	1				
1884	143	57	40	—	—	—	—	38	27	48	34
		—	—	42	29	15	10				
1885	192	85	44	—	—	—	—	61	32	46	24
		—	—	67	35	18	9				
1886	177	76	43	—	—	—	—	61	34	40	23
		—	—	59	33	17	10				
1887	210	97	46	—	—	—	—	76	36	37	18
		—	—	71	34	26	12				
1888	158	103	65	—	—	—	—	33	21	22	14
		—	—	56	35	47	30				
1889	108	55	51	—	—	—	—	24	22	29	27
		—	—	29	27	26	24				
1890	145	74	51	—	—	—	—	34	23	37	26
		—	—	39	27	35	24				

Mission used this term (and it may have used it inconsistently), "removals" referred to patients who left its care on their own initiative or that of relatives, friends, or other responsible persons. For reasons discussed in Chapter 4, patients and their families often preferred living at home to care in an institution.[30]

The change in the mix of patients must have contributed to the rising improvement rates, but probably also important was medical self-deception. With no established criteria to guide them, with no x-ray or bacteriological studies, and with probably limited skills in physical examination, enthusiastic physicians could easily overinterpret symptomatic improvement and exaggerate their claims, just as the Rev. Mr. Duhring had suspected. Food, rest, nursing care, and a little financial help may have restored the health of a few patients, but for many of them, as subsequent years would demonstrate in other institutions, the apparent gains were often both temporary and illusory.

As the clergy increased their support for curative treatment and reduced their burden of home care, physicians accommodated themselves to the care of advanced cases. Although they still complained intermittently that these patients could not benefit from medical treatment, that they used too much of the nurses' time, that they depressed the spirits of other, less ill patients, and that they increased the Mission's death rates in comparison with those of other institutions, they recognized some benefits from admitting such cases. Many patients lived in deplorable conditions, physicians acknowledged, and to give them comfort or possibly even to prolong their lives the Mission should accept them. If it did not, where but the Almshouse could the patients go?[31]

During the mid-1890s, rising anxieties over the contagiousness of consumption gave the Mission's physicians an even more convincing rationale for institutionalizing advanced cases. Poor consumptives in particular, argued the five visiting physicians in 1894, endangered not only their families but also the community. Because bad home conditions increased susceptibility, they explained, "one person in indigent circumstances is a much more dangerous focus of contagion" than were others who, though similarly diseased, lived in "comparative comfort and affluence." The danger alone justified the expense of institutionalization; consumptives were now a menace. Any amount of money spent to keep such "centres of infection" under sanitary control in a hospital, asserted Dr. Angney in 1895, "is not spent in vain."[32]

Between 1876 and 1900, the City Mission's Home for Consumptives had changed significantly. While it still retained its original goals—the saving of souls and temporal relief—medical goals had gained important support. Physicians who claimed that they could prolong life and protect the community from infection had begun to compete successfully with the clergymen who offered comfort, relief, and hope of salvation. The location of care was shifting from homes to institutions, and the new Home was becoming a hospital. To the moral and social dangers associated with the poor in the 1870s, a new danger had been added—the germs that the poor carried in their bodies. Although the needs of poor consumptives probably remained much the same over this period, their image in the eyes of the people who wanted to help them was changing: from pitiable persons in spiritual and physical want to patients who might be cured, to potential beneficiaries of experimental remedies, and to sources of infection. It was in this later context that Dr. Flick and his friend Father John Scully started their own society for the consumptive poor.

A Crusade for Prevention: The Free Hospital for Poor Consumptives

Flick had dreams of his own for the care of poor consumptives. He knew the disease was contagious, he thought he knew how to prevent it, and he knew of the suffering that dying consumptives endured. Perhaps he dreamed of being a hero, of accomplishing something noble, or, as he had promised after his own recovery, of paying his debt to God. In 1894, Flick shared his dreams and concerns with Fr. Scully, pastor of St. Joseph's Church, and the priest agreed to help. He enlisted the support of two large sodalities, the League of the Sacred Heart and the St. Vincent de Paul Society and, in February 1895, a joint committee organized itself as the Free Hospital for Poor Consumptives. Its initial efforts were based at St. Joseph's, the oldest Roman Catholic church in Philadelphia, just two blocks from the House of Mercy. Perhaps the work of the City Mission helped to stimulate Fr. Scully's interest in the project. Roman Catholics had been steadily growing in number among the Mission's consumptive patients and now accounted for about a fourth of them, second only to Protestant Episcopalians.[33]

Like the City Mission in its early years, the Free Hospital directed its work toward poor and deserving consumptives with advanced disease. Visitors, most of whom were women, assessed the worthiness of applicants, and physicians confirmed the patients' medical condition. When an applicant had no physician and was very ill, visitors called upon Flick to go to the patient. "Will you kindly visit the case of Mr. Hugh Foren," wrote Miss Mary L. Coleman on January 2, 1896. "He seems to be worthy and destitute. . . . Mrs. Harte and I visited him this afternoon."[34]

The Free Hospital did not provide care in the homes of its patients; it paid instead for hospitalization. Although Flick and Fr. Scully wanted their own institution and looked for a suitable house in 1895, they had to settle for second best. For five dollars a week per patient, their society (as they and others commonly called it) paid hospitals to care for its patients and to segregate them from nonconsumptives. Flick made the first such arrangements with the Rush Hospital and with St. Mary's Hospital, one of the three Roman Catholic hospitals in the city. When worthy applicants exceeded the number of beds available, Fr. Scully persuaded Archbishop Ryan to use his influence. St. Mary's responded favorably, and Sister Mary Borromeo, sister superior of St. Agnes' Hospital, agreed to accept some consumptives there. During the next few years, Flick persuaded University Hospital and German Hospital to take a few patients. He also arranged for some of the more favorable cases to go to the country, especially to Gabriels, a new Roman Catholic sanatorium recently opened in the Adirondacks. Most frequently, however, he turned to St. Agnes'.[35]

Resistance to taking poor consumptives was strong in the general hospitals of Philadelphia, and in accepting them Sr. Borromeo had to resolve some conflicting interests. Flick, pressed by numerous applicants, sometimes sent to St. Agnes' more patients than the sister had agreed to receive. They not only filled the space allotted to them but spilled over into additional wards, where other physicians objected to their presence and where their coughing annoyed neighboring patients. When men and women, acutely ill with typhoid fever or pneumonia, needed admission, a hospital superintendent found that clogging the wards with chronically ill consumptives was difficult to justify. On the other hand, there were economic considerations. Sr. Borromeo bore the fiscal responsibility for the hospital and executed the job with considerable skill and success. She undoubtedly recognized the economic stability that payments from the Free Hospital gave to her young and struggling institution, opened only a decade before. By 1899, these payments accounted for 19 percent of the monies collected for patients' board at St. Agnes' and almost 10 percent of its total receipts. Although five dollars a week might not have covered the cost of a patient's care, it met the hospital's standard charge for a bed in its wards. When demand for admission was low, a continuing income must have been welcome.[36]

Persistent pressures to find still another bed for a consumptive occasionally exploded into an altercation between Sr. Borromeo and members of the society's staff. "There is no earthly use of your sending any more people to St. Agnes' Hospital," exclaimed Adele G. Tack, one of the visitors, on January 9, 1899. Sr. Borromeo had just refused to admit Joseph

Cassidy, and only "after the biggest kind of fuss" had she relented. Tack, exasperated by the encounter with "her serene highness," wanted nothing more to do with St. Agnes', at least for a time. The sister superior, after reviewing her records that evening, defended her position. St. Agnes' now had twenty-five of the society's patients, she explained, considerably more than the ten to twelve to which it had agreed. In conscience, she could do no more. "There is so much sickness now and we have so many pressing applications for acute cases, that I really feel I am not doing justice to them by filling up the wards with consumptives." About two weeks later Sr. Borromeo, yielding to Flick's persuasion, agreed to take four more of the Free Hospital's patients. "You really are the biggest beggar going," she wrote to Flick. "When I told the sisters of your pleadings and your pitiful face they agreed to make room, though we now have nine on cots. . . . However you must not tax me again, until some of our present number go."37

Flick, like the City Mission, faced a painful choice. One of the problems that neither organization had anticipated was the partial recovery of presumably dying patients. They lingered in an institution, occasionally for years, perhaps too incapacitated to survive without help but less needy than others who were nearer to death. In April 1899, when the number of consumptives at St. Agnes' had risen to twenty-eight, Flick suggested the discharge of ten of the Free Hospital's patients, thus making room for the dying. Sr. Borromeo complied with his suggestion.38

Despite the difficulties in securing accommodations, the Free Hospital's resources and its ability to pay for the care of patients grew impressively from 1895 through early 1902. Moneys spent annually for the maintenance of patients rose during these seven years from $1,912 to $10,597, while the annual number of persons treated rose from 40 to 267. During this growth, and probably to facilitate it by appealing to a wider group of contributors, the society separated itself from its church connections. It incorporated independently in 1897.39

Flick's fundraising appeals for the Free Hospital between 1899 and 1901 sounded two of the major marching themes for the growing campaign to combat tuberculosis. First, consumption was contagious. It could "reach the home of the rich man through the occupations of the consumptive poor," read the back cover of the annual report in 1900. "A consumptive letter carrier brings contagion in your mail; a consumptive car conductor hands it to you in your change; a consumptive saleswoman ties it up in your package; a consumptive cook contaminates your food; a consumptive maid implants the disease in your children; a consumptive mechanic contaminates your house." But the consumptives themselves were not to blame; people should pity and help them. Their suffering was indescribable, and, as Flick expressed it in 1899, they were "outcast from Christian charity," blocked from relief "by indifference, fear or loathing," their fate worse than that of lepers. They had to work until they died, or starve.[40]

Countering fear and despair, Flick in his second theme offered action and hope. Consumption was now preventable. "If every consumptive in the land could at once be placed in a hospital, tuberculosis would be stamped out in a few years." In a hospital, consumptives could be made innocuous. Flick called upon contributors to join in the great crusade: "Charity, philanthropy and science here join hands to entice you on. . . . What a boon to the future men and women to be exempt from the ravages of the great white plague! Is there a greater victory in store for science than to get control and bring under subjection a disease which, from time immemorial, has been death to one-seventh of the human family! Join the crusade against tuberculosis, and you thereby gratify the noblest instincts of your soul."[41]

The third theme of the campaign—that consumption was curable— was barely discernible in the society's early annual reports. In the summer of 1901, however, the Free Hospital, like the City Mission before it, was to take a major step toward curative goals. It was to open a camp for incipient cases in the mountains of eastern Pennsylvania, where poor men and women could benefit from the hygienic regimen offered by a sanatorium. Wherever the care was offered and whatever the goals of the caretakers, the patients had their own ideas of what they wanted. Poor consumptives were not in a strong bargaining position, but many of them were not entirely helpless either. The relationship between caretakers and patients cannot be reduced to simple control and submission.

4. Life as a Patient

The men and women who were helped by the City Mission and the Free Hospital had personal strengths, desires, social relationships, and responsibilities. Although their poverty limited their ability to shop for treatment and care with the ease of more affluent patients, they still made their own judgments, decisions, and choices. They bargained with their caretakers, thanked them effusively, and sometimes rebelled. Some patients, finding that their needs and desires fit nicely with the care provided, appreciated the food, the shelter, and the kind attention that they received. Others, however, grew discontented; they felt unwanted, misunderstood, or even maltreated. Institutionalization disrupted their personal habits, their daily interactions with friends and relatives, and the countless decisions—large and small—that once had ordered their lives. Further, the care that was offered did not always come soon enough or last long enough, and seldom gratified one fundamental yearning of the sick—that somehow they might get well.

The Network of Support

When consumptives could no longer work, they turned if they could to their families. Brothers, sisters, parents, and even more distant relatives, though frequently poor themselves, paid their rent, helped to feed them, or took them into their homes and cared for them. A husband, even when poor, could often support an invalid wife, but when the man—the chief breadwinner in most households—became incapacitated, the consequences were often disastrous. A woman's earnings could not match a man's, and if she had to work outside the home she frequently left her husband and children without care. In 1879, for example, the wife of twenty-six-year-old R. P., one of the City Mission's patients, could earn only $1.25 a week by washing. This sum, together with "a pittance from his mother, a poor widow" who also washed for a living, had to support the man, his wife, and their three children. Twenty years later, a similar situation faced by Martin Fox and his family precipitated an application to the Free Hospital. Because "his wife is compelled to go out washing to procure bread for himself and the children," Fox had no care at home.[1]

Life in a large and expanding city often disrupted traditional family ties. Migrants and immigrants, uprooted from their native environments, took time to reestablish their social networks, and men sometimes had to leave their families in order to find work. For wage-earners of all kinds, a change in employment often necessitated a change in residence. Although the city had developed a horse-drawn trolley system in the latter half of the century, most workers could not afford the daily expense of commuting; instead, they moved to within a mile or so of the job and walked.[2] In addition to these disruptions, accidents and acute infectious diseases took their inevitable tolls, and widows, orphans, the maimed, and the disabled tried to survive.

Consumptives whose family support had been lost through these and other misfortunes had to find other sources of help. Friends, neighbors, and even strangers cared for them or supplemented their meager resources, at least for a time.[3] A few consumptives were eligible for the aid of benefit societies—a form of insurance that paid small weekly allowances for limited periods.[4] Organized charities offered their own particular forms of assistance. A church parish or the St. Vincent de Paul Society, for example, provided some aid to destitute consumptives at home. The Charity Organization Society helped to get work for the wife of Mr. Ghiotti when he entered St. Agnes' Hospital, and an "old mother" came from the Little Sisters of the Poor to care for Mrs. Gallagher's five small children. When Mrs. McClelland's physician told her that she could not live for more than another month, she decided to enter a hospital and arrange for the care of her children; the Society to Protect Children from Cruelty offered its help.[5]

Beyond such charitable assistance lay the Philadelphia Almshouse and Hospital (or Blockley, as it was often called), but to self-respecting men and women the prospect of becoming a patient there was repugnant and grim. Its overcrowding, its cheap and inferior food, the shame of becoming an inmate and a pauper, and the risk of becoming teaching material for doctors and medical students all made potential patients wary of the place. As clergymen, physicians, and others tried to find care for consumptives in whom they were interested, they expressed some widely shared reactions: "Is there a hospital other than the one at the Almshouse to which he could gain admission?" "He has been for a short time in the Philadelphia Hospital, but does not want to return there." "Our people have a terrible prejudice against the Almshouse." "Robert Flannaghan . . . shrinks from Blockley."[6]

Attitudes Toward Hospitalization

Despite such views of Blockley, many consumptives came to a point in their lives when they needed a refuge or wanted to go to a hospital. They could work no longer, families could not support them, nobody was at home to take care of them, friends grew tired of the burden, and boardinghouse keepers wanted their rooms for somebody else. Perhaps the network of support had been weak from the beginning and broke under the strain of continuing illness; perhaps a casual laborer or an unmarried domestic had no network at all. As visitors for the Free Hospital reported to Flick, "The man is a stranger here and without a home." "The husband has almost no work, and uses even the very little money they have very badly." "He has no one to look after him the sister who should do it being a worthless character and now the Constable is to put them out of their home."[7]

Dismissal from one institution sometimes necessitated the search for another. When a voluntary hospital admitted a poor consumptive—perhaps because of another diagnosis—it often tried to limit the stay. St. Joseph's Hospital accepted Frank Dale as a free patient in 1900, for example, but when he was found to have consumption the sister in charge had a talk with him. The hospital did not allow contagious patients, she explained, and if he lived for more than four or five weeks "he would have to get out." When officials of an institution for the blind found that Annie Quinlan, aged seventeen, had consumption, they responded in similar fashion. "They turned her out of It yesterday," Thomas Kearns reported to Flick. "She is blind and consumptive. . . . Her Father and Mother are dead. She has no home. . . . She is now at her uncle's house stopping. . . . [He] is a poor man and has no means to keep this girl."[8]

As their lives ebbed, some of the applicants to the Free Hospital turned to Roman Catholic institutions for religious solace, or at times others anticipated that distressed and dying patients might find it there. For "an old man, living in a sailor's boarding house," for a down-and-out and abusive drunkard, and for a single woman in "Protestant, or at least non-Catholic surroundings," spiritual attention seemed just as important as physical comfort or medical attendance. "It would be a great Charity if you could secure his admission to [St. Agnes'],", wrote Fr. Bradley, "as he is . . . badly in need of Spiritual Succor." Please admit this man from the penitentiary to St. Agnes', requested Mary L. Coleman. Mrs. Fassitt, who had referred him, "seemed to favor it so much and hoped the care of the Sisters would obtain for Lee a good death." Some of the visitors for the Free Hospital, like those for the City Mission, drew spiritual rewards from their work with dying patients. "Augusta Conroy . . . died at the Hospital last week," B. C. Feran reported. "She became a Catholic a few days prior to her decease. One more saved."[9]

Hope for their bodies, not for their souls, stirred in the hearts of other applicants to the Free Hospital, just as it must have for patients at Chestnut Hill. "Can a young man named Wm Comley . . . be readmitted to the Rush Hospital[?]" asked Dr. Henry Fisher. "He was there for a few weeks as a free patient but was discharged, he says, because they claimed he was incurable. He thinks differently . . . and is very anxious to go back to a hospital so that he may gain strength enough to visit . . . the West in the Spring."[10]

In spite of any advantages that hospitals offered, some consumptives, backed by their relatives, balked at the thought of going there. They started to feel a little better, they were managing at home, or, worsening, they became too sick to move. They tried to bargain for a more desirable situation. Howard Greenwood's sister-in-law, for example, refused to go to St. Agnes'; she thought it would do her no good. If she could not get into Rush, she would not go anywhere. Charles Lapetina dreaded St. Agnes' because one of his friends had died there; he wanted to enter the Pennsylvania Hospital instead. For a variety of reasons, patients and their families did not want to be separated. Sarah Kelly, though partially mute, sick, and entirely alone when her mother was out at day's work, told one of the Free Hospital's visitors, that "her mother would not part with her." Mrs. Lynch, in contrast, was "most anxious to go to the Hospital." She was "in a miserable state," getting "neither rest or nourishment," but her husband was "cranky about her leaving him and the children" to the care of his mother-in-law.[11]

Although possible payment for hospital care did not affect the decisions of the truly destitute, it must have shaped the choices of the few applicants who still had some income or savings. When patients or their relatives could afford to, the Free Hospital expected them to pay at least part of the cost of the patient's care, and a charge of three dollars a week, for example, could make family members hesitate. Could they manage the expense? How long would they have to pay? Would care in a hospital prove worthwhile? Would they still have money to bury the patient? Agents of the Free Hospital and Sr. Borromeo understandably tried to avoid the cost of disposing of patients' bodies. If visitors from the Free Hospital believed that families could pay, they sometimes extracted from them a promise to bury their relatives before they agreed to admit them.[12]

Institutional Environments

Despite hesitations and doubts, by choice or the force of circumstance, on foot, by rail, or by horse-drawn ambulance, poor consumptives came to the few institutions in Philadelphia that would accept them. Although the various places involved in the work differed in important ways, they all offered shelter, food, nursing care, medical attention, congregate living, and a certain degree of regimentation.

A man admitted in the 1890s to the House of Mercy at 411 Spruce Street, for instance, entered a modest, three-story, brick rowhouse that was "airy, cheerful and homelike, though exceedingly plain and almost poor in its appointments." There he joined a group of about twelve patients— fifteen when the house was overcrowded—and he shared a room with one or more of them. Each man had a chair and an iron bedstead with woven wire springs. Open windows in the bedrooms and halls assured good ventilation throughout the house. Few patients were bedridden, and most could go to the dining room for their meals. When the weather was suitable, the men were encouraged to sit out in the "roof garden"—a fifteen-by-eighteen foot platform that also served as a drying place for the laundry. It had been made cheerful by boxes of growing plants. To take care of the patients, the Mission hired two nurses—one for day and one for night work—together with four servants. A matron supervised the house-hold, and both clergymen and Dr. Angney paid regular visits. Although the City Mission published no rules for the House of Mercy, it probably had them, and the location itself must have had a settling effect on the patients' behavior: the Mission's offices were just downstairs.[13]

A woman who went to the Home for Consumptives at Chestnut Hill entered a very different environment. In the mid-1890s she was assigned to a room in one of the three stone cottages, each of which could accommodate about fifteen patients. She probably had a room of her own but may have shared one with another patient. The room, illuminated by gaslight, was

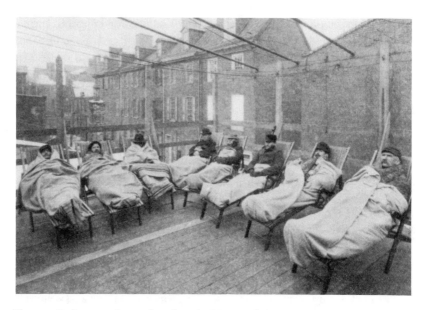

Figure 1. Patients on the roof garden, the House of Mercy, in mid-winter. From the *Annual Report of the Philadelphia Protestant Episcopal City Mission* 36 (1906). Historical Collections, College of Physicians of Philadelphia.

neatly furnished with an iron bedstead, a dresser, and small tables, on one of which rested a basin and pitcher. Many of the rooms had open fireplaces, not so much for heat, which was supplied by a central unit, but for ventilation. A patient might spend much of her time in the sun parlor, where she could, if she wished, enjoy the view, read, sew, knit, or visit with another patient. If well enough, she was expected to walk about outside. As in the House of Mercy, most patients were not confined to bed. For their meals, the women walked through glass-enclosed corridors to an attractive dining room in the Home's central building, where they were served an "ample although plain diet." Once a month, lady visitors or other volunteers gave special entertainments that helped to relieve the tedium of sickness and confinement. Sometimes the ladies sent their carriages or sleighs to give some of the patients a drive through the country. In 1895, when the Home could accommodate forty patients, it had a staff of five day nurses and two night nurses "with seven servants and two men." Two resident physicians, both women, attended the patients medically and could turn for weekly advice to visiting physicians. Patients who could were expected to help in the nursing and in other light duties. Other rules

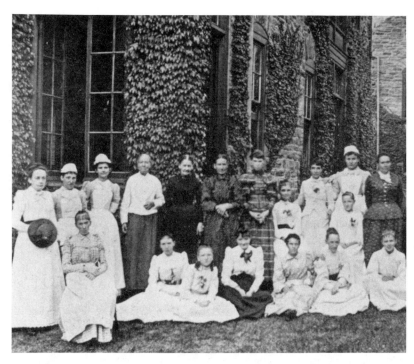

Figure 2. Patients and staff at the Home for Consumptives, Chestnut Hill. From the *Annual Report of the Philadelphia Protestant Episcopal City Mission* 24 (1894). Archives, Episcopal Community Services, Philadelphia.

stipulated lights out at 10:00 P.M., decorum toward others, attendance at daily prayers, and "No LIQUORS, PROVISIONS nor MEDICINES" other than those authorized by the physicians.[14]

A consumptive admitted to St. Agnes' had a rather different experience. St. Agnes,' neither a house nor a converted country estate, was built by the Sisters of St. Francis as a hospital and officially opened in 1888. Its large, three-story stone building in south Philadelphia could accommodate about two hundred patients in the late 1890s—some of them in single or double rooms, but most of them in wards. In 1898, two of these wards were reserved for consumptives and one was reserved for typhoid cases. If the consumptive wards resembled the medical ward illustrated in the hospital's reports, its beds were arrayed down two sides of the room, each separated from the next by a space roughly equal to the width of one bed. A straight chair sat at the foot of each bed, a religious image adorned the otherwise plain walls, and light came from the four globes of the gas fixture that hung from the ceiling. The hospital changed to electric light in 1899. Almost certainly, the patients were served their meals in the wards; they would not have been welcome in other areas. The sisters themselves, together with their postulants and some male attendants, did almost all the work in the hospital, including the care of patients. During the first few years of the hospital the sisters did not have formal training in nursing, but after the St. Agnes' Training School began in 1894 they worked and learned as pupil nurses. Medical care probably came from one of the four or five resident physicians, with periodic supervision by the attending staff. In a hospital where surgery was performed, where patients arrived by ambulance and patrol wagon, where typhoid fever was treated by icewater baths, and where income from private patients was needed for institutional survival, many more urgent and demanding situations must have distracted the caretakers away from the poor and chronically ill consumptives.[15]

Gratitude and Dissatisfaction

Regardless of where the patients went, hospitalization brought comfort, kindness, and hope to some of them and their families. Mrs. Mary L. Morrison, for example, deeply appreciated the care that her brother received at German Hospital, which accepted a few of the Free Hospital's patients. During the final weeks of his life, she found him "comfortable and contented there," the staff "sympathetic and gentle." And to Mrs. Josie C. Collom the care at Chestnut Hill was everything she might have hoped for: "I like it very well   Dr's Coh[e]n and Bacon say my case is a very hopefull one so I pray and hope to God that it is   my throat is beaing treaty by Dr. Watson   he say, my voice will come back again   it is improving very slow Doctor but Dr Bacon and her asstant are so good and kind   they try to make every thing plasent for the pation   We have had t[w]o intertaiments since I have been here."[16]

There was something about being sick in a hospital, however, that discontented some people, made them suspicious and restless, and led to rebellion. Perhaps it was loss of their independence, lack of control over their lives, loss of their self-respect. Perhaps at times they were indeed mistreated or neglected. "I wrote to you some time ago About taking My husband to the Hospital And you did so thanking you very Much," wrote Mrs. Wm. F. Laird in 1901.

But they are Not treating him right   he,s Not as well Now as when he
went   they wont give him Medecine And wont Alow Any out siders to take
him Any

We have two small Children And i have to work out for our living but i will
try and get him Medicine if you will Alow it, Also he is Not getting Very Much
to eat

Not only him but others   i was told last saturday when i was there that the
Dr that is there dont want those Patients there so they are trying to starve them
to death

Francis Fisher experienced similar problems at the Rush Hospital, where
he and his fellow patients felt neglected. They could not get the medicines
that they expected and could not get the food that they felt their illnesses
required. "It occurs to me," he confided to Flick, "that patients from [the
Free Hospital] society is not wanted." Both he and another patient had
departed from Rush.[17]

Religious incompatibilities sometimes helped to explain the dissatisfaction. Catharine Golden left the Episcopal Hospital because the people
there, she believed, were ridiculing her scapulars and St. Anthony's Cord.
Michael J. McCaffrey removed himself from the House of Mercy, where his
relatives, "very bitter Protestants," had persuaded him to go, because he did
not want to attend the religious services there. The rules at Chestnut Hill
forbade public religious services except for those provided by its chaplain or
his surrogate; other religious advisors, including priests, could make a visit
only if a patient specifically requested one and was granted official permission. "This is a protestant place," complained Cecilia Healy. "I have never
heard mass since I been hear [sic]   that makes me very unhappy as I am
very tired of it   I feel that I am in danger of loseng my soul."[18]

More commonly, patients yearned to be at home, believed they were
needed there, or were asked to come home by their relatives. They grew
homesick; they left to care for a sick child or a sick sister, to nurse an invalid
wife or mother; they wanted to try to work again; or they wanted to die at
home, not in an institution. Florence R.'s husband took her home from
Chestnut Hill because he could not be separated from her, and Ella F. was
removed after she tried to kill herself.[19]

Desire for a drink lured some of the patients out of the hospital, where
liquor, unless prescribed, was against the rules. Intoxication was a problem
familiar to the sisters at both St. Agnes' and St. Mary's, and although many
such lapses were tolerated, repeated offenses could lead to dismissal. In 1900,
the sister in charge of the Free Hospital's patients at St. Agnes' reported to

Charles W. Naulty, secretary of the society, that she had had to dismiss Henry Devere for drunkenness and disobedience. Devere was well enough to walk about in the open air, she noted, but every night he returned to the hospital intoxicated. At first she had overlooked this behavior and then she had forbidden it, but nothing had done any good. Devere "was in the habit of going out early in the morning, scaling the fence, obtaining liquor and bringing the same into the other patients while the Sisters were at Mass." Naulty, who himself had given Devere some money after his dismissal, lost patience and thought that the man should be sent to the Philadelphia Hospital. It was not the Free Hospital's purpose to take care of such people, he declared angrily, reflecting the typical view of private charities; other, more deserving persons were "only too glad . . . of being placed under our care."[20]

Just as alluring as drink was the notion that a change of some sort might alter the downward course of an illness. In 1888, Superintendent Durborow recognized this feeling in many consumptive patients:

> [The disease is] tantalizing and deceptive. All are familiar with the manner in which they [the patients] express themselves:—"If I could get rid of this cough," "If I only could get rid of this trouble in my throat," or "of this shortness of breath," etc., "I'd be all right," they say, when all around can see that already their case is one [in] which the disease has made great advances.
>
> The sufferers from it are filled at times with vain and delusive hopes,— seduced by fancies that change of some kind would effect a cure, and yet, in most cases, even . . . [under ideal circumstances] they fade and weaken, and at last drop into untimely graves.[21]

Mrs. Regina O'Leary, one of the Free Hospital's patients who had been admitted to Rush, wrote to Flick on September 11, 1900:

> Dear Sir
> I am at Hospille now 4 weeks getting weaker and not stronger   tond you think if I was at the Mountians it would be better for me   you have been so extra kind to me and I tond like to empose on you so much   I think if i was at the mountians that I would get better   i have diearrea neraly all the time and never had it till i went to Rush Hospille . . . please write and let me no what I have to do   sooner i get better i will be able to help your society   alwas will remember you in my poor prayers and Holy Comunions.[22]

Life and Death in an Early Sanatorium

For a small percentage of its patients the Free Hospital could grant such wishes. In Flick's efforts to increase his society's capacity, he had arranged for a few of the less seriously ill applicants to be admitted to sanatoriums away from the city. Chief among these during this period was Sanitarium Gabriels, a new establishment that the Sisters of Mercy had opened in the Adirondacks in 1897. On December 2, 1900, Mrs. O'Leary wrote her first letter from Gabriels: "Dear Friend   I tond no how to thank you enough . . . i arrived safe . . . everything is for a person health up here   i sat out all day long   i will do all in my power to get well   when i set at the Grotto i remember you . . . i can't but pray for you night and morning for all you have done for me . . . God will reward you in due time."[23]

Gabriels had several advantages for patients of the Free Hospital. In addition to its private rooms, the entertainments, the food, and the "most sociable and pleasant sisters," as the patient Katie Leahy described them, the healthful reputation of the Adirondacks must have given them hope. Just a few miles away lay Saranac Lake, where Dr. Trudeau's sanatorium was establishing its reputation, and Gabriels enjoyed the same pure air and climate and a somewhat higher altitude. Gabriels, like Trudeau's, declared its intent to accept only early cases, not the advanced ones that seemed so depressing at Chestnut Hill or St. Agnes.' Although intent did not necessarily assure reality, the healthy look of the patients at Gabriels impressed Katie Leahy; in her judgment only two or three of them looked sick.[24]

Distance from home, however, could prove troubling. For a poor person the cost of the railroad fare could prohibit the trip, and even if families or friends raised the money the trip itself could be frightening, especially, perhaps, for a young and inexperienced woman. Patients were a long way from friends and relatives, and if they felt worse or, for instance, developed a hemorrhage an additional worry surfaced: would weakness prevent them from ever getting home again? A sanatorium could not consistently avoid the seriously ill, nor could all of its patients avoid heartaches and anxieties.[25]

Twenty-three months in the life of Annie E. Hackett illustrate some of the comforts of sanatorium life, some of its limitations, and some of the conflicts between the interests of an institution and those of its patients, especially when the patients were poor and very sick. Annie Hackett first wrote to Flick from Gabriels on August 24, 1899:

> I cannot find a word fit enough to thank you for your great kindness of the past months. I feel as though I owe you something I will never be able to pay. I have found the scenery of the mountains, something beyond mention, and as for the air, I can also say the same. . . . I have improved a gread [*sic*] deal, for example: I weighed 94 on my arrival, now weighing 104, a gain of 10 pounds. This is considered good. . . .
>   The only thing I find hard, is to breathe. . . .

The Sanitarium has been crowded ever since I came. The table-board is excellent, and the Sisters are kindness itself. . . .

The only thing I dread is to think of going back and, get sick due to the difference of air. . . .

Yours very Respectfully
A. E. Hackett[26]

On December 23, 1899, she wrote again:

I am feeling very much better, gaining in weight and strength. However, it is to you that I owe my life, had it not been for your great kindness to me, I would not be living to day. . . . I trust Our dear Lord will give you the reward which you Justly deserve. I will not forget you on Christmas Morning in my humble prayers. . . .

Very resp. Yours
Annie E. Hackett[27]

Annie remained at Gabriels through the winter and early spring, but she knew that she would not be allowed to stay there indefinitely. By May 8, 1900, she faced some anxious questions about her future:

[I] ask your advice on the one Great subject "myself." I was examined by Dr. Carr of New York Sunday. He told me, I was doing well, but that I would have to remain in the mountains. . . . Dr. Lamb tells me . . . I would be able to work by June. I have secured a position as waitress, at Rainbow Inn, 3 miles from here. . . . I have never done anything in this line, and I fear I will find it hard at first. . . . Dr. Hallock a Lung Specialist of Saranac Lake . . . told me, the disease was nicely rested, but he found a little trouble on the appex [sic] of the right lung. He told me, that if I remained in the mountains I would soon be entirely cured. . . . I told him my future prospects, of staying in the mountains, he then said, he would advice me to obtain a position as Child's Nurse. So, now, I am unsettled. . . .

Now Dr. will you please write me what you think I had better do.[28]

Sallie Morgan, a patient at Gabriels who had secured the waitress job for Annie, tried to enlist Flick's help in keeping her at the sanatorium for the summer. Dr. Lamb, the physician at Gabriels, however, thought that Annie should leave. He "is desirous that the summer boarders about to arrive shall not find . . . patients who have been here so many months without being cured," Morgan explained, "as it would be a discouragement to them. It is simply a matter of business and convenience." Dr. Lamb's opinion prevailed and, on the advice of the sisters, Annie accepted an offer of employment. The sisters thought her fortunate to get work that permitted her to be in the open air a great deal, but Annie took a less sanguine view of the move.[29]

June 30, 1900

I have left the Sanitarium and am now living . . . [in] Utica, N.Y. . . . I am doing light waiting, assisting housekeeper. . . . I do not think I will like it, but will keep it for a while, until something better turns up. Am keeping fairly well. . . . I am very lonesome after The Sanitarium, everything seems strange to me   quite a change from the mountains. This place is somewhat out of the City, so I think it will be better than going to Phila. I had an offer of a clerical position but was afraid . . . it would be confining. I only hope I will not get sick again. . . . If I ever get rid of my cough I will be thankful.

Instead of the formal closures that Annie had used in her previous letters, she ended this one "your Thankful patient."[30]

On July 9, Annie wrote to Flick from Clayville, New York. Desperate now, she even forgot to sign her letter. The work in Utica had proved too hard, requiring "a much stronger person," she believed, and through the Woman's Exchange she had found another position. It involved doing housework and caring for a helpless woman invalided by rheumatism. When assisting the woman out of bed that morning, Annie had apparently hurt herself and was now experiencing "intense pains" through her waist.

What am I going to do. I am really not able to work. I fear I am much worse than I was. I am getting very pale and thin. I cannot sleep and cough all night, as well as during the day. It is quite difficult for me to walk, as my breath is getting so short. . . . Do you think you could let me go back to Gabriels, for a little while, until I get rested, and some strength. I have not had any nurishment since I have been away. I have suffered so much I am not able to suffer anymore. Please befriend me, as I am so sick and lonely, without one to talk to and in such a place   I have to leave here by Sat.—and as yet have no place to go. If I could go back to the mountains I would try after a little to get something to do. . . .

Please let me hear from you before Sat.[31]

This time Flick responded favorably to Annie's plea, but Gabriels was crowded and the sisters could not immediately find a room for her. "We will . . . take Miss Hackett," Sister Kieran replied to Flick on July 14, "though we'd prefer she would try to brave it out; and stay at her post during the summer."[32] Annie, meanwhile, feeling depressed and forsaken, turned to a priest for support. Religion, not medicine, was able to help her.

July 11, 1900

Your kind letter received this morning. I also received one from the Sanitarium, and they have no room for me at present. . . . I will do the best I can, though I am really not feeling strong. I have been so heart sick, and lonesome, that life at times, has been quite a burden. Last evening, my spirits gave way, and I thought best to seek the parish priest, and confide my troubles to him. I did so, and found him to be very kind and nice. You cannot imagine what a relief it was to talk with him, and to know that we always no matter how desolate, have a friend or brother in a priest. It is indeed one of the many fine things concerned in the Catholic Faith. I do wish I could return to Phila. I would give anything to see some one I know; you have been more than kind, and I do wish I could in some way repay you. . . . So then for the present I will continue to work, until I hear from Gabriel's. If I feel anyway better, or able to work, I will not go back; if I can get along with out it. I have not enough to go back to Phila. and would like to earn this amount or over before returning if I am able. Do you not think if I could get a position as Child's nurse in the Country—in Phila, I could get along? . . .

> Thanking you for your kindness in befriending me,
>> Believe me always
>> Your little friend
>> Annie Hackett[33]

No further word came from Annie until she wrote from Gabriels on April 17, 1901:

You cannot imagine how glad I was . . . when I received your kind offer, for I was all done out. . . . I have had a great many ups and downs, since Xmas, but, I have put my trust in God, and I know *he* won't forsake me. I wish you could write me Sometime, as I am quite friendless now. I hope I will soon gain back my name as Prize Patient. So, say a prayer for me that I will Soon be well.

Extend to the league my sincere gratitude for their kindness.

> Annie Hackett[34]

Annie never regained the tenuous hold on health she had had the year before, and on July 20, 1901, the Sisters of Mercy questioned Flick about her future. Annie was too ill, they believed, to stay at Gabriels.

Can you not let us know what decision you have arrived at concerning Miss Hackett. She is failing rapidly, and we would like to have her removed before she becomes too weak to travel.

Though we would be glad to do so, we cannot give her the care she would receive in a place fitted for those who are very ill. Then, the appearance of one so ill, has a depressing affect on the others.

Please let us hear from you as early as possible.[35]

On July 24, 1901, Sr. Kieran sent a telegram reporting Annie's death. James McNamee, a fellow patient at Gabriels, wrote to Flick the following day:

I suppose . . . you have heard the sad news of Miss Hackett's death. It was indeed a shock to everyone. But, since her arrival, she has been gradually failing. For the last couple of weeks she has complained of a pain in her right side: but she was afraid to mention pain to the Doctor. Indeed the night she died, she was at supper and on her way to her room, she dropped from weakness. Mrs. O'Leary, who is a great friend of the sick, urged her to tell the Doctor. She did so the night before her death. He gave her a pill and said it would pass away. But, alas! she passed with it. R.I.P.[36]

The Sisters of Mercy gave further details on July 29:

Like you we did not realize that Miss Hackett was so near her end though we knew she was failing. She kept up till the last—was in the dining room for her meals the day before she died. In the evening she was taken with a weak spell, and becoming worse we had her prepared for death. She knew she was dying and even longed to go. She seemed to suffer a great deal, but was conscious till the end.

We were glad to do what little we could for her, but it was hard to see her die and be buried among strangers. Please let us know if you wish her clothes etc. sent on to you.

If you so desire we can give them to some poor people here.[37]

During the summer in which Annie Hackett died, the Free Hospital was planning a new venture: a camp of its own in the mountains of Pennsylvania, the White Haven Sanatorium. News of this development reached Gabriels in July 1901, and the society's patients there were eagerly anticipating a change. "I am so glad that your sanitarium will soon be finished," wrote Mrs. O'Leary on July 10; "then I can repay you for your kindness to me   i will sew make beds or nurse the sick   hope to bee a great help to you and the society yet." A week later James McNamee requested admission to the new sanatorium. Although he had improved very much since his arrival at Gabriels, he reported, he had been losing weight for two or three weeks and "I feel that a change would benefit me considerably." McNamee added a postscript to his letter: "All the guests here from Phila-delphia, are anxious to go."[38]

In December 1901, Mary A. Becker, another patient who had gone to Gabriels, questioned the logic of the Free Hospital's methods. For less money than the society spent on institutionalization, she suggested, it could pay for a person's care at home. Becker supported her opinion with her own example. She had used all of her remaining money on her journey from Gabriels, and neither she nor the cousin with whom she was staying could afford to have her prescription filled. What she now proposed was basically the home relief with which the City Mission had started its work in 1876.

> She [the cousin] only has a weekly salary of $14.00. . . . With that she has to supply heat, light, feed and cloth seven children, besides furnish the necessaries for the house.
>
> She has already put herself to a great deal of inconvenience on my account by giving me a room to myself, to do it she has taken three children in her bed and two sleep with the father; and I cannot expect her to board and get me medicines and other necessaries gratis?
>
> Was thinking whether the Society for Free Hospital for Poor Consumptives could or would pay her three dollars per week. it takes that amount to furnish me with 3 qts of milk and 1/2 doz. eggs per day, milk amounts to .24c and eggs .18c per day; making .42 cts.   in a week those two articles alone amount to #2.94 [*sic*] not counting anything else.
>
> At Gabriels they paid $7.00   at a Hospital it would cost $5.00 would it not? I would feel a great deal more at ease if they paid a little for me while I am here; this way I feel as if I am robbing the children, they all need shoes and she cannot get them on account of this extra expense.[39]

Whatever the values and problems in Becker's proposal, Flick and his colleagues were moving in just the opposite direction, toward institutionalization. Their next step was the White Haven Sanatorium, which, like Gabriels, was meant not for people like Annie Hackett but for those with early disease.

5. A Camp in the Mountains: The Beginnings of the White Haven Sanatorium

Throughout much of the United States, care of the tuberculous sick was beginning to shift to sanatoriums. After 1885, when Edward L. Trudeau opened the Adirondack Cottage Sanitarium, others followed his example. In 1891 Dr. Vincent Y. Bowditch, son of Henry I. Bowditch, started the Sharon Sanatorium just eighteen miles from Boston. Bowditch was challenging some conventional wisdom by establishing his institution at a low altitude and near the seacoast, but results there seemed heartening. Other eastern establishments followed in states such as Connecticut, New York, and Maryland. In Massachusetts, the legislature began to build a hospital for advanced consumptives but, persuaded by the favorable reports from Sharon, decided to change its purpose to the curative treatment of early cases. This institution—the first state sanatorium in the nation—opened in 1898. Meanwhile, sanatoriums were also appearing in resort towns of the West and South.[1]

Starting in 1893, Flick and his Pennsylvania Society for the Prevention of Tuberculosis tried to promote a sanatorium in Pennsylvania, to be run by the state or, when that effort failed, by the Society with state assistance. They even selected a desirable site on Green Mountain, in the town of White Haven. Its climatological conditions were favorable, its two railroads made it accessible to patients, and S. W. Trimmer, a local physician, offered to give the Society more than two hundred acres if it developed the site within two years.[2]

Facilities in a sanatorium did not need to be elaborate; Trudeau had started with a single tiny cottage. Even so, the Society lacked the necessary funds and, despite repeated lobbying, failed to get support from the state legislature. Precedents for state support of medical institutions abounded in Pennsylvania. Not only did the state pay for the care of some of its insane, among other afflicted citizens; it was also appropriating increasing amounts of money to assist voluntary hospitals throughout the commonwealth. The appropriations process was thoroughly political—even recklessly lavish and corrupt, according to some observers—but people who believed that consumption was contagious felt that state action was now required.[3]

The Free Hospital for Poor Consumptives, frustrated by its too few beds and its lack of control over treatment, decided to make the effort itself. The Pennsylvania Society supported the idea and, together with the Philadelphia County Medical Society, sponsored a meeting to consider and publicize the issue. Speakers discussed the need for two kinds of institutions: rural sanatoriums for incipient cases, and urban hospitals for those with advanced disease. While the care of advanced cases was a local responsibility, they asserted, the state should support a sanatorium. In addition to simple humanitarianism, the state should do so for two reasons: consumptives endangered the public health, and their loss of income and their prolonged dependency drained the public economy. Benjamin Lee, secretary of Pennsylvania's board of health, concurred with this opinion. State support of hospitals "simply for the relief of suffering and healing of diseases is . . . a flagrant misuse of public funds, and leads to serious abuses," he declared in the fall of 1900. "But once admit that consumption is an infectious and therefore a preventable disease, and presto, the whole situation is changed. . . . That which would before have been an unwarrantable and vicious use of the public treasure now becomes an imperative duty . . . of the state."[4]

With this kind of backing, Flick began a campaign to steer an appropriations bill for a sanatorium through the state government. He wrote appeals for the newspapers, he and his colleagues pressed the legislators for favorable votes, and the Free Hospital sponsored at least two letter-writing campaigns to politicians. The bill worked its way slowly through the Board of Charities, the House of Representatives, the Senate, and the governor's office. Although the requested $110,000 shrank to $50,000 during this process, the Free Hospital won its first fight for governmental assistance by July 1901. The money, to be spread over two years, included $40,000 for buildings and equipment at White Haven and $10,000 for the maintenance of dying patients in Philadelphia. Financing the maintenance of patients at the new sanatorium depended on the Free Hospital and its contributors.[5]

Getting Started

As the prospect of starting a sanatorium drew closer, Flick broached the possibility of the superintendency to Elwell Stockdale, his patient who had gone to Germany and Davos for treatment. After a year in each place, Stockdale had returned to the United States and now, much improved, was completing his cure in Colorado. Having worked as a salesman before his long illness, the twenty-eight-year-old Stockdale had never been affluent and was starting to look for a suitable position, preferably out of doors. Flick's offer was doubly welcome: the young man needed the work, and during his treatment he had often thought of starting his own sanatorium. "When you get ready to go ahead hope you will let me know," he responded to Flick on June 22, 1901; "guess I would come back gladly for such a job for I am awfully lonely here and time hangs heavy and with all going out and no income is a big drain on a small capital."[6] He and Flick agreed on terms of employment, and Stockdale, returning east, went to White Haven. "My first trouble has arrived," he wrote to Flick on July 31, after inspecting the small farmhouse in which he was to live; "I find the house is a nest of bed bugs and germs."[7]

The town to which Stockdale had come lay on the west bank of the Lehigh River, not far from the anthracite coal fields of eastern Pennsylvania. Approximately half a mile south and a little west of the town's center, Green Mountain rose to a height of seventeen hundred feet, almost six hundred feet above the river. Part way up its eastern side lay the Trimmer farm, a crescent-shaped, sloping plateau of cleared land on which stood a "very dilapidated" four-room farmhouse and a "tumbled-down old barn". These became the consumptives' camp in the mountains of which Flick had dreamed in the 1890s—the White Haven Sanatorium. Dr. Trimmer had changed his mind about donating the 215 acres of land, as he had once offered, and the Free Hospital had to buy it for twenty-five hundred dollars. The price was considered fair by friends of both parties involved in the purchase.[8]

Flick was eager to get started, and Stockdale bustled about to prepare the place for patients. Electric lights were installed in the barn and farmhouse, both buildings were cleaned, and beds, mattresses, linens, and chairs were ordered from Wanamaker's department store in Philadelphia. A small range was placed in the farmhouse's "very primitive kitchen," and "a table and a few benches were made out of old boards for dining-room furniture." Meat, eggs, potatoes, and flour could be obtained from local farmers, the new superintendent reported to Flick, but "prices here for fruit and vegetables are ruinous." Early in August Stockdale moved into one room of the farmhouse and the cook into another, and on August 8 the first three patients took up residence in the barn.[9]

The Free Hospital intended to limit the clientele of its new sanatorium to those who had early tuberculosis but could not afford to pay for their own board. Because all patients had to live in the barn—at first on the threshing floor, then in the hay mow—they also had to be male.[10] Patients with early disease, physicians believed, would benefit not so much from the medical treatment or nursing care of a hospital but from the plentiful food, fresh air, and regulated rest and exercise that a sanatorium could provide. Although Flick visited the sanatorium and saw the patients there every two weeks, the tasks of implementing the regimen and caring for the men fell principally to the superintendent.

Stockdale undertook his new responsibilities with energetic enthusiasm. From his personal experiences as a patient, both in Philadelphia and abroad, he had acquired a thorough knowledge of the hygienic regimen and of the discipline it involved. As a man who had faced the likelihood of his own death yet had markedly improved under medical supervision, he, like Flick before him, had acquired a faith in the treatment that had seemingly saved his life.

The regimen at White Haven included one large meal daily, as much milk and as many eggs as the men could tolerate, and life in the open air. During the early months of his superintendency, Stockdale frequently reported to Flick on the patients' progress:

Aug. 15th 1901 . . .
The men are doing fine—temp normal and pulse good—one man had 17 glass milk and 8 raw eggs yesterday and another 14 and 8—I find by being there and urging them on they take more.

Aug. 18 1901 . . .
Montanye came yesterday . . . his temp and pulse are normal and think we can make a good case—his weight is way down—will you send his prescription?
The others are in fine spirits over the three who gained so much and am urging them on hard at milk and eggs—one had 20 glass yesterday another 18 . . . we will make some of these other sanatoriums feel sick.

Monday [August 26, 1901]
The chairs are fine and [I] now insist on their staying out all clear days. . . .
. . . Hamilton had dysentery for a couple of days and it made him lose one of the pounds he gained. Haywood only gained 1 lb. his 2nd week—so have insisted on them both taking more milk—all who take 15 glasses are allowed a cup of tea for supper. . . .
Reynolds put on 4 more lbs and is my star man so far.
McNamee and Lengel will be out of Tonic tomorrow.[11]

On September 1, Stockdale listed the fourteen patients at the sanatorium and their weekly weights since admission. The average gain for a patient's first week, as the superintendent computed it with great precision, was $5 \, ^{88.7}/_{100}$ pounds. During the second week, the men gained an average of 2 pounds; the third, 2 1/4 pounds. The sanatorium had achieved these excellent results, he noted, at costs that compared favorably with those of other institutions. A patient's food, on the average, came to $.50 a day, including $.26 for milk and eggs. If one added the weekly sum of $.75 for medicine, the grand total was $4.25 per week. "You see we are well within what the hospitals charged and guess they did not give eggs or so much milk and possibly no medicine," Stockdale observed proudly. "At Gabriels rates we are way under and then your rate for administration will not increase as long as we are here and I can easily take care of 35 patients." Because the Free Hospital was depending on Providence for help in paying its bills, as Flick expressed it, this accomplishment must have been a great relief.[12]

Coping with the Patients

Stockdale's medical responsibilities went well beyond the patients' diet. Despite the Free Hospital's intention of sending only early cases to White Haven, nine out of ten men who arrived there had advanced disease. Those with early tuberculosis had not applied for admission, and pressure to accept the others "was too great to be withstood."[13]

The men with advanced tuberculosis frequently had symptoms that demanded medical attention, and some of the patients developed other kinds of illnesses. They had colds, night sweats, hemorrhages, and fever, and Dr. Trimmer thought that Hamilton had malaria. Carberry was doing poorly. Heath had slept on the damp grass and developed a fever of 102°. Stockdale painted his chest with iodine and gave him some quinine, but these measures had brought no improvement. On October 11, 1901, the superintendent reported that Heath's fever persisted and now "he vomits all his food and the place smells awful. he hardly seems to be fit to do without lots of attention. Carberry gets no better. has bad sweats he also vomits all over the place and now has some pain in the appendix. Dr. Trimmer is looking after both. Think I will fix up the feed room as a bed room and put them in there where they could get sunshine all morning and be more quiet." A week later, Stockdale was "getting discouraged" with both patients. "Made them all take a full bath this morning the place smelt so mean." Carberry continued to do poorly, felt wretched, and by November 6 was begging to go to a Catholic hospital. "He needs nursing,"

Stockdale explained, "and while the boys are awfully kind to him yet there are many comforts we are unable to give him. If you think this is all right let me know what day to send him and will get him off on the morning train."[14]

Before any such arrangements were made, Carberry suddenly worsened, as Stockdale reported on November 8:

> Have passed a couple of awfully anxious days and nights and have had a mild taste of what a doctors work must mean.
>
> When I returned from Wilkes Barre Wednesday at 4. oclock found everything in great state of excitement. . . . Carberry they though[t] was dying. had terrible chills and bad hemorrhage and thought his time had come. John was off for Father Bergrath. So I took his temperature and pulse and they showed 104.6 and 130 He looked certainly like a dying man. So I treated the bleeding first with our medicine [probably nitroglycerine] and ice on chest and succeeded in checking it. . . . [Then] went after his fever and got it down to 103° by bed time. later to 102° . . . kept sponging him. . . . [Today I] think the worst is over and How I wished you were nearer. Had Dr. Synder [*sic*] come up and look at him and he said nothing more could be done than I was doing. Said it was congestion and a little pneumonia. . . . Think I can take care of him. Am giving him beef tea every 4 hours—he is much better now.

By November 16, calm had returned for a time to White Haven. "All are well here," Stockdale reported. "Heath is a wonder. his past 4 weeks gains have been 4, 7, 8, 5 1/2—Hard to beat it."[15]

Stockdale had to contend with the men's behavior as well as with their illnesses. Almost as soon as he had settled his patients in their quarters, some of them left the sanatorium. John Haywood left in September. So did Reynolds, who just the month before had earned the title "star man." "It appears to have been, as you say, a matter of discipline," wrote his brother, a physician, to Flick. "I am afraid the youngster has done himself an injury by his impetuosity." James McNamee, who had been so eager to come from Gabriels, also departed in September, but hoped his brother could take his place. Jay M. Brown left too. "I regret that I felt too miserable to undergo the exposure of the life at the camp," he explained to Flick; he simply felt unequal to it.[16]

The responsibilities and attractions of home called some of the men away from the sanatorium. One man's father needed his services back in Philadelphia, for example, while sexual need pulled another. It seems he could not get along without his wife, Stockdale noted, "and every morning he adjourned to the stable and abused himself." Of the forty-four men who left White Haven between August 1901 and the end of February 1902, with or without medical approval, 41 percent remained there for less than a week and another 30 percent remained for less than a month.[17]

The rigors of life at White Haven partly explained the short stays. Regardless of the climatological enthusiasms of some physicians, the autumn weather on Green Mountain tested the faith and determination of the men who lived there. The cold winds blew across the barren plateau in through the doors of the unheated barn and through the cracks in its walls. Even Stockdale, who had accustomed himself to the cold, noticed the chill. "Weather is still mean and damp," he reported on September 18. The previous night he had let "the boys" into the farmhouse after supper to play cards; "it was such a mean dismal night. it surely does get awfully lonely at times but guess one can get used to it." "Have had some awfully cold nights and some have 4 blankets," he wrote on September 21; "my room is like an icebox in the mornings. with the bare floor. Am still taking a cold tub every morning." On October 24, Stockdale wrote to Flick again: "The two men you sent yesterday are leaving today. not enough luxurious from what I hear. the man who came by mistake Sunday also left. same reason. . . . Then the man Frease [*sic*] from Haze[l]ton—looked like a Jew—disappeared early yesterday morning and went home—so we have 3 beds.[18]

Freas himself gave an account of the situation in a letter written on October 28 to Mrs. Eckley B. Coxe from nearby Drifton. Mrs. Coxe, the widow of a wealthy coal-mining magnate, was a benefactor of the sanatorium.

> I wish to inform you of the unbearable treatment that is being imposed on those poor misfortunate patients at the Sanitarium for poor Consumptives at White Haven Pa   I was a patient at this Sanitarium and was driven away by the unbearable treatment of the Supt. Mr. Stockdale. . . . I was a patient . . . for 10 days and would under oath Say I Slept warm but one night while there . . . the Same . . . with all the other patients and yet you are made to believe the patients are all comfortable. . . . Am writing this letter in the hopes of benefiting those other misfortunate patients at the Sanitarium by telling you the true State of affairs. . . . The next time you make a visit . . . go out and See the patients without an escort.[19]

Stockdale defended himself against the charges. Freas had "had two heavy blue blankets which are same weight as the usual <u>pair</u> of blankets and one of the Drifton blankets," he asserted on November 7, "also a Spread and overcoat which they all use. . . . Some are quite warm with 2 blankets," he explained. "Some of the others complain of cold and are given another." Hamilton, for example, had four blankets, a spread, and an overcoat and

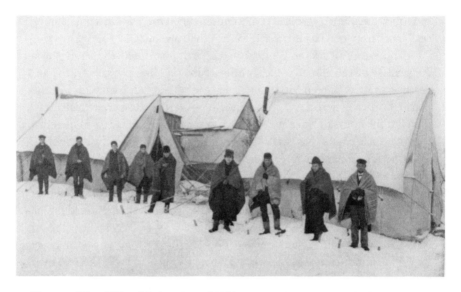

Figure 3. "Tent Life 28° Below Zero," White Haven Sanatorium. The barn is in the background. From the *Annual Report of the Free Hospital for Poor Consumptives* 6 (February 1904). Historical Collections, College of Physicians of Philadelphia.

still felt chilly on some nights. "I say if they wont keep him warm, nothing will and any more would weaken him." As to the charges of cruelty, if making the men "stick to their cure is cruel I plead guilty. They—some of them—feel quite abused at times (I hear) that I wont permit them to bum around the kitchen fire and in the house or barn." The men were supposed to stay outside; his best cases stayed there until bedtime. "[I] can honestly say that with all the money I spent for my cure, I never had any comfort more than these men."[20]

Dr. Henry M. Fisher, who took an active interest in the Free Hospital, reported his own observations to Flick on November 21.

> My sister Mrs. Eckley Coxe writes that "She never believed that there was any ground for the accusation of cruelty made by the man Freas," but I did think and still think the experiment a doubtful one. The climate of that bare and exposed hill, swept by every wind of heaven is very different from what life in a pine forest would be. Yesterday morning Mrs. Charles Coxe and I drove down there and in the warmest part of the day, at noon, with the sun shining bright outside. There was ice on the floor of the barn and in all the tin basins that had been standing there. A great chill pervaded the place. No doubt the steam pipes that they are beginning to put in may temper the air somewhat,

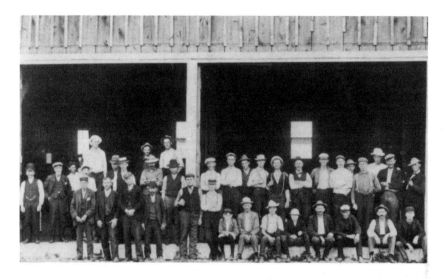

Figure 4. Patients at the door of the "barn pavilion," White Haven Sanatorium, ca. 1903. The windows are new. From the *Annual Report of the Free Hospital for Poor Consumptives* 6 (February 1904). Historical Collections, College of Physicians of Philadelphia.

but meanwhile I feel sure that the poor fellows there must suffer. It would need really <u>Arctic</u> outfits to make them comfortable and their clothing is by no means sufficient. I took down a lot of warm undershirts and Miss Becky Coxe sent some outside flannel shirts. I told Mr. Stockdale to order some tin foot warmers for the beds and this I hope will help a little.[21]

The sanatorium soon saw some progress in solving the heating problem. On November 29, Stockdale reported to Flick that "Thanksgiving was a howling success." Stockdale's parents, the cook, and John had waited on table and cleaned up afterward "so all the boys had to do was eat." Moreover, the ice cream and the four turkeys that Mrs. Coxe had sent were "gorgeous," "the boys were all in high spirits," and the heat was on in the barn. It was "working o.k.," he added, "but will be better when I get the place properly fixed."[22]

Heating the barn proved unexpectedly difficult. On January 1, 1902, Stockdale reported "a fine cold night last night   Bed room hit Zero at last. hard to beat that don't you think? Barn was 18° above and it seems impossible to keep the heat in. the heater works all right but the wind gets through." The blanket question, moreover, was "becoming a vexed one," and Stockdale feared what the board of directors might think of the rate at which he was buying them. Some of the men now had five blankets, and "when a man departs his are seized at once. I don't like to take them away from a man as he would then say it was cruel. . . . I sleep under two with perfect comfort," he added, "and when that colored man was there I had to give one up and only had a single one and was never cold."[23]

The Free Hospital, despite its continuing shortage of funds, had to improve its living conditions if it was to keep its patients and achieve its preventive goals. By the first of March, it had scraped together the money to weather-board and line the barn, lay a new floor over the old one, and install some windows to let in the sun.[24]

Fundamental to life at a sanatorium was discipline. Patients had to comply with the medical regimen in order to get better, physicians believed; they had to take special precautions to prevent the spread of infection; and they had to adapt to living in a group, cooperating with others as needed and, if they were well enough, sharing the work. Among Stockdale's many tasks was maintaining this discipline both fairly and wisely. His "boys" were often helpful. After the flurry of departures in September 1901, he reported to Flick that the "discipline is now A.I. and could not be improved on. The ones [who have] been here for sometime soon break in the new ones."[25]

Before long, however, disciplinary problems recurred, and Stockdale had few methods of enforcement other than discharge from the sanatorium—a measure that worked directly against the purpose of the institution. On October 1 he felt obliged to send Larkins home. "He has always been shirking his work since being here," the superintendent reported, "and today refused to help with the wood. We have rotten 2 × 6's to saw that a child could do, with our two hand saw, but he said he would rather leave." Late in December, Stockdale suggested to Flick that the men be divided into two clubs, each with rules of its own, so that potential shirkers and rule-breakers could be controlled better. By early February 1902, however, this system seems to have proved a failure. The two leaders of the clubs could not control their men. "Wardrop makes no effort to keep them out. . . . Butler also is helpless. . . . I will have to lock the doors of [the] barn and let Butler keep the keys."[26]

Around Christmastime, moreover, Heath had been detected spitting in the dining room, and the floor was caked with dried sputum. Because all the men knew of this discovery and Flick had recently lectured on the hazards of such behavior, Stockdale recommended "his immediate dis-

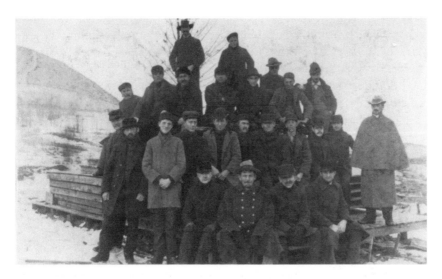

Figure 5. "The Men's Working Squad," White Haven Sanatorium. Elwell Stockdale is standing at the far right. From the *Annual Report of the Free Hospital for Poor Consumptives* 6 (February 1904). Historical Collections, College of Physicians of Philadelphia.

charge especially as he has since boasted we dont dare remove him. Dont sympathize with him Dr. he is not worth it. . . . He is a low depraved man and has simply done all in his power to demoralize our conduct." By December 29 Stockdale had modified his opinion, probably in response to a letter from Flick. "There is no question but what he deserves punishment," commented the superintendent, "but it may be that kindness will hurt him the worst and will give it a trial. It would only worry me awfully if he was sent away—not on his account, but his health and his family." The resilient superintendent, who had been sick and in pain himself through much of the fall and winter, added a characteristically optimistic paragraph: "Then again the rest of the boys seem so happy and contented and do any thing I ask of them so I should be thankful enough for their loyalty to me and not let one exception spoil our happy life here."[27]

While Stockdale gradually transformed the barn at White Haven into a "pavilion" that could accommodate forty men, the Free Hospital still needed facilities for women. By paying the board of a few women patients it was able to "stimulate into existence two private sanatoria in Pennsylvania," as the fourth annual report expressed it; both opened late in 1901. One was the short-lived Bide-A-While in Perkiomenville; the other was Sunnyrest, which Stockdale's parents opened across the river from White Haven. Mrs. Regina O'Leary arrived at Sunnyrest on December 6, 1901, the first of the Free Hospital's patients on record.[28]

Some of the troubles at the men's camp also appeared at Sunnyrest. Mrs. O'Leary, for example, who "reports she has your permission to visit the sisters chapel any time she chooses," was going off in the afternoons and promenading through the town. Moreover, Flick had agreed to admit a gravely ill consumptive whose care demanded a great deal of time. Her throat was so bad, Stockdale reported, that she could not even swallow a soft egg. Finally, a few days after Christmas, the dying woman was transferred to St. Agnes' Hospital in Philadelphia. "I feel I should call your attention to Mrs O Leary," wrote Stockdale to Flick in reporting the transfer. "Whatever her faults are and I fear many yet she deserves the greatest of credit for her attention to this woman. She simply had to give her attention all the time and when you know she [the woman] was devoured with lice you can imagine how hard it must have been."[29]

Boarding a few women patients at Sunnyrest and Bide-A-While was only a temporary expedient, and in the spring of 1902 the White Haven Sanatorium prepared to receive them. In May, Stockdale reported that hospital tents measuring fourteen by fourteen feet could be obtained—cheaply—for twenty dollars each. One tent could easily accommodate four beds, and large openings at front and back assured good ventilation. Costs of the shelter and necessary equipment came to less than thirty dollars per patient, as Stockdale pointed out in an itemized list:

Tent	20.00
4 beds	43.00
8 blankets	14.00
12 sheets	6.00
12 pillow cases	2.15
4 milk cups	1.00
4 basins	1.00
floor	10.00
8 towels	1.75
Table	2.50
soap cups	.40
4 steamer chairs	11.00
	4)112.80
	28.20

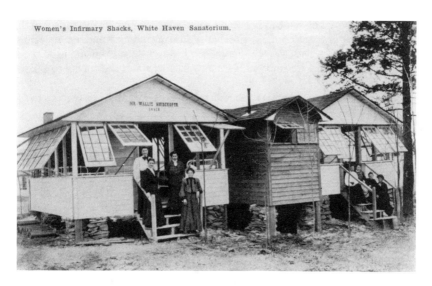

Figure 6. Women's shacks, which replaced the tents at the White Haven Sanatorium. From a post card taken from the *Annual Report of the Free Hospital for Poor Consumptives* 5 (February 1903).

By June 4, three women and a nurse had moved into tents at White Haven. Mrs. O'Leary may have been among them; on May 15 she had written to her "Kind friend" Dr. Flick, asking for a position there. Whoever the women were, they probably unsettled the male community that Stockdale had developed with his boys. "[I] assure you," the superintendent reported to Flick, "they keep me busier than my 50 men."[30]

As the women arrived at White Haven, more than the patients created problems for Stockdale; now there was also the nurse. Miss Margaret G. O'Hara, a graduate nurse who had had tuberculosis herself, agreed to come to White Haven for the summer, probably to gain experience with its therapeutic techniques. She differed from the superintendent as to the best methods of running a sanatorium. Inevitably, their courses collided, and Stockdale exploded with anger on August 20, 1902:

> I am having my life pestered out on a/c of my insistance that the rules of the place be lived up to. Miss OHara can see no sense in them   she says and claims her friends, which apparently consists of every man woman and child in White Haven, are insulted by being asked if they have colds. . . .
>
> Now am I to see the place is conducted as an institution and the rules laid down are lived up to or is she running the place and our Board's rules silly etc. To her mind it is a picnic grove with always guests to supper at our expense.

> No rules has any sense in her opinion and I want you to let me know can she authorize people to come at all times and in any numbers and that they must not be asked the usual questions and am I to be insulted here in my office for seeing our rules are enforced. I have swallowed about all I intend to and for sake of peace have said nothing. . . .
>
>   I am sorry to bother you about all this but if we want the place to go to the deuce she will soon put it there.[31]

There is no record of Flick's response to Stockdale's exasperated outburst, but O'Hara's summer tenure was probably coming to its natural close. During the following spring she established her own private sanatorium in Philadelphia and, with numerous referrals from Flick and other physicians, made a great success of it.

Stockdale, meanwhile, stayed at his post, persistently trying to improve the expanding sanatorium and keep its inhabitants under reasonable control. His troubles had not abated. "Louis Mandato had his pocket picked." After an unsuccessful search for the missing goods, someone found them in a closet used by the superintendent—"no doubt . . . placed there by the guilty one," of whose identity Stockdale felt certain. The water closets filled up and froze solid during the winter, the springs ran dry in August, and three of the women wandered off the sanatorium property and into a house of "disreputable character" that they mistook for a candy store. They were seen, and the event could reflect badly on the institution. When Stockdale punished one of the women for leaving the grounds and thus breaking the rules, she left the sanatorium.[32]

Growth and Promotion of the Sanatorium

Despite such problems, demands for care at White Haven grew steadily. A year after the sanatorium opened, its capacity had risen to eighty patients, and Flick reported over a hundred more on the waiting list. New applications flowed in, and a few previous patients begged to be readmitted despite their past transgressions. John Campbell, for example, wrote to Miss Rebecca Coxe in May 1902, hoping that she would intercede on his behalf and persuade Dr. Flick to overlook his having left White Haven without permission. "The doc[t]ors in Hazleton," he explained, "will not do anything for a poor person if they have no money."[33]

The waiting list and the fact that patients could place their hopes in the primitive camp at White Haven resulted partly from the Free Hospital's own publicity. Stimulating a demand for care in the sanatorium and establishing the effectiveness of its regimen were undoubtedly both essential to the future of the institution; without them, both state support and charitable contributions would have faltered or ceased. Fundraising itself provided one method by which the Free Hospital could gain attention. Contribution boxes, first distributed in Philadelphia, now appeared in the stores, hotels, and saloons of other cities, inviting their clients to give a few coins to the cause.[34]

Fundraising appeals took a sanguine view of the effectiveness of treatment. "The twenty cases in our camp at White Haven are rapidly improving," read an appeal letter in the fall of 1901. "Ninety per cent of them will recover and return to lives of usefulness." By March 1902, the Free Hospital's claims had grown a bit more guarded but still glowed with optimism. "The experiment . . . seems to indicate that we may hope to cure at least seventy-five per cent. of the patients whom we shall send to White Haven," read the annual report. "How easy is the task of curing tuberculosis when the proper conditions for the care of patients are given!"[35]

Probably more important in influencing public opinion were the newspaper reports. Flick had long known how to use the press to good advantage, and successful treatment of the dreaded consumption undoubtedly made a good story. Articles praising the sanatorium appeared in the papers. The Sunday edition of Philadelphia's *North American* on October 13, 1901, devoted two-thirds of a page to the sanatorium. The story, entitled "CURING CONSUMPTIVES, AND SEEING THEM GROW FAT IN A MONTH, AT THE FIRST OPEN-AIR SANITARIUM IN PENNSYLVANIA," described a "merry band of consumptives" who had "thrown physic to the dogs with a touching faith in the power of Dame Nature." The "once miserable wrecks of humankind now go about the day's business rejoicing in every hour of it. . . . The 'boys' are a happy family." "CURED OF CONSUMPTION," announced the *Philadelphia Record* on March 17, 1902, in a style familiar to those who scanned the paper's advertisements; "Dozen Convalescents Coming from White Haven, INSTITUTION NEEDS MONEY, Thousands of Afflicted Could be Restored to Perfect Health by Early Treatment at the Mountain Sanitarium." And "CURED CONSUMPTION IN SEVEN WEEKS," proclaimed the *North American* on March 21. Max Wirtschafter had gained twenty-seven pounds at White Haven and had just returned to Philadelphia. "'[I] was cured of consumption . . . by heroic open-air treatment,'" he declared, and "'never felt better or stronger in my life.'"[36]

Stockdale participated in promoting the sanatorium and raising funds for it. "Came down here early this morning," he wrote from Easton, Pennsylvania, in the fall of 1901, "and have fully stocked the place with our boxes—22 in all—also called on the Editors of the two newspapers here and they will give us a good article . . . so guess Easton people will know what they are for." The superintendent promised to "pursue the same course at other places." In March 1902 he queried Flick as to Peter Schmitt's sputum report. "Am going to send him to Dr. Johnson," he explained, "and get his paper [to] give it a big 'Ad' and want all particulars. Will do same with [Warren] Nagle at Allentown."[37]

If Stockdale had a stake in the sanatorium's success, so did the railroad company, which, like its counterparts in the West, joined in boosting local enterprise. "You will be pleased to hear the L.V.R.R. [Lehigh Valley Railroad] has had a man here taking photos," Stockdale wrote to Flick in November 1901. "Their idea is to boom it as a health resort and use our results to prove it. Our property may thus increase in value if the boom was a success."[38]

Results indeed looked promising. Of the 184 patients who were discharged from White Haven between August 8, 1901, and February 28, 1903, after staying there for more than a week, 60 percent were considered improved or much improved and another 24 percent were thought to have had their disease arrested. An average weight gain of fourteen pounds per patient seemed to attest to this success.[39]

The course of tuberculosis could not be assessed easily, however, and purported improvements such as these were not necessarily genuine or sustained. On April 1, 1902, just one week after Stockdale had sent Warren Nagle home to Allentown, where he hoped to publicize his cure, Nagle's father reported that Warren was doing poorly. "He had a night sweat lately and other unfavorable symptoms," and the family physician found a "sore spot" on his right lung. "Dont think that we are finding fault," Mr. Nagle wrote, but the doctor said "we should return him to you until the weather was settled and he thoroughly healed." In January 1903 Dr. Solomon Solis Cohen, a respected Philadelphia physician, reported to Flick that John Conlin, who "states that he was in the White Haven Institution for nine months, and was discharged <u>cured</u> six weeks ago," had active disease with "extensive softening of both lungs." Several other patients from White Haven had turned up at the Rush Hospital, Solis Cohen continued, and, like Conlin, had asserted that they "had been discharged 'cured.' If the fault lies in careless expressions on the part of the superintendent . . . it might be worth your while to see that a more circumspect announcement is made to patients when they are dismissed."[40]

In the fall of 1902, Flick himself acknowledged that the gains at White Haven might be temporary. Many patients had left the institution as soon as they had felt able to work, and he feared that a majority of them would sicken again when they encountered the hardships of life outside. His support of sanatorium methods, however, remained strong. "Tuberculosis is curable under the most primitive conditions," he declared, "provided the patient is kept out of doors and given plenty of the right kind of food." Incipient cases recovered quickly, and some of the chronic cases could also be cured, at least if they stayed long enough.[41]

Working Toward Institutional Stability

Demonstrating that patients wanted admission to the sanatorium and that they improved there, although necessary for institututional stability, was only part of the task. The Free Hospital also had to economize on expenditures, raise additional money, please its supporters, and meet medical standards that physicians would find acceptable. Between the fall of 1901 and the winter of early 1903, the sanatorium made notable gains in meeting these sometimes conflicting objectives, but its efforts were to continue and change direction for many years afterward.

Improvements in the sanatorium increased its capacity to ninety-eight patients and made it a bit more livable. Workmen built a washroom in the barn, enlarged the farmhouse kitchen, and constructed a porch around two sides of the house so that in suitable weather the patients could take their meals there. Stockdale designed a kiosk—a long, wooden, porchlike lean-to—where the men could rest in the open air yet be sheltered from the wind. More than fourteen thousand seedling trees were planted, an artesian well was drilled, and three sturdy brick cottages—each able to accommodate sixteen patients—were built on the windswept plateau. The cost of maintaining a patient, however, was kept low: $5.42 per patient per week during the fiscal year ending in February 1902, and only $4.65 the year afterward. Stockdale and Flick, who both tried hard to economize, were very proud of the accomplishment.[42]

A few generous benefactors, most notably Mrs. Eckley B. Coxe, Miss Rebecca Coxe, other members of their family, and Henry Phipps, a wealthy industrialist, contributed to the success of the institution. The Coxes not only gave coal, blankets, clothing, hot-water tins, food, and monetary support; they also took personal interest in the patients, and on occasions of special need, sometimes intervened on the side of a patient's welfare. Phipps, who admired the economies with which Flick was accomplishing so much, contributed substantial amounts of money.[43]

The expectations of the men and women who supported the institution financially put pressures on Flick and Stockdale. The Coxe family took special interest in the patients' comfort. As the second winter at White Haven drew closer, heating the barn (or the pavilion, as it was now called) became worrisome. "I am sure we will make a big mistake and lose some of our best friends if we do not put heat in the Pavillion [sic] this winter," Stockdale warned in September 1902. "Some how every one that comes from the Coxes are all interested in the Pavillion . . . and to take out the heater already there and not replace it would put us in bad favor with them." Henry Phipps, a shrewd businessman, although interested in the patients' welfare, was also concerned with results. "How is the Hospital getting along?" he queried in mid-October. "How many men have you cured sufficiently to enable them to go back to their duties?" Flick's answers, though not recorded, satisfied the businessman. After the two men met the following week, Phipps sent Flick one thousand dollars for heating the barn.[44]

Pressures from politicians who anticipated favors for past or future support of the sanatorium were just beginning, but Pennsylvania's system of making biennial appropriations for each competing hospital made them inevitable. Even before the sanatorium had opened, the governor had tried to get one of his old friends appointed to the board. Flick had refused. Within a year, as White Haven's waiting list lengthened, legislators started trying to influence the selection process to favor their constituents. Political requests of this kind encroached on the Free Hospital's authority to run its own institution and raised a fundamental question for its future: could it continue to attract politically authorized money without bowing to political control?[45]

As the sanatorium enlarged its capacity, moreover, physicians within the organization grew increasingly concerned that Flick's strict economy was impairing medical safety and perhaps even the institution's respectability. Patients were growing in number, most were sicker than had been anticipated, a few had died, and Flick's biweekly visits seemed inadequate to meet the needs. During the winter of early 1902, two physicians from the region, Charles H. Miner and Henry M. Neale, agreed to supplement his visits, but both were busy men, neither had had special training in the disease, and Stockdale, among others, was worried about the medical coverage. Although Dr. Robert P. Elmer, a young consumptive physician, served as resident physician for a short period late in 1902, the amount of work he could do did not resolve the problem.[46]

A distressing event around New Year's Day of 1903 probably helped to force a confrontation between Flick and the five physicians on the Free Hospital's medical administration committee. Miss Allison, one of the women patients who, having improved, were serving as matrons in the sanatorium, suddenly developed a high fever, became desperately ill and, despite every effort that Stockdale could muster, died within a few days. Dr. Elmer resigned during the episode. Flick, nevertheless, resisted the committee's appointment of a new resident physician, apparently on the grounds that it was too expensive. On January 14 Guy Hinsdale, chairman of the committee, defended the committee's action. "Our failure to have a resident physician has been severely criticized," he asserted, and "the weekly visits of the attending staff are not adequate." Hinsdale believed that the necessary money could be raised for the resident's salary; he had collected ten dollars for the purpose that very morning. To save money, he advised, the Free Hospital should curtail the admission of advanced cases to city hospitals and slow the acceptance of patients into the new cottages at the sanatorium. Competent medical care was more important than a large number of patients.[47]

Flick was upset by the letter, Hinsdale was adamant, and the resolution of the conflict was a mixed victory. The sanatorium did hire a resident physician, and the number of advanced cases admitted to city hospitals declined markedly and then ceased altogether the following year. The number of men and women admitted to White Haven increased even further, however, more than compensating for the decline. The Free Hospital, like the City Mission before it, had chosen to shift its limited resources away from the care of dying consumptives and toward the care of the presumably curable. While Hinsdale succeeded in realizing two of his recommendations, Flick retaliated. He dropped both Hinsdale and a second physician from the medical administration committee. By the end of February 1903 Hinsdale's name no longer appeared on the Free Hospital's board of directors or on any of its committees. Flick disliked discord within his organizations, and if he could not correct it peacefully he tried to remove the source.[48]

The camp in the mountains, shaped by both internal and external pressures, was changing into a proper sanatorium. A separate development in Philadelphia hastened this metamorphosis. In 1903 Flick, with a sizable gift from Henry Phipps, opened an institute for the study, treatment, and prevention of tuberculosis. This organization, unlike the sanatorium, needed patients with advanced disease. Its purpose was scientific investigation, not the more popular cure of early cases.

The prospect of the institute's new hospital interested Mrs. Regina O'Leary, who was now back at home in Philadelphia. "Thanking you for your fatherly friendship in the times past," she wrote to Flick on January 27, 1903, and "hoping to be of some service to you and the sick," Mrs. O'Leary wanted to work there.[49]

Part II

New Systems of Care, 1903–1917

6. Research, Training, and Patient Care: The Henry Phipps Institute

On the evening of January 9, 1903, Flick invited reporters to his home on Pine Street to hear an announcement: the industrialist Henry Phipps would establish in Philadelphia a research institute for the study, treatment, and prevention of tuberculosis and would endow it with at least one million dollars. For the rest of the month, Flick's mail swelled with good wishes and praise for the new enterprise. "Your energy and courage have had their reward at last. What a pleasure it will be to you to see your hopes of helping the poor and sick realized!" "The application of medical principles on an American scale . . . marks an epoch in human progress much more than the production of grain or cotton or steel." "Future generations will bless your name."[1]

A research institute that included the care of patients and the prevention of disease was new in turn-of-the-century America. Although medical research was thriving in Germany and to a lesser extent in France, it had attracted little support in the United States from either government or philanthropy. During the latter years of the nineteenth century, however, there were modest but definite signs of change. American physicians who had studied in Europe were returning home, eager to take advantage of their new learning and to improve medical education and practice in the United States. A few university medical schools, major hospitals, and health departments were beginning to establish laboratories for purposes that included research, evaluating individual patients, and protecting the public's health.[2]

Bacteriology offered the most immediate promise. During the 1880s and 1890s, European scientists had successfully linked one disease after another to its causative microorganism: typhoid fever, malaria, tuberculosis, cholera, diphtheria, and bubonic plague, to name a few. Although therapeutic rewards were still few, bacteriology led to new understanding of the body's immune system. In the mid-1880s Pasteur developed a vaccine against rabies, and in 1891 Behring and Kitasato produced an antitoxin against diphtheria. Although Koch's tuberculin had failed, preventive vaccines for many diseases seemed just a matter of effort and time.[3]

The promise of medical science coincided with changes in wealth and attitudes in the United States. After the Civil War, a number of men had amassed fortunes from their industrial enterprises, and in 1889 one of these, Andrew Carnegie, published two influential articles that became known as the "Gospel of Wealth." While Carnegie defended men's right to accumulate wealth, he urged that they spend it to benefit humanity. Among the worthy ways to use such monies, he cited hospitals, medical colleges, laboratories, training schools for nurses, and other institutions that would relieve suffering and prevent illness.[4]

In 1901, John D. Rockefeller contributed an initial twenty thousand dollars to establish the Rockefeller Institute in New York City—one of the nation's first and most prestigious organizations for medical research. No one knew then how best to organize such an endeavor, and Rockefeller started by offering small grants to existing laboratories. In May 1903—four months after Flick's announcement in Philadelphia—the Rockefeller Institute purchased land on which to build its own laboratory. Its hospital opened in 1910.[5]

The Phipps Institute thus emerged at a time when physicians and philanthropists felt increasingly optimistic about research but had few models to guide them in how to proceed. Flick had a broad and ambitious plan. By linking the care of patients to medical research, he believed that tuberculosis could be exterminated. Like the Free Hospital, the White Haven Sanatorium, and even the City Mission by the late 1890s, the Phipps Institute aimed to check the spread of infection by segregating consumptives. The Institute, however, would go further than this. Out of its dispensary and hospital would come the materials for the scientific laboratory, and from the knowledge accumulated in all three places there would develop some new answers to the old disease.

The Institute offered a new reason to support the care of patients and new rewards for those who did the work. To the earlier goals of saving souls, relieving bodily suffering, and curing consumptives was now added the hope of conquering the disease through scientific investigation. The opportunities involved in the work attracted and rewarded physicians who saw, among other advantages, a chance to advance their careers. Through training, certification, and other benefits, the Institute also persuaded a group of tuberculous women to become the organization's nurses. Physicians, nurses, and the Institute's patients were drawn together in a relationship that asked a price of each but promised something to all.

Henry Phipps and the Institute

Henry Phipps, the man who had contributed to the White Haven Sanatorium the year before and now supported this new venture, was born in Philadelphia in 1839. The son of an immigrant English shoemaker, he moved with his family in 1845 to Allegheny City, now part of Pittsburgh. His father reestablished home and business, and in 1848 made the acquaintance of another poor immigrant family newly arrived from Scotland—the Carnegies. Mrs. Carnegie supplemented her husband's meager income by binding shoes for Mr. Phipps, while Henry and his older brother John became friends with the Carnegie sons, Tom and Andrew. At the age of thirteen Henry started work as an errand boy, at seventeen he became an office boy, and by 1861, when he was twenty-two, he acquired an interest in an iron forge and manufacturing business. The business thrived during the Civil War and merged with a Carnegie company after the war. Phipps continued as a partner of Andrew Carnegie in the iron and steel business until 1901, when they sold their interests to the United States Steel Corporation. From this transaction, according to the *New York Sun*, Phipps received one hundred million dollars.[6]

Phipps, now in his early sixties, increasingly focused his attention on using his wealth for humanitarian purposes. Unassuming, modest, even shy in his public appearances, he brought to his philanthropic endeavors the characteristics that had made him successful in business: cautious conservatism, painstaking attention to detail, unwillingness to take an important step before he had thoroughly studied its probable consequences, and a distaste for unnecessary expenditure that tinged his extraordinary generosity with frugality.[7]

As Phipps looked about for suitable philanthropic projects, Francis J. Torrance, a successful Pittsburgh businessman who served as president of the State Public Board of Charities, told him of Flick's work at White Haven. In his characteristic manner Phipps quietly investigated ways to approach the problem of tuberculosis. He studied articles that Torrance had requested from Flick and was much influenced, he acknowledged later, by *The Nordrach Treatment*, a book written by an English chemist, James A. Gibson. Gibson, who described himself as a consumptive cured by the treatment, gave a ringing testimonial to Nordrach, Dr. Otto Walther's sanatorium in the Black Forest of Germany. Walther's regimen, which resembled Brehmer's, Dettweiler's, and now Flick's at White Haven, consisted of pure country air, large amounts of nourishing food, rest and exercise, and strict medical supervision. Gibson also advised that sana-

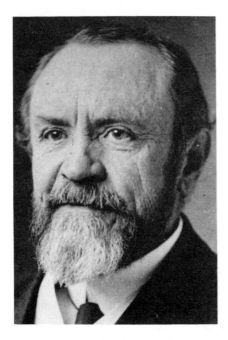

Figure 7. Henry Phipps. University of Pennsylvania Archives.

toriums be constructed cheaply, and that a Medical Training Sanatorium be founded in which physicians could learn the new methods.[8]

After a number of months, Phipps decided to meet with Flick and inspect his work. On a wet, slippery day late in April 1902, the two men met at White Haven and picked their way carefully around the primitive institution. Phipps seemed interested, polite, but reticent during the visit, while Flick, as he reported, felt distressed, fearing that the wealthy industrialist "might be scandalized at our attempt to start a sanatorium with such inadequate resources." Early the next morning, however, a special-delivery letter from Phipps arrived at Flick's home. "It really surprises me how much good you are doing with so little money at your command," Phipps observed. "It is very creditable to your management. If you had been a business man in any line you would have been a serious competitor." He enclosed a check for twenty-five hundred dollars for the Free Hospital.[9]

During the next several months, the two men communicated sporadically. Phipps thought of starting a sanatorium on Long Island, but Flick would not consider moving to New York. Flick had hopes of opening a clinic in Philadelphia but, although Phipps offered to back it, they could not get clear title to the desired property. Flick, moreover, became ill in the fall, probably with a reactivation of his tuberculosis. Phipps offered to give more money to the Free Hospital if Flick would take a rest and sail with him to Europe, and Flick at last agreed. During the voyage across the Atlantic and their subsequent visits in England and France, the two men formulated their ideas for what would become the Henry Phipps Institute for the Study, Prevention, and Treatment of Tuberculosis.[10]

The fundamental goal of the new Institute, as Flick announced it in January 1903, was the extermination of tuberculosis, chiefly through preventive measures. The Institute would include a hospital for the isolation and treatment of patients with advanced disease, laboratories for scientific research, and a dispensary in which to treat and instruct patients whose disease was somewhat less advanced or who would not or could not enter a hospital. The Institute's staff would study the cause, treatment, and prevention of tuberculosis and would disseminate new ideas as widely as possible, thus, Flick believed, stimulating the crusade.[11]

Flick, now forty-six and nearing the peak of his career, lost no time in getting started. At 238 Pine Street—in the slums of old Philadelphia—he found temporary quarters for the new organization, and on February 2, 1903, he opened the doors of its dispensary. Because Phipps was to pay the rent from the first of the month, Flick—the medical director—insisted that the work begin at once.[12]

The building, a four-story brick structure, had not been occupied for years; it was scarcely fit for use on opening day. The intended dispensary occupied the first floor. Dr. Joseph Walsh, one of the first to work there, found it "dirty, cheerless and chilly," with bare floors, bare walls, and only a few chairs. Physicians found it impossible to examine their patients properly while other men and women waited in the same room. Nevertheless, patients crowded in at a rate of twenty to thirty a day, soon exceeding the Institute's capacity. The doctors tried to work while carpenters, building partitions around them, created an office, consultation rooms, a waiting room, a drugstore, and a laboratory.[13]

The hospital, which took a little longer to ready, occupied the three upper floors of the building. Each floor—twenty-six feet wide and sixty feet deep—consisted of one large front room, two small back rooms, and a stairway. Flick and his workers created the wards for advanced consumptives by furnishing each of the three front rooms with sixteen or eighteen beds, some chairs, and a dining table for those who could walk about. Windows in front and along one side of each ward, together with a ventilator over a rear door, provided "natural ventilation," while three

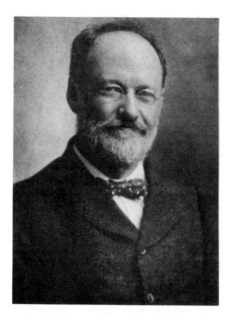

Figure 8. Lawrence F. Flick, ca. 1904. From Cecilia R. Flick, *Dr. Lawrence F. Flick As I Knew Him* (Philadelphia: Dorrance, 1956). Historical Collections, College of Physicians of Philadelphia.

electric fans on each floor helped to stir the air during the hot summers. One of the small back rooms on each floor became bathroom and linen room; the other was used as a kitchen. A small, low-ceilinged house behind the main building provided space for the laundry, the sterilizing room, and an autopsy room. In addition, the nurses ate in a small dining room there, and a corner was furnished for the head nurse. The entire transformation cost about twelve thousand dollars. The hospital opened on April 20, 1903, and patients filled the wards as rapidly as they could be accommodated.[14]

The Medical Staff

To care for the patients and to undertake the anticipated research, Flick wanted a group of highly qualified physicians who were clinically competent and had also had some "preliminary training for original research and advancement of medical science." American medical schools of the time produced few such graduates. Although the Johns Hopkins University had opened its medical school with these goals in 1893, most schools still admitted ill-qualified students and lacked the facilities to train them well in either laboratory sciences or the care of patients.[15]

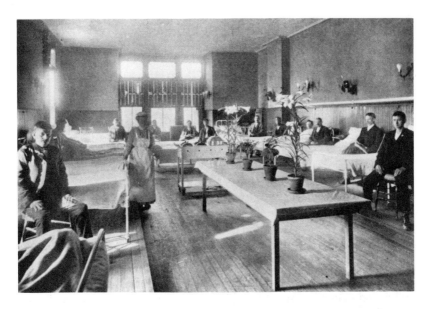

Figure 9. Men's ward at the Henry Phipps Institute. From the *Annual Report of the Henry Phipps Institute* 1 (February 1904).

Most of the physicians whom Flick attracted to the Institute graduated from the medical school of the University of Pennsylvania, but even this school did not recruit or prepare its students for the role that Flick had in mind. It did not require a high-school diploma for admission until 1897. According to George W. Norris, an early member of the Phipps staff who earned his medical degree at the University in 1899, "'some of the entrants could hardly more than read or write.'" Furthermore, the medical school had just emerged from an educational system based largely on lectures and was only beginning to integrate the new laboratory sciences of bacteriology and clinical pathology with bedside teaching. Physicians who had graduated only a few years before the Phipps Institute opened probably had little, if any, exposure to these sciences. David L. Edsall, who graduated in 1893 and later joined the Phipps staff, recalled how seldom bacteriology was used during his internship in Pittsburgh. His chiefs had "'never once asked for an examination for tubercle bacilli,'" despite the fact that the disease was frequently suspected.[16]

Although deficiencies in medical education restricted the number of men qualified for work at the Institute, they also made a position there more attractive. Young physicians could supplement their education at a time when alternative postgraduate opportunities were scarce. They could become expert in physical diagnosis of the chest, gain experience in new laboratory procedures, and possibly publish a paper or two. The work was a step in professional advancement.[17]

Work at the Institute, however, carried risks, most obviously that of infection. "It was often suggested to me," Norris recalled, "that I needlessly was jeopardizing my life by spending so much of it in ministering to highly infectious tuberculous patients." For Norris, at least, there were also political hazards to his career. The Phipps Institute, he observed, was "a new and unknown organization," and many of Philadelphia's outstanding practitioners looked askance upon Flick's penchant for publicity. " 'If you expect a future position on the teaching staff of the Medical School of the University of Pennsylvania,' " Norris had been advised, " 'don't become too much of a "Phipps Man." ' "[18]

A physician also had to consider the prospect of spending time with very ill and dying patients. The work was sometimes depressing and painful, as at least one of the early recruits acknowledged. On December 27, 1904, Ward Brinton wrote the following note in a patient's chart:

> A cold damp day, penetrating—bad for lungs. Patient feels very badly and looks much worse—cold all the time, shivering. Sits with head bowed— Hands between his knees with swollen joints and heaving chest. Despair in every line.
>
> Is quite hopeless about himself and says he will not live until spring. . . . He gasped for breath and in his agony tore at his shirt front and whilst he gasped his eyes seem[ed] blank and with his staring eyes in a leaden skin he seemed more like a subject from Dante's Hell than aught else I know.
>
> And then he babbled incoherently of wife and children and of their helplessness and almost raved against his Maker for his giving him such suffering of weakness and of dull dread unhopefulness.
>
> And nothing can be done, no, absolutely nothing that I know. And when I feel my own weakness to help him I am ashamed to face the dying man's eyes, to offer words of hope and encouragement for he knows I lie.[19]

Despite the risks and unpleasantness Flick succeeded in attracting physicians, and by early February 1903, when the Institute's dispensary opened, he had appointed three of them to help with the work. One of these was Joseph Walsh, who had taken care of some of the Free Hospital's patients during his residency at St. Agnes' Hospital. The staff grew through active recruitment and an informal network of interpersonal contacts. Men who had been appointed encouraged their friends to apply or recommended their assistants for positions. By the end of the first year the staff had grown to fifteen physicians, by the end of the second year to twenty-nine, and by the end of the fourth year, 1907, to its peak of thirty-seven. None of the clinicians among them devoted their full time to the work. Many held other part-time appointments, and most made their living through private practice.[20]

Between February 1903 and February 1908, forty-four physicians joined the staff of the Institute for varying lengths of time. Thirty-one of them served as general physicians and thirteen as specialists in fields such as pathology, bacteriology, otolaryngology, and genitourinary surgery. They were a young, fairly homogeneous group of men, 80 percent of whom had graduated in medicine from the University of Pennsylvania. Another 16 percent had graduated from Jefferson, Flick's alma mater. At least one-fourth of the men had enriched their medical education by additional study in Europe.[21]

The general physicians and the specialists differed slightly in age, in experience, and probably in the advantages that they saw in their work. The average general physician was approximately thirty years old when appointed, and had been out of medical school for about five and one-half years. Just over half of these men had graduated only two to four years before their appointments. At this stage in their careers, most of them were not yet fully established in practice; they had time to do some extra work and acquire added clinical experience. The specialists were slightly older, averaging thirty-three years of age, and had been out of school for roughly ten years. Somewhat further advanced in their careers, they were increasing their expertise in tuberculosis, and perhaps establishing contacts with other physicians who might later refer some private patients to them. George B. Wood, a laryngologist, for example, later wrote appreciatively of the "abundant clinical material for the perfection of [his] intralaryngeal technique." The clinical experience gained in his five-year affiliation with the Institute "was a most important acquisition to my knowledge," and the opportunity to work there "a most important stepping stone to whatever success has come to me in later years."[22]

Among his staff Flick needed some senior men with both specialized training and established scientific reputations. These would give leadership to the research and credibility to the Institute. By the late summer of 1903, Mazÿck P. Ravenel agreed to join the staff as assistant medical director, with an annual salary of three thousand dollars. Ravenel was an experienced bacteriologist who had graduated from the Medical College of South Carolina in 1884 and had also studied at the University of Pennsylvania, at the Pasteur Institute in Paris, and at the Institute of Hygiene in Halle, Germany. In October 1903, Flick reported to Phipps that Ravenel was "all that can be desired." He had also recruited David L. Edsall, a physician whose biochemical studies at the University of Pennsylvania were then attracting favorable attention. Edsall, Flick wrote, was "a man of great ability, who has won considerable reputation for himself along a certain line of work which I am anxious to have done at the Phipps. He is one of the men whom we must anchor to the Institute by . . . a fellowship with a salary attached." In addition, Flick was eager to attract Courtland Y. White, a pathologist. "When I have secured him I will be quite content with our equipment for scientific work and I do bel[i]eve we will have the best organization for this particular purpose in the world." White joined the staff in 1904.[23]

The Medical Work and Its Rewards

The work of the clinicians on the Phipps staff included the care of patients in either the dispensary or the hospital. A man assigned to the dispensary spent two hours there twice weekly. Although the environment was simple, even crude, Flick wanted to make it attractive to patients, thus encouraging the sick to come in the first place and to attend regularly on a biweekly schedule. To accomplish this objective, each physician was assigned his own group of patients and took responsibility for their diagnosis, treatment, and instruction in preventive measures. A physician assigned to the hospital wards accepted the continuing care of about seven patients with advanced disease. The clinical work carried with it no direct remuneration, but every year from 1903 through 1905 Flick arranged for a Christmas honorarium of about two hundred dollars for each man.[24]

In addition to the clinical work, staff members were expected to participate in research. To Flick's disappointment, some of the men lacked the time, the skill, or perhaps the inclination to involve themselves deeply in it. In 1906, with Phipps's approval, Flick converted the yearly honoraria to small fellowships and began to assign specific research projects to members of the staff. H. R. M. Landis was expected to study occult blood in the stools of tuberculous patients and explore its relationship to gastrointestinal ulcerations, for example, while William B. Stanton, along with several colleagues, was asked to investigate the pathology and bacteriology of pleurisies and pulmonary cavities. Each of these two men was expected to work for at least three hundred hours on his project and receive two hundred dollars in return.[25]

As Flick envisioned the mission of the Institute, the clinical work had to match the laboratory work in exactness and scientific value. Out of man's accumulating knowledge, he believed, came his power over disease, and that knowledge came from bacteriology, pathology, clinical observation, and veterinary surgery. Each patient's history and each physical examination constituted a portion of that growing body of information, and from its totality would emerge new and important understandings. Tuberculosis, he asserted confidently in July 1904, was "about to be exterminated from the earth."[26]

Staff physicians caught some of Flick's enthusiasm and worked diligently on their clinical skills and records. With care and persistence they pieced together the best possible formats for collecting information about their patients, and medical committees scrutinized each record for accuracy and completeness. While physicians sometimes grumbled about the time required for paperwork and committees, they also took pride in their accomplishments. "The principle . . . is that of giving the maximum amount of study and care to the individual case," explained Albert P. Francine to the state medical society in 1906. "There is no hospital in this country nor Europe . . . where every case is so accurately studied both clinically and pathologically, and where the records are so admirably symmetrical and so carefully kept as at the Phipps Institute."[27]

Pride in a good performance, increased knowledge and skill, professional advancement, and participation in the exhilarating crusade to exterminate tuberculosis all helped to reward the physicians at the Institute. So did the honoraria or fellowships and the occasional gifts of books from Henry Phipps. Of all the rewards that they remembered and wrote about, however, one predominated—the Monday evening staff meetings. Among the subjects discussed at these meetings, the correlation of physical findings with the pathological changes found at autopsy evoked the most vivid memories. By a curious alchemy of scientific enthusiasm, physicians transmuted the ultimate failure of medicine—the death of a patient—into the gold of knowledge and collegiality.

The case of every patient who died and came to autopsy at the Institute was presented at the Monday evening meeting. The responsible physician had to draw on a blackboard a meticulous diagram of what he had found on physical examination and then predict the abnormalities that the pathologist would report. Any discrepancies between the clinical picture and the pathological findings had then to be explained by the physician. "No patients were more thoroughly, carefully and repeatedly examined than those in the wards of the Phipps Institute," recalled Frank A. Craig, "especially when they were seriously ill." The system, physicians believed, benefited the patients as well as the doctors. "No slipshod diagnoses, and the treatment of patients had better be good," asserted George B. Wood. "It sharpened one's wits to know that you had to give the whys and wherefores to a bunch of lions 'waiting to tear you to bits.' But with all of this give and take, the frequent getting together . . . developed a spirit of comradeship and understanding that made us united and loyal in our enthusiasm for the good work . . . and some of the personal friendships started there lasted throughout our lives."[28]

Policies of the Institute helped to ensure that physicians would get these rewards. Patients admitted to the hospital for treatment had to meet three criteria: they had to have reached an advanced stage of tuberculosis, they had to be poor, and the nearest responsible relative had to give written permission for an autopsy in case the patient should die in the institution.[29]

The Patients

Most of the patients seemed to accept the autopsy requirement. "Oddly enough," George Wood recalled, "this rule did not seem to have any depressing effect on the patients themselves. . . . I remember once, as I passed through a ward, hearing one poor, scarcely alive, disease-ridden human relic say to the patient in the next bed, and with a grin on his face, 'I'll bet you ten dollars I'll beat you to the cutting-up room.'" Acceptance, however, was not unanimous. John Gallagher, an early patient at White Haven, for example, tried to get into the Phipps Institute every year from 1903 through 1905, but his wife consistently refused to "Sign the document." Father Heaney found himself "at a loss what to do" about a friend who needed hospital care. "I am afraid I would scare both him and his mother into an immediate collapse," he wrote to Flick in 1904, "were I to show them that blank."[30]

Once patients had entered the institute, with documents properly signed, they and their families could circumvent the agreement. When family members sensed that the end was near, they sometimes took the patient out of the Institute so that he or she could die at home. The people likely to object to autopsies belonged to one of three groups, observed

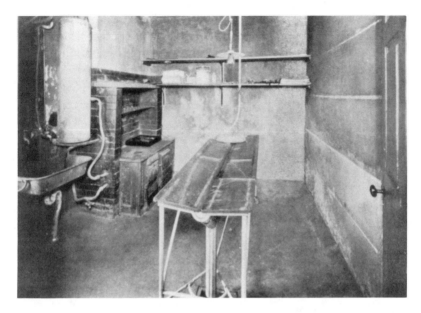

Figure 10. The autopsy room at the Henry Phipps Institute. From the *Annual Report of the Henry Phipps Institute* 1 (February 1904).

Joseph Walsh in 1908: "First, the Hebrews, since it is definitely against their belief; second, the Irish who have a great sentimental regard for the dead bodies of their friends; third, the colored people, who fear that the permission to do the autopsy carries with it the sure death of the individual."[31]

In making their decisions about hospitalization, patients and their families undoubtedly weighed conditions at the Institute, insofar as they understood them, against their situations at home. The place offered shelter, food, nursing attention, treatment, and even hope. If a doctor wanted to give a patient creosote to see how it affected his kidneys or offered to inject his larynx when he had an intractable cough, who would be likely to object? "When I stood in your wards I could not help thinking of what a man said to me once," wrote Dr. Edward L. Trudeau after a visit to the Institute in 1903—"'Dr they say there is nothing to be done for me but I wish somebody would try!'"[32]

A profile of the patients emerges from data collected by the Institute. Of those who either entered the hospital at Phipps or visited the dispensary from 1903 through 1909, 90 percent lived in Philadelphia. Between 40 and 50 percent of them, however, had been born in another country, as had roughly two-thirds of their parents. Fifteen percent of the patients, most if not all of them Jews, came from Russia, while 8 percent came from Ireland and smaller proportions came from Germany, Italy, England, Austria, and other countries. They were relatively young: 16 percent twenty years old or younger, 62 percent between twenty and forty, and 15 percent between forty and fifty. Males, outnumbering females, constituted 59 percent of the group. Most of the patients came from the working classes—laborers, factory hands, tailors, and clerks, for example—and through 1905 close to half of them still worked, despite their disease. They had few alternatives. They earned low wages, they had saved little, and fewer than 10 percent of them had sick benefits of any kind. More than half had dependents to support, usually children or elderly family members. By June 1903, enough of them had entered the hospital to occupy all of its fifty-two beds, and names of others filled the waiting list for several years.[33]

The Nurses and a Training School for "Cured" Consumptives

Finding reliable nurses to work in the hospital proved unusually difficult. In 1903, trained nursing in the United States was still fairly new, and only in the previous two decades had schools proliferated to meet the demands of the burgeoning general hospitals. Many of the new schools had not sustained the high standards of skill and deportment envisioned by nursing's early leaders, and no official agency regulated licensure or practice. In trying to recruit nurses for the Institute, Flick confronted two additional problems: few had been trained in tuberculosis, and most were afraid of contracting the disease.[34]

Nurses faced arduous and disagreeable duties in almost any setting, but work at the Institute brought with it particular kinds of danger and unpleasantness. Although some of the patients could walk about and even make sputum boxes out of paper, others, in the last stages of consumption, became quite helpless. By coughing or vomiting, they repeatedly soiled their clothing, their beds, and even the walls, floors, and furniture near them. Such patients could be kept harmless, according to Flick, only by the "careful and vigilant supervision" of competent nurses. This meant "frequent changing of bed-clothes and body linen, and scrubbing of floors and furniture. Everything must be kept spotlessly clean," and every particle of broken-down tissue must be removed before it dried. "The nurse may at any moment have to scrub the floor or turn washerwoman in an emergency," Flick observed, "and to be a good nurse for tuberculosis, she must do it with alacrity and good humor."[35]

The behavior of some of the nurses first employed could not be tolerated. During the summer of 1903, the Institute's night watchmen began to complain: the nurses entertained gentlemen callers when on night duty, created "considerable racket up stairs," made off with supplies from the kitchen and laboratory, and failed to respond to some of the patients' calls. Two of the women, who had been out drinking with male companions, returned one Sunday night and went into the "diet kitchen where they made loud noise laughing and throwing cantalope rind at each other." "When the institute first opened we were forced to take any nurse that we could get," Walsh observed. "We got," Flick noted sourly, "the scum of the profession."[36]

Fortunately for the Institute, there emerged an alternative source of workers—women patients from White Haven. One of them, Mrs. Margaret Cole, gave the first service of any kind in the building: she "devoted herself heroically to cleaning it up and putting it into condition." Subsequently, two other women joined her, one of them Mrs. Regina O'Leary, whose wish Flick had again granted. Both women, "out of gratitude for what had been done for them at White Haven," as he expressed it later, "devoted themselves in the most slavish manner to the interests of the new Phipps Institute in spite of all restraint that could be put upon them." In the early summer of 1903, as the nursing situation worsened, Flick asked Elwell Stockdale to find some additional workers from among the patients at the sanatorium. On July 14 Stockdale sent his first four "girls" to join the other three women as ward-maids. In persuading them to leave White Haven, he reported to Flick, he had found that their "only fear was that they may not be able to stand the work." Stockdale believed they could perform well and would continue to improve as long as they kept up their milk and eggs, but he left the workers a loophole: "I have promised these girls that if they should find the work too much for them we would immediately take them back."[37]

Two weeks later, one of the new recruits, who Stockdale believed would not exaggerate, wrote a personal letter to Miss Murphy at White Haven. The work at Phipps was "terrible." She was worked from eight in the morning to eight at night without any stop, and the women had to do much of the nurses' work as well as cleaning the wards. One of the women was about to leave, and the others might do the same. "I know if they are compelled to work so hard," Stockdale cautioned, "we would never be able to send you any more." In August, the pattern of work at Phipps was altered. Some of the women were shifted to clerical duties, while others began to alternate between working as ward-maids and visiting dispensary patients in their homes. By making home visits, Flick pointed out, the women would profit from getting outdoors.[38]

The women did well in their work, and Flick, pleased with their accomplishments, soon saw in it the answer to the Institute's nursing problem. Like others responsible for staffing hospitals, he decided to inaugurate a training school for nurses, but this one would differ by taking as pupils only those women who were recovering from tuberculosis. During September he discussed the idea with the medical staff, and the new school opened with eight pupils on October 1, 1903. The women who had served as ward-maids were exempted from the usual month of probationary service.[39]

Mrs. O'Leary probably never entered the school. She "wanted to die a martyr to the cause," as Flick expressed it, "and in spite of all that could be said or done, insisted upon working in the most unselfish manner in the services of the institute . . . until she had won for herself that coveted crown." At the age of forty-two, she died as a patient there on January 12, 1904, "happy to her last moment that she had been able to do something for the cause."[40]

The training school at Phipps, like many nursing schools of the time, offered a two-year program of practical work and instruction. In return for their labor, the pupils received board, lodging, ten dollars a month, plenty of milk and eggs, and the chance of bettering their lives in the future. If they completed the program, they received a certificate. In turn, the Institute benefited from the training school: the pupils' work probably cost no more than that of their predecessors and it was surely superior in quality. According to Flick and some of his colleagues, women who had had the disease made better nurses for other consumptives: they were unafraid of infection, they had greater sympathy with the afflicted, and they were heartening to the patients by their very example. Flick took pride in training the women and in creating a new occupation for "cured" consumptives.[41]

The reciprocal interests of the pupils and the Institute, however, hung in precarious balance. Suitable women were few and hard to attract, pupils dropped out of the school, and the Institute never achieved stability in its nursing staff. The nursing directress and the physicians in charge of the Training School Committee issued repeated and urgent appeals for additional pupils during the subsequent years.[42]

The Dispensary

The pupil nurses at the Institute worked in both the hospital and the dispensary; each area played an important role in prevention. The hospital, in Flick's opinion, segregated advanced consumptives during the stage when they were most infectious, but hospitals were costly, their beds few, their interventions late, and patients—unwilling to leave their homes or work—often refused to go there. A dispensary, on the other hand, could reach many more people at lower cost; members of the staff could treat patients with early disease in addition to advanced consumptives; and, most important, Flick believed, staff could teach the patients and their families how to prevent the spread of infection.[43]

Instruction began the moment a patient entered the dispensary.

> As each patient comes into the waiting-room he is handed a spit-cup, and during his stay is taught to use it. When he goes away he is given a tin spit-cup holder, a bundle of paper cups, and a bundle of paper napkins and paper bags to take home with him. He is also given a set of rules on a large cardboard to hang up in his house, and on a folder to carry in his pocket. Every time he comes back to the dispensary he is given a new supply of preventive measure material, and is further instructed in its use.[44]

The rules stipulated just how patients should use these materials, and added some further precautions against infecting others. If a man had a moustache or beard, for example, he should shave it off or crop it close lest germs linger there. All patients should avoid handshaking and kissing. "These customs are dangerous to you as well as to others. They may give *others* consumption; they may bring *you* colds and influenzas which will greatly aggravate your disease and may prevent your recovery." It was up to the pupil nurses in their role as inspectresses to reinforce these rules.[45]

Although "well-to-do and enlightened" people might find circulars sufficient for their instruction, Flick believed, "the poor and ignorant" should be taught by demonstration. Trained inspectresses should visit the patients at home, review their instructions, and show them how to comply. "Tactful, kind supervision by a well trained woman," Flick wrote optimistically in 1904, "soon brings the most ignorant consumptive under control." A year later, he sounded a bit less sanguine. "Considerable pressure is brought to bear on patients to induce them to practise preventive measures when they seem reluctant to do so," he wrote in the second annual report. "When, ultimately, they are found to be intractable, they are discharged from the Institute."[46]

Discharge from the Institute could pinch a patient's welfare in several ways. In addition to spit-cups, rules, and instructions, the dispensary provided both milk and low-cost medicines to those considered needful. In 1904, after trying to deliver milk under its own auspices, the Institute established two milk stations where inspectresses distributed up to three quarts daily to qualified patients. "A little help in the early stages of tuberculosis . . . frequently is all that is necessary to bring about recovery," Flick observed in 1905. "Just a little more food, a little more rest, and a little more fresh air than the patient can get with his own resources, are all that are necessary to turn the scales." Such assistance should be properly timed, however, and it must not be excessive. It should be "just enough to hold up the family in self-respect and not enough to pauperize it."[47]

The rules of the Institute instructed the patients in healthful living as well as in modes of prevention.

> Sit out of doors all you can. . . . Always sleep with your windows open. . . . Avoid fatigue. . . . Go to bed early. . . . Don't eat pastry or dainties. They do not nourish you and they may upset your stomach. . . . Take your milk and raw eggs whether you feel like it or not. . . . Keep up your courage. Make a brave fight for your life. Do what you are told to do as though your recovery depended upon the carrying out of every little detail.[48]

Inspectresses helped the patients make the necessary adjustments—to camp out on the roof, for example, to sit on the porch in the sunshine, and, in order to shield the family from danger, to sleep alone.[49]

Within a few years, the inspectresses assumed two additional functions. By assessing the economic status of patients' households, they helped to determine how much assistance the patients really needed or whether they deserved to be helped at all. This kind of assessment served two purposes: it prevented the Institute from wasting its resources, and it helped to forestall medical criticism. Physicians of the time were characteristically sensitive to charitable activities that might draw away their paying patients. At the same time, the inspectresses looked for other members of households who showed early manifestations of tuberculosis. These they encouraged to come to the dispensary for examination and possible treatment. In turn, the physicians in the dispensary selected from among the patients those most suitable for the hospital.[50]

The dispensary, in summary, had its own important functions in treating patients and preventing the spread of disease. It also served the other parts of the organization. By attracting patients to the Institute, it helped to assure the supply of "clinical material" for both the hospital and the laboratory. The dispensary, moreover, functioned economically. Maintenance of a patient there, Flick estimated in 1905, cost roughly $.85 a week, compared to $9.33 for care in the hospital.[51]

The opinions of patients can only be guessed at from institutional statistics and an occasional letter. That the dispensary remained crowded attests to its value, and many doubtless appreciated the aid and attention. "Dear Nurse," read a letter in 1907, "wont you please come two see me as I . . . have been so sick since I have been down two the Instute . . . I will be very thankful if some nurse will come two see me as soon as it is conveninte as I am very nearly helpless—I am Mrs Mc Laughlin . . . I live in the Front Attic and at present I cannot go up or down stairs."[52]

Inevitably, however, attention created conflict and misunderstanding, as Mrs. John Schick made clear in 1909:

> And doc, I now right to you to tell you, that you sent 2 nearses here to see Katie MiCarty and I would like to know, if you can tell who sent you a letter about my doarter.   If they wanted to say any thing about her why, was they not lady, or man enueff to say some thing to me a bout it, doctor   I have got both doctor priest and sisters to look after her. I had my doarter down to 3. and pine st [the Institute's address] and waited a half day and then she got so bad that I had to bring her home, I would like to you to tell your's nearses to pleas not bother a bout my business, for there is only one cure for my child and that is in heven.[53]

In spite of the Institute's problems, Flick established his basic organization within only a year or two. Although the Phipps Institute did not offer sanatorium care for incipient cases, the Free Hospital helped to fill this gap at White Haven. As soon as the Institute could find more satisfactory quarters, Flick felt sure, it would become a model for the world.

7. Achievement and Disappointment at the Institute

Linking the care of consumptives to scientific research in the hope of exterminating the disease was a bold but risky strategy. For the gamble to work, the Institute needed to show success—something to gratify the man who was paying for it and to make it seem like a sound investment. By concentrating on the care of advanced and dying consumptives, appropriate as this might have been to the Institute's research, few cures could make the treatment of patients seem worthwhile. The laboratory made no new discoveries that would treat or prevent the disease. Given the state of medical knowledge, high expectations of research were premature.

Further, the treatment of chronically ill patients over long periods of time became more onerous than Flick had anticipated. Even when the dispensary helped patients materially, many of them died and contaminated their environments in the process. The effort, therefore, failed to check the spread of infection. The patients' continuing use of the Institute's aid, however, aroused in Flick the widely shared anxiety that assistance bred dependency. As he recognized the limitations of the dispensary and the abuse that its services seemed to invite, he turned to institutionalization as the preferable method of preventing the disease. Only in hospitals, he concluded, could poor and advanced consumptives be controlled.

Although the Phipps investment produced no new treatments and no major scientific advances, it had an impact through education and publicity—odd results, perhaps, for a research institute, but appropriate to the needs of the time and natural in view of Flick's abilities. The Institute trained a cadre of physicians and a group of consumptive women as nurses, and it helped to promote the campaign against tuberculosis.

Henry Phipps, recognizing the need for change, transferred the organization to the University of Pennsylvania in 1910. Flick lost his directorship. The University, interested chiefly in education and research, reduced the Institute's commitment to patient care. It gave Phipps a somewhat different return on his money but, over the next decade, was no more successful than Flick had been.

Differences and Uncertainty

The Institute's rapid early development masked a fundamental difference between Flick's goals and those of Henry Phipps. While Flick wanted to prevent and exterminate tuberculosis, Phipps wanted to cure it. It was the hope of curing consumptives in a country sanatorium that had attracted him to Flick's endeavors, and for most of the first year he kept returning to this idea. "Mr. Phipps will not be satisfied with mere isolation of consumptive patients," explained George E. Gordon, his secretary, in a letter to Flick in May 1903; "he is most anxious that the main effort shall be directed toward the cure and reclamation of those who have a fighting chance for life." That meant a sanatorium where the "pure air, ample room for exercise, and so many pleasant diversions (to say nothing of the lower cost of land)" would all contribute to the patients' recovery. To Phipps, "as to most people," Flick later observed, "a house full of dying consumptives with a lot of enthusiastic medical men trying to extract a boon for humanity out of them was a melancholy sight not well calculated to pull fifty thousand dollars a year out of one's pocket." By repeated persuasion, however, Flick managed to hold Phipps to the announced goals of the Institute, at least through the first year.[1]

Early in 1904, efforts to find a new site for the cramped Institute rekindled the smoldering conflict. From the start, Flick had considered the quarters on Pine Street a temporary expedient, and for much of the year a realtor had been searching for a larger, more suitable site. Early in January 1904 he seemed to have found one, but Phipps hesitated. The magnitude of the laboratory was now the major question. Phipps had consulted some "eminent physicians," foremost among whom were probably two men from Johns Hopkins, William Osler, professor of medicine, and William H. Welch, first dean and professor of pathology. The men had advised caution, as a letter from George E. Gordon revealed. In thinking over the proposed buildings, Gordon wrote on January 6,

> I have felt somewhat concerned as to whether . . . we are not giving too much prominence to the Laboratory and Scientific Department. . . .
> I know it is your hope that Mr. Phipps may be credited with having inaugurated and made possible the research which may develope [sic] an absolute cure for tuberculosis, and while I am not able to speak of the relative merits of a scientific or philanthropic course, I think Mr. Phipps should know clearly what you expect will be the requirements of a Laboratory. . . . For instance: How much ground, and what would be the cost of the building— how much for equipment; how much for maintenance; supplies; Physicians' salaries; fellowships, etc. Also given an assumed income of, say $50,000.00

what proportion of this amount would you devote to Laboratory work, and of what relative importance is it, keeping Mr. Phipps' original purpose in mind?

With so many Hospitals, Medical Colleges, Universities, etc. thoroughly equipped for Laboratory work, do you not think these are sufficient—in other words, isn't the field well filled?[2]

The inquiries touched a weakness in Flick's capacity to lead the Institute. Although he had remarkable abilities to organize, promote, and publicize, he was neither a scientist nor a man trained to plan and manage a laboratory. His responses were vague—unlikely to satisfy the cautious, meticulous Henry Phipps. While the medical director replied to some of Gordon's questions, he gave few details for the proposed laboratory other than estimates for total expenditures and medical fellowships. The laboratory buildings, equipment, maintenance, and so on, he wrote, could "be made as little or as big as you want to make it." Instead of specific plans, Flick outlined his vision of the Institute's role and influence. No man's wealth, however large, he asserted, could have any effect on tuberculosis "unless thousands and hundreds of thousands of others are thereby stimulated into activity." Mr. Phipps's money should be made to "reach much farther than a few hundred poor people in Philadelphia. To make it reach to all parts of the world it is necessary to have a laboratory in which work can be done which will attract the attention of the world." It was not so much a question of searching for a specific cure, he continued, but of determining the best methods to treat and prevent the disease. No other laboratory was doing this kind of work, and no institute without a laboratory could educate the world.[3]

On February 2—the first anniversary of the Institute—Flick sent to Phipps a congratulatory message in which he hailed the goodness and happiness that would pour from the Institute's work. The conquest of tuberculosis, that "death dealing monster," would shield millions of mothers from loss of their children and husbands, save them from charitable institutions, and prevent the inevitable crime that accompanied dependency. Phipps replied to the letter but made no commitment.[4]

On February 5 Flick wrote again, this time giving vent to some of his pent-up feelings. "'Hope deferred maketh the heart sick,' and I am beginning to experience this disintegrating influence of deferred hope upon our organization," he confessed. "I have gathered around me the best medical talent of this City and I have been able to gather it because of the prospects which our Institute held to talented young men for advancement in reputation. One of the greatest difficulties I have had in getting the men I wanted

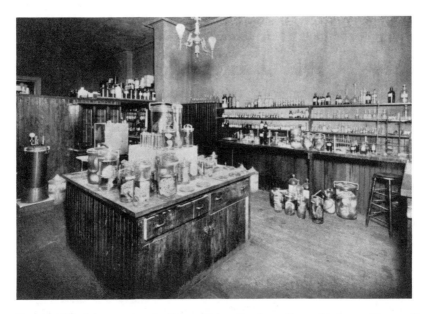

Figure 11. The laboratory at the Henry Phipps Institute. From the *Annual Report of the Henry Phipps Institute* 1 (February 1904).

has been my inability to show them a material guarantee of the permanency of our undertaking."[5]

Tensions mounted through February, and toward the end of the month Flick, Phipps, and Gordon met in New York and resolved their differences. "The charity end of our work appealed to him most," Flick observed, referring to Phipps, "and on this[,] judgment was unnecessary. It was a matter of heart." The physicians whom Phipps had consulted, however, had shaken his confidence in the laboratory. "The scientific end was a matter of reason and on this he wanted to feel his way." The disagreement ended in compromise. Laboratory investigation continued at the Institute, but permanent quarters were further delayed.[6]

The Search for a Curative Serum

In the summer of 1904, new scientific developments appeared to vindicate Flick's faith in the laboratory. Because the Institute could show little research of its own during the first year, Flick had invited a series of distinguished men in the field to lecture in Philadelphia. Among them was Edoardo Maragliano, a physician from Genoa who, like some other European physicians, was trying to develop a serum or other immunological method of treating tuberculosis. Although Maragliano had to cancel his trip at the last moment, Flick read his paper at the Phipps Institute on March 28, 1904. "All my researches . . . for more than fifteen years," Maragliano asserted, "lead me to state: (1) *That it is possible to produce a specific therapy for tuberculosis*; (2) *that it is possible to immunize the animal organism against tuberculosis as is done in other infectious diseases, and that there is good reason to hope for an antituberculous vaccination for man.*" [Maragliano's emphasis][7]

Maragliano's serum differed from Koch's tuberculin. While tuberculin was injected to stimulate an active immunity in a patient's body, the serum produced a passive immunity transferred from an animal. The Italian physician first prepared a substance from tubercle bacilli and their "secretions," and next injected it into cows, horses, or other animals until their immune systems had produced circulating antitoxins and antibodies. He then withdrew some of the animals' blood, separated out the serum, and administered it to experimental animals or to patients. By either injecting or feeding this serum, he believed, immunity was transferred to the second subject. His results seemed very encouraging.[8]

Maragliano's paper created excitement at the Institute. Bacteriological advances in the past two decades had prepared physicians for just this kind of announcement. "The whole subject [of bacteriology] was new," Dr. Joseph McFarland recalled; "miracles were being performed . . . and every day new miracles were hoped for and expected. . . . If diphtheria and tetanus could be prevented or cured by the serum of immunized horses, why not tuberculosis . . . ?"[9]

Within two days, Flick arranged for Mazÿck P. Ravenel, the assistant medical director of the Institute and a competent bacteriologist, to go to Genoa and study Maragliano's methods. Phipps supported the plan and even urged a quick departure. Ravenel arrived in Genoa late in May 1904, and on June 12 sent an enthusiastic letter to Flick. The men in Maragliano's laboratory were treating him cordially and he had mastered the techniques of producing all the necessary toxins and fluids for the animal work. He had given five injections of the serum to two rabbits and had just bled one of them. In nine days, the blood had "acquired an agglutinating power of more than 1 to 150. If agglutination goes pari passu with immunity, this short period of treatment had raised the resistance of those rabbits to a high degree." Ravenel was also attending the free clinic with Dr. Figari three times a week. One woman whom they saw there had been unable to stand before treatment, but now after only four weeks of injections "she *walks* to the clinic. They prescribe nothing else and the family is poor. . . . There can be no question, I think, of the action of the serum on animals," Ravenel concluded, "and this being true, I see no reason why it should not act well on man."[10]

Flick received this report with enthusiasm and passed the good news along to Phipps. In August, the Institute spent $150 for serum to treat from twenty to forty patients and thus get a head start on the research until Ravenel could produce his own. Quarters, of course, were an obstacle. "I hope something has been done about the grounds and buildings," wrote Ravenel from Paris in August. "I dread trying to do good bacteriological work in the cramped quarters we now have, but we must get started at once." Tactfully, Flick broached the question to Gordon and Phipps in September, and this time won approval. By the end of October 1904, the Institute had a new laboratory in a nearby rented house. Meanwhile, Ravenel completed a tour of European laboratories and was joined for part of the trip by Leonard Pearson, a leading veterinarian enlisted for the bovine part of the work.[11]

Both men were back in Philadelphia by September 6, and within a week or so physicians at the Institute began to use the purchased serum on patients. Word of it had already leaked to the public. "I see by to day's paper," wrote Andrew Innis to Flick on September 1, "that you are going to try another method to beat consumption. I am a victim of tuberculosis, but I feel satisfied and willing to try this new treatment, if wanted, I will go first. . . . I am anxious to get better and will try anything." Flick tried to avoid publicity. "The newspapers have been hot after us for information," he reported to Phipps later that month, but he had cautioned members of the staff not to divulge anything until they can "speak definitely and upon scientific basis."[12]

The medical director, however, could scarcely contain his eagerness. "If the serum is worth what it appears to be worth," he wrote to Gordon, "we probably can manufacture it for sale and get enough revenue . . . to not only pay Ravenel's salary but to have some income for the Institute." With both Pearson and Ravenel behind it, "we could [probably] put serum into the market on a very creditable basis and perhaps could control the market of this country." Phipps approved of making the serum, but thought of the market differently. If the serum should prove promising, he suggested to

Flick, its sale would be large, but for a limited time only. Then "welcome competition comes in that will fill the field I hope to the benefit of humanity."[13]

Early clinical trials of the purchased serum dampened the hopes of the three physicians who used it, but in 1905 and 1906 Ravenel proceeded with making his own. Thirty-seven patients from the Institute received the injections, as did a small number of private patients. As physicians observed the results, enthusiasm for the treatment waned, and early in 1906 Flick responded gloomily to an inquiry about it. Although the Institute had spent much time and money in studying Maragliano's serum, he wrote to Dr. Walter Reynolds, it could not yet draw conclusions. "You may readily infer from this that its value . . . is not very marked to say the least." Later reports confirmed the worst: the serum was risky as well as useless.[14]

No one could have known then that search for a serum was futile. Regardless of agglutinating power or any other kind of antibody found in the serum, immunity to tuberculosis lay elsewhere, in the cells of the body. Unlike serum, these could not be therapeutically transferred. The medical breakthrough in the treatment of tuberculosis was to take another form—drugs that inhibited or killed the bacilli. The first of these was not discovered until the 1940s.

The Dispensary: "Like Bailing Out the Sea"

If Flick had been overly optimistic about finding a cure for tuberculosis, he also overestimated the ability of a dispensary to treat consumptives and prevent disease. Medicines, milk, and instruction proved to be puny forces against the disease and against the socioeconomic conditions in which the patients lived. In a series of steps from 1903 through 1908, Flick's confidence in the dispensary and his sympathy with the patients gradually changed to restriction and blame.

Ever since the dispensary had opened, crowding had plagued the work and, in Flick's opinion, had impaired its scientific value. In order to help as many people as possible, physicians had taken shortcuts, had made incomplete or erroneous observations, and had even treated patients without first taking a history. Because of so many patients, moreover, expenses were exceeding the funds allotted. Flick had allowed expenditures to rise, he explained to Phipps in December 1903, because "the poverty and distress of the poor people who appeal to us are so great that it is difficult to say no."

Nevertheless, he had recently limited the number of patients seen each day and had established a waiting list. "I can quite understand the great pressure upon you to help the poor people, and you are the best judge to what extent the work should go," Phipps replied, but he added a note of futility. "It is almost like bailing out the sea."[15]

Flick's action reduced the numbers of patients in the dispensary and improved the scientific work, but costs still troubled him. Material assistance in the form of milk and preventive supplies was straining the budget. In early 1905, however, he still defended the expenditures. To get patients well and to keep them well without such assistance were both impossible, he asserted, and proper instruction protected others from a first infection.[16]

While Flick recognized that the poor could not always follow instructions, he did not then blame them. "On account of home conditions and great poverty it is next to impossible to maintain discipline with such patients in their homes," he observed. "They often will not sit out in the open air because they have no convenient place to sit in. They will work when they ought to be at rest, because they have some one depending on them. They will not take the diet. Even when supplied with milk, they will divide it up with other members of the family rather than use it for their own recovery. This is particularly true where there are small children in the family." Flick, a devoted husband and father, often used the family image in his rhetoric. "What sadder picture of human suffering can one conjure up," he asked a year later, "than that of a starving child asking for bread from a starving, disease-stricken father? or of a heart-broken old man or woman accepting a morsel from a disease-stricken son or daughter?"[17]

By early 1906, however, Flick was starting to recognize the cumulative burden. Almost a third of the patients treated in the first two years were returning for further care in the third year. "There is necessarily a limit to the time during which material assistance can be given," he cautioned. "A pension list soon springs up if patients are carried too long. . . . [It] absorbs all the resources of the Institute and prevents the extension of the benefits of the work to new patients."[18]

Despite this concern, he still expressed sympathy for the plight of poor consumptives. Statistics for the year ending early in 1906 showed that 47 percent of the patients worked. "Why they work can be read out of the table on income and sick benefits," Flick wrote in the annual report that year. "Work is the alternative of starvation. . . . Sick horses are not permitted to work, and sick cats are . . . humanely cared for. Sick brothers and sisters, however, not only are permitted, but are compelled to work even at la-

borious occupations. How strange that there are no societies for the prevention of cruelty to human beings!"[19]

During the next two years, however, the Institute's statistics gave
further cause for concern. The proportion of patients who worked fell from
47 percent to 26 percent and then remained low at 28 percent. Early in 1907,
Flick blandly attributed the change to the educational campaign that was
promoting rest as part of the treatment but, early in 1908, he reacted
differently. "It would seem that our influence upon the community has
been for idleness, if the patients tell the truth," he observed. "It is possible
that some may have misrepresented the facts in order to get aid, but it is
more probable that many have taken up a life of idleness because they have
received assistance. This brings out a feature of the dispensary work which
will have to be carefully studied and weighed."[20]

Of the aid given to patients, milk was the most popular among recipients and the most costly to the Institute, and the distribution of milk, Flick
now argued, led to abuse. "There is danger of pauperization in it," he
warned in 1908. "It even encourages dishonesty." Some of the patients sold
their milk; others asked for it when they could have bought it themselves.
Even a patient's neighbor supported these points in an unsigned postcard:
"As you give Tessie Neerenberg milk so it is wrong for doing that because,
her son makes $10 per week and her husband $12 and the milk that you give
her she sells and she also has a photograph and $100 worth of furniture . . .
and if you would like to find out the real truth you can see it all upstairs."[21]

In January 1908, the Institute inaugurated restrictions on milk. Joseph
Walsh, who had become assistant medical director of the Institute after
Ravenel resigned in 1907, had been collecting data on patients who received
milk over long periods, and now began to notify their physicians of the new
policy. "Louis Addler, a patient of yours at the Phipps Institute, has been
getting milk for thirty-six weeks," read the typical letter. "Our usual period
for giving milk to one patient is not more than six months." When Dr.
E. H. Goodman questioned Flick on behalf of a patient, Flick clarified the
intent of the new rule. Although six months was not a binding term, he
explained, a patient who has "received milk for six months ought by that
time to be restored to a condition of health in which he can help himself." If
not, "his case is probably not a curable one in a dispensary. . . . If in your
judgment the patient needs a little longer assistance it is proper that you
give it but if you are merely pensioning the man and making an object of
charity of him without a possibility of his recovery the milk should be
stopped." During the next two years, the annual number of patients receiving milk dropped by one-third.[22]

Flick carried his criticisms beyond the issue of milk and attacked the dispensary itself. "Theoretically it is a perfect measure," he argued in 1908, but "in practice it is defective." The therapeutic value of the dispensary was limited. Although teaching resulted in "healthier living and greater resistance" and although patients improved, survived longer, and might "even get well," most of them "ultimately become advanced cases, serve their turn as sources of seed-supply for new cases, and die." Further, dispensaries could not effectively prevent tuberculosis because they could not safely manage the chief source of infection—poor consumptives dying at home. Their families could not give the necessary supervision, nor could the dispensary staff because of prohibitive costs. Dispensaries already consumed "too much of the available resources of the crusade, and they should at once be cut down and restricted to their proper sphere." If dying patients were to be made harmless, they must be isolated in institutions, and in furthering this effort lay the chief value of the dispensary: it fed the hospital as well as the sanatorium. The dispensary, finally, lay vulnerable to abuse. "Undeserving alms obtained under false pretense have a very demoralizing influence upon the public," he concluded in 1910, "and in carrying out a great movement like the crusade against tuberculosis pains should be taken not to degrade and demoralize where it is sought to improve and build up."[23]

Flick, who in 1888 had suggested that governments pension poor consumptives, was changing his views with remarkable speed. Gone was his radical idealism, and gone were the emotional pleas to relieve the suffering of the sick poor. The poor consumptive, once a deserving object of pity, had become an economic burden, made idle, dependent, and even dishonest by the assistance received. This new image was strikingly similar to that used by charity organization societies during the latter part of the nineteenth century. Andrew Carnegie had warned of creating dependency in his 1889 "Gospel of Wealth."[24]

Actual costs of care at the Institute seem insufficient to account for Flick's changing opinions. Although some of the patients undoubtedly did misuse their assistance, reported statistics show no increasing drain on the Institute's economy. From 1905 through 1907 the proportion of new patients receiving milk did rise but then decreased, along with the number of quarts supplied. Total cost of the aid showed little change—roughly eight to nine cents per patient per day. In 1907, inspections became a bit more numerous but averaged a meager 3.4 visits per patient per year. In 1904, Flick had publicly recommended that poor consumptives be inspected once a week.[25]

Flick's change of mind must have had other explanations. It was probably not so much what the dispensary had cost but what it would cost to make it effective that helped to turn Flick against it. Demands for care were too high, and the Institute could not meet its own expectations. To make a very ill or dying patient harmless at home would require almost constant supervision, not an occasional visit. That would be too expensive and, because of the Institute's shortage of pupil nurses and the geographic dispersion of patients, clearly impossible. Besides, it might not even suffice. The "unhygienic conditions," the "insufficient air space," and the lack of basic necessities in the homes of the poor all seemed to make the effort impracticable. Flick had been wrong in thinking that medical instruction, together with a little material aid, could overcome these obstacles. His rhetoric responded to institutional necessity. Unconsciously, perhaps, he may have been trying to shift the blame for the failure from himself to the patients. At any rate, he needed another solution. The centralization of poor and advanced consumptives in hospitals, by comparison, now seemed economical, feasible, and indispensable for proper control.[26]

Growing pressures on Flick from additional sources probably contributed to the increasingly shrill quality of his commentary. In addition to problems at Phipps, the White Haven Sanatorium was facing financial difficulties, as Chapter 9 will describe, the state was threatening Flick's leadership, and state-sponsored dispensaries were beginning to encroach on the Institute's territory. Probably some of Flick's criticisms were really directed at them. It was the state government, more than the modest dispensary at the Phipps Institute, that was giving free care to tuberculous Pennsylvanians. While trying to cope with all these problems, Flick also had to make a living in private practice: he accepted no salary as director of the Institute.[27]

Despite Flick's verbal attacks on the dispensary, the numbers of persons treated there remained stable through early 1910. In addition to prevention and treatment, the dispensary had a third and essential function: it supplied patients to the hospital, and the hospital in turn supplied materials for the laboratory. As one way to attract patients, the Institute continued to distribute milk.[28]

Promotion and Education

The Institute's failure to find a cure for tuberculosis and Flick's disillusionment with the dispensary had few effects on the pursuit of two additional, interrelated goals—disseminating knowledge and stimulating the crusade against tuberculosis. Although Flick was not a laboratory man, promotion and publicity were two of his strengths, and he used them to good advantage—locally, nationally, and internationally. "Flick's natural flair for justifiable publicity," as Walsh later characterized these activities, "made the Phipps Institute internationally known in three years."[29]

The chief vehicle with which Flick hoped to reach the scientific community and beyond it was the annual report. Into these reports he packed extensive reviews of the work of the Institute, and staff physicians published their research there. Through this medium, all the carefully compiled clinical data, neatly tabulated and summarized, reached the public annually. The first report "will be a valuable document," Flick wrote to Gordon in 1904, "and ought to be placed in the hands of every scientific man in the world." With Phipps's money, he planned to distribute one thousand copies to "newspapers, magazines and medical journals throughout the world," and thousands more to "professors of the medical colleges and some of the Universities and to all of the principle [sic] workers in the tuberculosis problem." Of the five thousand printed copies, each numbering 265 pages, he planned to distribute four thousand at once and hold the remainder in reserve. Perhaps, he suggested to Phipps after sending him two hundred copies, "some of your wealthy friends" might be "thereby induced to take a hand in the crusade." If only such men could inform themselves of a "practical method of applying money to the cause," he added, they would willingly give to it.[30]

Lectures provided another means of reaching the public. During the first year, when Flick was still organizing the Institute's staff, he invited men from outside the city to give the lectures. Some distinguished men responded to his invitations, including William Osler, Edward L. Trudeau, and Hermann Biggs, chief medical officer of the New York City Health Department and leader in the municipal control of tuberculosis. Flick made certain that their presentations attracted the proper attention. Advance copies of Trudeau's lecture, for example, were sent both to European and American medical journals and to newspapers throughout the United States. The publisher Charles M. Lea congratulated Flick on the success of his efforts. He had attracted "the attention of the entire medical press to the Phipps' Institute," Lea noted, "as was shown by the editorials of all the leading weeklies."[31]

After the first series of lectures, Flick decided to shift responsibility for future ones to the Institute's own men. This change would accomplish a double purpose, he explained to Gordon: it would help the staff's physicians and give them standing in the community, and it would also carry on the educational campaign. Flick could "have lantern slides made for illustrated lectures and put our staff into the lecture field all over the country"; each man would receive a small honorarium for his work. Phipps approved the plan. "Every man of the staff was called upon constantly to give popular talks," recalled Frank A. Craig, "in schools, churches and industrial plants."[32]

From 1906 to 1908, an international undertaking of extraordinary dimensions consumed increasing proportions of Flick's energies. As early as 1902, when he and Phipps were still planning the Institute, he had envisioned a way it could "'give a strong impetus to the Crusade Against Tuberculosis'"; it could bring the International Congress on Tuberculosis to the United States for the first time. In his original announcement of the Institute in 1903, Flick had reported that preliminary arrangements for the Congress had already been made. First, however, a national committee had to be formed to sponsor the project. The organization that finally attracted the Congress was the National Association for the Study and Prevention of Tuberculosis,* established in 1904.[33]

Flick, a leading participant in founding the National Association, was appointed in 1906 as chairman of its Committee on the International Congress. He and his committee planned the sessions, raised the money, and created a vast network of supporters from every state in the country. They enlisted the aid of the U.S. Congress, which not only appropriated twenty-five thousand dollars for federal contributions to the exhibition but also gave another forty thousand dollars so that the new National Museum might be put in condition to house the many displays. Dr. Henry G. Beyer of the U.S. Navy took charge of arranging the 438 contributions sent by organizations and individuals from both the United States and abroad.[34]

Five thousand delegates and representatives attended the Congress, which opened in Washington in September 1908. During the six-day meeting, participants attended lectures on almost every conceivable aspect of tuberculosis: its pathology and bacteriology; its diagnosis and treatment; the hygienic, social, economic, and industrial aspects of the disease; and the proper role of government in controlling it. Speakers included scientists, physicians, economists, government officials, nurses, and social workers. Robert Koch himself addressed the group, and President Theodore Roose-

*In 1918, the NASPT shortened its name to the National Tuberculosis Association. I will use National Association for either name.

velt spoke at the closing ceremonies. Transactions of the meetings filled eight bound volumes. One hundred fifty thousand visitors viewed the exhibition, while hundreds of thousands more saw it later in New York and Philadelphia. Although the efforts and tensions involved in organizing the event exhausted Flick, the Congress itself proved a triumph. It was widely credited as having stimulated the nation's organized fight against tuberculosis, just as he had intended. The achievements of the Phipps Institute, moreover, gave him considerable pleasure: its exhibits won six prizes.[35]

Delay and a Change of Direction

As time for the Congress approached, however, conditions at the Institute caused its medical director increasing embarrassment and dissatisfaction. Flick, his staff, and the patients still occupied the old, inadequate quarters. Although Flick in 1904 had rented a house where the nurses could live and attend classes and had rented a second house for the laboratory, the main building remained a problem. For this, neither he nor the realtors could find an appropriate substitute. Late in 1907 a suitable site finally seemed within reach, but as realtors squabbled over prices Phipps still hesitated. By January 30, 1908, Flick could no longer bear the situation. "The delay in completing this real estate transaction and putting the Institute on a permanent basis," he wrote to Gordon, "has a very disconcerting influence upon my organization here and makes it exceedingly difficult to keep up the esprit de corps of the staff. . . . I do not believe that either you or Mr. Phipps realize how much of a damper this delay has been upon the zeal and ardor of our organization and how it handicaps me in developing the scientific end of the Institute." The timing of the delay, he pointed out, was particularly unfortunate. "With the coming gathering of men from all parts of the world we are placing Mr. Phipps in a somewhat embarrassing position." The whole situation would be "exceedingly difficult to explain to the prominent foreigners" expected to visit.[36]

At last, in February 1908, the Institute acquired title to new properties at 639 and 641 Lombard Street in Philadelphia. Seven months later, however, visitors from the International Congress saw no evidence of progress except for the architectural plans the Institute had placed on exhibit in Washington. Although planning continued, Phipps made no decisions on building, and Flick, preoccupied by the Congress, had less than his usual time to devote to the Institute's affairs. Further, five key members of the staff, holding among them thirteen committee positions for the Congress, necessarily shifted their energies toward it.[37]

While Flick and his staff considered the Congress one of their greatest successes, the work and excitement involved in it could not conceal the Institute's troubles. From 1906 through 1908, resignations were multiplying; they further impaired the research effort, which had never been strong. By 1909, too few papers had been written to justify publishing an annual report. Joseph Walsh, who edited the reports, suggested to Charles J. Hatfield in July that they skip a year, thus combining the sixth and seventh volumes. By this time, Walsh acknowledged, the reports had already fallen a year and a half behind.[38]

Through the summer of 1909, Flick continued to press for new facilities. Otherwise, he wrote to Gordon, the Institute would have to abandon its scientific work and either lower its flag or content itself "with pure charity work." On October 29, Gordon announced the fateful decision: Phipps would neither erect new buildings nor make the Institute permanent. He would, however, continue to support the Institute as it was then conducted. Flick, in response, tendered his resignation. He suggested that either of two qualified men, Joseph Walsh or Charles J. Hatfield, might be persuaded to take the directorship, and that any of three organizations might offer it a suitable permanent home: the Free Hospital for Poor Consumptives and White Haven Sanatorium Association, the Jefferson Medical College, or the University of Pennsylvania.[39]

Before taking his next step Phipps consulted with other physicians, most notably William Osler, who by this time had retired from Johns Hopkins, and William H. Welch, the most influential proponent of scientific medicine in the country. According to Theodore H. Ingalls, who more than forty years later became director of the Institute, these "eminent scholars" gave Phipps advice entirely consonant with the scientific reform of American medicine. If "continuity and quality of function, research direction and staffing were to be maintained at a high level, the Institute should be part of the medical operations of a great University." On November 26, 1909, Phipps asked Welch to explore the possibilities of establishing relations with the University of Pennsylvania, and on December 6 he sent a definitive proposal to Provost Charles C. Harrison. He offered to "erect a building to be used for the study, treatment, and prevention of tuberculosis, along the lines established by the Henry Phipps Institute . . . and to give fifty thousand dollars per annum for six years, from and after the completion of the building," in order to operate and maintain it. Should the University accept the proposition, Phipps also "requested that the University authorities offer the Medical Directorship to Dr. Lawrence F. Flick." The Board of Trustees unanimously accepted the terms of the proposal.[40]

Provost Harrison and two other University officials met with Flick on December 16. The "University was prepared to offer him the Medical Directorship of the new organization," as Harrison reported to Phipps, "or such other position in it as might assure his continuation in the work." In what Harrison described as a "most kindly" conversation, Flick declined to commit himself and allowed his resignation to stand. Harrison then told him that, as soon as the University's trustees had considered the new organization, the plan would be submitted to him and "a further invitation extended to him to take such part as might be agreeable." Flick accepted this offer. On December 23, the medical staff of the Institute passed a resolution and forwarded it to Phipps. The physicians reaffirmed their allegiance to Flick as medical director, praised his "stimulating personality and heroic self-sacrifice," and strongly recommended that he be retained in his post.[41]

No new invitation, however, was ever submitted to Flick. On January 7, 1910, Harrison wrote to Gordon that Flick had finally decided to withdraw from the Institute, but when the University announced its appointments Flick was unprepared. Despite his resignation as medical director, he was probably secretly hoping that Harrison would offer him some kind of position, as the provost had indicated on December 16. The day was the low spot in his life, his daughter Ella recalled. "It was luncheon hour and my father was lying on the couch in his study, shading his eyes with his hands as he oftentimes did when he was very tired. 'Are you ill?' mother asked in her direct way. 'No,' he answered. 'Something has happened,' she said. 'What is it?' 'Phipps Institute appointments were made today,' he quietly replied, 'and I was not included.'"[42]

Under University Auspices

Although the University undoubtedly welcomed the financial support of Henry Phipps and whatever prestige the Institute may have enjoyed, its own goals were chiefly research and teaching. The bargain implicit in University auspices, therefore, meant a significant change in the Institute's work. The responsibility for the care of tuberculous patients, University leaders believed, belonged to the state and municipal governments, not to the University. Patient care could be linked to teaching and research, of course, but it had to fit into the budget. Although Phipps increased his yearly support from $50,000 to $54,000 in 1913, the Institute still had to control its expenditures.[43]

In June 1910, the University took charge of the Institute. All the physicians had resigned so that the University could reorganize as it wished, and the new medical staff—small by previous standards—consisted of eleven men. One of the early Phipps men, H. R. M. Landis, became director of the clinical department. Paul A. Lewis left the Rockefeller Institute to direct the laboratory, and Alexander M. Wilson, secretary of the Boston Association for the Relief and Control of Tuberculosis, took charge of a new sociological department. Social workers took over some of the home visits previously made by the pupil nurses, and a few of the physicians branched out into sociological experiments that included an open-air school for children, a study of housing conditions, and a supervised shirtwaist factory where consumptives could earn their living by part-time work.[44]

Until 1913, staff members continued to function in the old quarters, but then they moved to a new building, specifically designed for their work, at 7th and Lombard streets. Henry Phipps had finally paid for the structure that Flick had wanted for so long. The five-story building included a wing for the laboratory, small wards for advanced cases, additional wards for incipient cases, and rooms on the first floor for the dispensary.[45]

Because of the change in auspices, however, parts of the building soon became obsolete. Most affected by this change was the hospital, which in 1909 had accounted for 52 percent of the Institute's expenditures. In 1910, the University reduced the number of hospital beds in the old building from fifty-two to twenty-five, and the new building opened with twenty-four. While expenditures for the hospital were thereby reduced to roughly one-third of total expenditures, costs remained a problem. By 1915, closing the twelve free beds for incipient cases seemed to be the only way to balance the budget. On July 1 Charles J. Hatfield, an early Phipps man whom the University had appointed as executive director of the Institute, announced that the space would be opened again for paying patients at a charge of fifteen dollars a week. Patients who paid for their care would enter into a bargain different from the one that was offered to poor people. First, they would not have to promise their bodies for research by signing an autopsy permit. Second, the other patients with whom they might mingle would be a bit different; black patients, who had been welcomed in previous years, would not be accepted in the paying wards. Despite these accommodations the new plan failed, and in 1916 the hospital closed.[46]

Dispensary services diminished but did not cease. In 1910, Landis reduced the number of sessions and changed two of those remaining to tuberculosis classes—a method of treating and teaching patients in groups. During the same year, Alexander Wilson recommended that distributions of milk to dispensary patients be stopped. Three social workers—"college women of experience"—helped to accomplish this task. Relief in the form of milk, Wilson explained in 1911, had been very liberal in the previous administration. "In some instances the milk had been considered . . . a bribe to induce patients to follow instructions and to report regularly at the dispensary. Gradually, by taking each case up on its merits and seeking the natural sources of help, and in not a few instances finding that no help was needed, the disbursements for relief in this form were reduced month by month." Annual expenditures for milk distribution dropped from $4,015 in 1909 to $615 eighteen months later, and only $100 was budgeted for milk for the subsequent year.[47]

Education continued at the Institute, but mainly at the student level. By 1911, twenty-five senior medical students at a time were spending their mornings at Phipps, where they learned to examine tuberculous patients. Student nurses from the Hospital of the University of Pennsylvania also went to the Institute but not without resistance. At the suggestion of Executive Director Hatfield and despite some student opposition, six student nurses started a two-month course at Phipps in 1914. They replaced all but one of the tuberculous nurses then employed there. Late in May 1915, the students rebelled. Complaining of long hours, menial tasks, and having to sleep in the same room with tuberculous patients, among other conditions, three students, backed by their classmates, refused to go to the Institute. The authorities investigated, corrected some of the conditions, and denied or explained others, and most of the students agreed to resume their work. A few were expelled or left the school on their own accord. Sometime during the year, the Institute's training school closed.[48]

Under the leadership of Paul Lewis, research at the Institute became somewhat less descriptive and more experimental. Lewis was particularly interested in dyes and other substances that might restrain the growth of tubercle bacilli. His ideas were closer than Maragliano's serum to the future breakthrough, but he was no more successful than Ravenel had been in finding an effective treatment. In terms of important research, Phipps's investment was still in advance of a fruitful time.[49]

Although Flick in his later life found fault with the altered directions of the Institute, he acted during the turnover with helpfulness and grace.

When the University formally opened its new building on Lombard Street in May 1913, he attended the ceremonies and delivered a speech.[50] Meanwhile, he still had the command of the Free Hospital for Poor Consumptives and its White Haven Sanatorium. Ths sanatorium, developing rapidly out of its primitive origins, was evolving some serious problems of its own.

8. Expansion at White Haven

Between early 1903 and early 1905, the camp at White Haven developed into a proper sanatorium with an enlarged capacity, a resident medical staff, and an increasingly complicated organization. It attracted more applicants than it could easily accept; its income grew, primarily through the state's assistance; and its care better satisfied the patients. Continuing ability to treat poor consumptives, however, depended precariously on factors that the Free Hospital could not entirely control. The sanatorium needed fiscal support from the state government without allowing the politicians to dictate which patients were admitted. To function within its budget, it needed patients who were well enough to work for their maintenance, not the incapacitated ones who required a great deal of care. The interests of a sanatorium often conflicted with the needs of the sick. For two years the Free Hospital managed fairly well, but only at considerable expense: it had to mortgage the sanatorium, overwork some of its patients, and abandon one of its original goals, the care of dying consumptives in Philadelphia.

Pressures and Choices in Patient Admissions

Inquiries about the White Haven Sanatorium often arrived in Flick's mail. Men and women heard of it through friends, advisors, and former patients, or they read accounts of it in newspapers. They wrote from places as diverse as Maine, Iowa, New Mexico, the almshouse in Harrisburg, and the mountains of western Pennsylvania. Elsie Listebarger read in the *Chicago-American* that six young ladies had been cured of tuberculosis at White Haven. The article "caused me to thinking . . . If I could go there too," she explained; "I am so anxious to get well." Relatives and friends inquired on a patient's behalf: "I have heard about your cures. I have a son . . . a niece . . . a very dear friend . . . with consumption. Can you find a place in your sanatorium?"[1]

Physicians, clergy, and other interested persons, adding their social and moral authority to such requests, begged Flick's attention to needy and deserving applicants. Writing on their own initiative or at the request of an applicant or a relative, they vouched for the goodness of patients and their families, the importance of a patient's recovery to the family's welfare, and their faith in the treatment at White Haven. They sweetened their pleas with promises of money or held positions that added extra persuasiveness to their requests. John J. Buckley, a pork packer from Chester, Pennsylvania, enclosed a "small contribution" with his petition, and Henry C. Lea assured Flick that, if the White Haven Sanatorium could take a certain man, "I will very willingly repeat my recent contribution of $100." Francis J. Torrance, president of Pennsylvania's Board of Public Charities, requested special consideration for two young ladies. It was Torrance who had interested Henry Phipps in Flick's work at White Haven, and now two of his wife's brother's nieces had consumption. James Elverson, Jr., general manager of the *Philadelphia Inquirer*, wrote on behalf of one of the newspaper's employees. "My father [president of the Inquirer Company] was very much interested in the Sanitarium . . . the last time the State appropriations were made," he noted. "Won't you . . . arrange for this man to be admitted?"[2]

Reference to state appropriations undoubtedly touched a raw nerve. None of the many entreaties exasperated Flick more than recurrent demands from politicians, and none were more ominous for the sanatorium's future. Funds from the state constituted the largest source of the Free Hospital's income, and many politicians believed that the sanatorium owed them special privileges. They asked that their friends or constituents be admitted to the institution or be advanced on the waiting list. In turn, they often promised future support or, if dissatisfied with Flick's response, threatened to withdraw it. Representative Theodore B. Stulb described the situation in April 1903:

> At the request of the Speaker of the House and a few members of the Press with several members of the Appropriations Committee, I would most favorably recommend to your careful consideration the application of Miss Edna Hoover . . . for your care and treatment at White Haven. . . . I trust that you will make an effort to stretch your rules so as to admit of her being taken under your care at once. I understand from the Speaker that he has written you on the subject and the delay in having her placed there has annoyed him considerable. As the matter of appropriation is now under consideration and as there have been reports made here that it is impossible to get a patient assigned to your care without a great deal of trouble, I would urge upon you the necessity of meeting this case and dis[a]busing the minds of those of whom you are asking the appropriation. . . . There are so many statements made that similar

cases come before your notice and have received like treatment, that it has really to a large degree endangered the appropriation asked for. If this is a State charity, those having charge of State appropriations feel that when a case is brought directly to their notice . . . they should receive immediate consideration.[3]

With a righteous obstinacy that often antagonized the politicians, Flick rejected all requests to admit patients out of turn. The Free Hospital was established to help "the poor, helpless, and deserted," he explained in the annual report of 1904, and "if cases were admitted through influence the poorest, most helpless and deserted would never gain admission at all." This rule had not been broken, he wrote to Henry F. Walton, Speaker of Pennsylvania's House of Representatives, after Walton had urged the admission of Lillie McCorkle, the niece of a select councilman in Walton's district. "To break it would mean the demoralization of our work and its abandonment by people who are devoting themselves" to it. "I would have to resign from the presidency [of the Free Hospital] . . . because the pressure would be such that my life would become a burden."[4]

The selection of patients was more than a matter of principle; it was a matter of power—power necessary to achieve the goals of the institution. If the sanatorium was to cure its patients, as it claimed it could, it had to control the kinds of patients admitted. It needed curable patients, not just the people who wanted to come, not just those who were deserving and needy or had influential connections. It needed the early cases, those who could recover within six months, as Flick defined the criterion early in 1903.[5]

Finding such cases, if they could be found at all, required medical judgment. To help in the task of screening applicants, choosing the most appropriate, and avoiding long, futile trips for those who were not suitable, the Free Hospital appointed examining physicians throughout the state. The examiners, who tended to view these appointments as symbols of their competence and aids to their practice, agreed to perform this duty without charging a fee.[6]

Choosing some patients and rejecting others inevitably led to anger and disappointment, but Flick defended the sanatorium's admission policy as both medically and economically sound. While even advanced cases could be improved by modern methods, he argued, it often took years of treatment, but early cases could usually be restored to health in a short time. "Four early stage cases can be cured during the same length of time which it takes to cure one advanced case," he asserted in 1903; "it is surely better charity to save the four lives than to save one life." Accepting more cases for shorter stays, moreover, reduced the long waiting period during which other applicants deteriorated to an incurable state. Early cases also had a better outlook after treatment. They could return home physically well, germ-free, and able to compete with others in the struggle for a livelihood. "So long as only a limited number can be taken care of," Flick reasoned, "it is commonsense to admit only those who can get well to remain well, in preference to those who, even if they are restored to health, will again have to fall back, because of the hardships of life over which they have no control."[7]

Patients with early disease were also economically advantageous to the struggling sanatorium. They were cheaper to care for than sicker patients; they needed less complicated facilities and less nursing care. They could also contribute to the cost of their maintenance. Although their poverty precluded their paying in dollars, they could pay with their labor, and the sanatorium's economy depended in part on their work. "Maintenance at White Haven Sanatorium is probably the lowest of any sanatorium . . . in the world," noted Flick in the 1903 annual report. "The cost of maintenance has been kept down by using the patients for the performance of certain duties which ordinarily are paid for in other institutions. . . . The cost of food has been kept very high, while the cost of labor and supervision has been kept very low. The economical administration of a sanatorium for the consumptive poor is of very great importance because of the large number of cases who need help."[8]

The expectation that patients contribute their labor was neither unique nor new. Poor patients in nineteenth-century hospitals often had long convalescences during which they could be up and about and help on the wards, and a number of tuberculosis institutions continued this practice through at least the first two decades of the twentieth century. The hygienic regimen did not preclude work. If a person had fever, a rapid pulse, emaciation, or pulmonary hemorrhage, virtually every knowledgeable physician would recommend rest, but many patients, even those with advanced disease, showed no such manifestations. For these cases, there were no agreed-upon medical rules that determined the proper proportions of rest and exercise; physicians had to make judgments without them. Complicating the medical uncertainty were the various psychological effects of rest and exercise and the social assumptions about the consequences of rest, especially on poor people who would have to resume a life of work after discharge. For these, some physicians asserted, work could add a sense of purpose to prescribed exercise, improve morale, prevent laziness, and gradually toughen the body to meet its future demands. Flick himself had worked during his own recovery.[9]

The Enlarging Sanatorium and Its Staff

Money saved through patients' labor contributed to the growth of the sanatorium, but more significant was the Free Hospital's success in attracting funds from the government. In 1903, the society mounted a statewide campaign for favorable legislation. Stockdale, who organized the patients at White Haven to participate in the effort, mailed at least thirteen thousand appeals for legislative support. Despite political resentments over patient selection, the Free Hospital managed to get a biennial appropriation of $110,000. Of this amount, $70,000 was designated for buildings and equipment and $40,000 for patient maintenance. Although private contributions dropped at the same time, total receipts sufficed to start a major expansion.[10]

Flick envisioned a sanatorium of three hundred beds, and between 1903 and early 1905 new construction altered both the appearance and the character of the institution. An administration building was started, a spacious new dining hall was completed, two infirmaries were built (one for men, one for women), two new frame cottages supplemented the three earlier brick ones, and "shacks" began to replace the tents. A shack was a rectangular frame structure that, like a tent, had canvas-draped windows for good ventilation and accommodated four patients. The sanatorium built additional kiosks for its patients, a new cottage for the superintendent, and important new utilities for everyone's benefit: a power house, an electric plant, a water plant, and a sewage system. By early 1905 the bed capacity had grown from 98 to 120, and a year later it reached 172.[11]

Expanded facilities and a larger number of patients increased the need for workers. The cook needed a kitchenman, and two firemen were hired to tend the power house, each on a twelve-hour shift. The list of employees early in 1904 also included a housekeeper, three matrons, two orderlies, and a stableman. Over the following year the staff grew further, from eleven to seventeen. Almost all of the employees were promoted from the ranks of patients. Flick and his colleagues believed that a job at the sanatorium offered patients a desirable transition to a normal life of work. Hiring them undoubtedly helped the Free Hospital too. Finding healthy, capable people to work for low wages at a sanatorium for consumptives was exceedingly difficult.[12]

To the matrons fell the responsibility of caring for the female patients and all the patients in the infirmaries. Some of the matrons had had prior training in nursing, but this was not essential. Stockdale looked for women who showed both aptitude and an agreeable refinement that would fit them into the "family" at the institution. The sanatorium paid its matrons an initial monthly salary of twenty dollars, along with board and lodging. Like other patients, some of the women worked without pay before taking official positions. In 1903, for example, Stockdale proposed that Miss Agnes Moss, both a patient and a trained nurse, be appointed as matron on June 1 "so there will be three attendants to 60 women. My idea is not to pay her until we are more flush and I think she will be glad to take hold gratis for the fact of getting on the 'Staff.' She will be just the nurse for our infirmary and it will give her a good training." In February 1905, the sanatorium listed five matrons on its staff and had spent $1,040 during the year on their salaries.[13]

Resident physicians completed the group of men and women who lived at the sanatorium and helped to take care of the patients. Like the matrons and most of the other employees, they were tuberculous. Between late 1902 and the end of 1906, eight men and one woman took the position for varying lengths of time. Each had graduated from a medical school in Philadelphia, usually just a few years earlier. Joseph Walsh, who served as visiting physician at the sanatorium and kept track of the residents, judged three of them to have early tuberculosis and six of them to have far-advanced disease. Some felt much improved during their terms at the sanatorium, while others had fever, hemorrhages, or incapacitating bouts of illness and fatigue.[14]

Despite the disabilities of the resident physicians, the Free Hospital found advantages in hiring them. In comparison with healthy physicians, they were probably more interested in the work and more willing to accept the terms of employment. The position usually carried no salary. In January 1903, after the medical administration committee had urged that the medical coverage be improved, Flick hired G. Justice Ewing to fill the post, with pay. In late March, however, when Ewing offered to stay at the sanatorium for another six months at the same salary, Flick tried again to economize. He made Ewing a counterproposal: instead of a salary he could have the privilege of seeing some private patients in the village, thus earning some money by part-time practice.[15]

At issue were two interrelated questions: how to get the needed

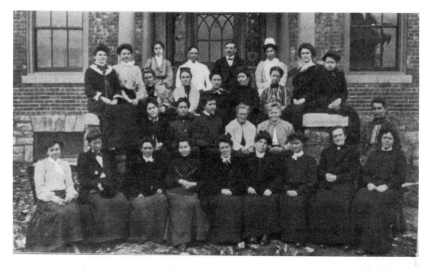

Figure 12. "Female Department With Staff" in front of a brick cottage, White Haven Sanatorium. From the *Annual Report of the Free Hospital for Poor Consumptives* 5 (February 1903). Historical Collections, College of Physicians of Philadelphia.

medical services for the sanatorium, and how to pay for them. Flick wanted the fees from private patients in the village to subsidize the care of the poor consumptives. Stockdale objected to Flick's proposal. The medical service was inadequate already, he observed. Ewing "gets no lab work done at all— It has been weeks since we have had a sputum or urine report of cases so if one man can not do the work fully as it is you can see what the result would be if he was to put time in at the Village each day." Stockdale reminded Flick of staffing patterns in German sanatoriums: "Your friend Dr. Walther [at Nordrach] claims no physician can look after more than 25 cases. . . . Falkenstein has 1 to 20. . . . The closer attention they get the quicker the improvement and do wish your medical Com[mittee] would come here and study the place for a day before deciding the matter."[16]

A compromise was apparently reached. There was no further mention of village practice and, at least for several years, no compensation was offered to the resident physicians except board, lodging, and treatment. Around 1908, however, when the Free Hospital needed to increase its resident staff, it began to pay fifteen dollars a month after the first six months of service and twenty-five dollars after the first year.[17]

For at least some consumptive physicians, work at the sanatorium seemed like a reasonable bargain. Sick and apprehensive about their futures, they could get subsistence and treatment without having to pay cash. They could also get training and experience in tuberculosis and be productive in their professions. The appointment "has brought about two very desirable things," wrote Mary E. Topham in 1904; "it put me into a line of work that I have greatly wished to be connected with and made possible my longer stay in a world that, for me, grows more interesting with every year." "I am improving in health," reported John J. Craig to Joseph Walsh after sixteen months of residency, "and am very happy and feel I am of some use." Six of the nine physicians who lived and worked at White Haven took advantage of their training and continued in the field after completing their residencies. For most, however, life was short. Seven of the nine died of tuberculosis—six years, on the average, after the end of residency.[18]

To the colony of tuberculous patients with its mostly tuberculous staff came one group of men who did not necessarily have the disease—the visiting physicians. The first two people appointed to this position were practicing physicians from neighboring towns, Henry M. Neale and Charles H. Miner. Starting in 1903, however, as the Phipps Institute developed, Flick recruited some of the Institute's staff to serve also at White Haven. By 1905, the visiting staff of the sanatorium had grown to nine physicians, seven of whom were associated with the Phipps Institute. Albert M. Shoemaker, an early resident physician who subsequently entered practice in the village, also served in this capacity, and so, still, did Neale. Each of the nine men visited the sanatorium for one day every two weeks. They consulted with the resident staff, examined the patients, made diagnostic judgments, and guided the treatment. They gave their time without compensation and paid their own travel expenses. Flick, as consulting physician for the sanatorium, made similar trips.[19]

The journey from Philadelphia to the sanatorium "was something of an event, especially in the winter time," Frank A. Craig recalled. Under the best circumstances, the trip by rail took three hours. After arriving at the White Haven depot, "it was necessary to ride on a rough farm sledge with boards laid across for seats and no protection from the wind and cold. Fur coats were a necessity. When the roads were too icy it was often necessary to stay overnight in the local hotel which was situated so close to the railroad tracks that, when in bed, the sound of a passing train made one instinctively draw up one's feet lest they be run over."[20]

The visiting physicians were not entirely unrewarded for their time and hardships. Although the Free Hospital never instituted village practice as a means of paying its resident physicians, a similar system helped to compensate the visiting staff. As the reputation of the White Haven Sanatorium grew, private sanatoriums developed in the vicinity, and the visiting physicians, in addition to their work with poor consumptives, frequently attended private patients there. Further, a staff appointment added to their professional stature, and caring for the less seriously ill patients at the sanatorium added to the clinical experience of those who worked at the Phipps Institute.[21]

From Camp to Bureaucracy

Growth of the sanatorium and its staff altered responsibilities and increased the complexity of the organization. Stockdale was freed from many details of patient care, but he had to supervise an enlarging band of workers, oversee the new construction, and cope with unexpected breakdowns in the water and sewage systems. He still had to ensure that food and medical supplies were purchased, the buildings and grounds were maintained, the laundry was washed and ironed, sputum was disposed of safely, the horse was tended, and patients were transported back and forth to the village depot. At times, everything went wrong at once. "This is about the worst week we have ever put in," he reported in September 1903; "all our strong men have been discharged, the horse is sick, one of our doctors went away so we are having about 26 hours a day work."[22]

Responsibility for maintaining discipline among the patients and assuring their proper regimen fell increasingly to others—to the resident and visiting physicians and to the matrons and other attendants who, hour by hour, implemented instructions, worked to maintain order, and helped to sustain morale. "The victim of tuberculosis approaches the sanatorium as a rule, broken, spiritless, dejected and not infrequently hopeless," Neale observed.

> The immediate duty of the attendant is to begin work in dispelling doubt, correcting false impressions and at the same time giving the patient a firm understanding as to the course of treatment to which he must now submit and what is expected of him during his stay.
> It does not require much time to convince the patient that he is now under closer supervision, and the rules to which he conforms aim to establish a system for conduct, a regularity in life for the perfection of which rigid discipline is absolutely necessary.

Once in the sanatorium, Neale continued, patients soon saw that the treatment was far superior to that of home. The sanatorium "insures more faithful compliance with the physicians' instructions because (1) the influence of relatives and friends is removed; (2) every facility is provided to make out-door life attractive, and in-door life as little a temptation as possible; and (3) a discipline is maintained by rules which are enforced by trained attendants."[23]

"Control and discipline are probably the most important factors in the successful treatment of the disease," asserted D. J. McCarthy, another of White Haven's visiting physicians. Any patient careless in expectoration or personal cleanliness might easily endanger others by reinfecting them with tubercle bacilli or spreading other germs that could help to destroy their lungs. Tuberculous patients, moreover, like those with nervous disorders, "must be carefully controlled," their every action "guarded by scientific principles," lest a simple violation of rules "transform an otherwise favorable case into an unfavorable one." Unless the patient could "be thoroughly controlled very early in his course of treatment, and made to appreciate how closely he must follow a rational routine scheme of life, and that he will be expected to sacrifice much in the way of personal desire, little hope can be extended to him." It was up to the physician, according to McCarthy, to cultivate in the patient a fighting spirit, willpower, and "the proper hope of cure."[24]

McCarthy's comparison of tuberculous and nervous patients highlights the close resemblance of the hygienic regimen to the moral therapy promulgated in nineteenth-century insane asylums. Removal of patients from their homes to a well-ordered environment, supervision by physicians and by vigilant yet humane attendants, and regulation of meals and activities were all methods that doctors believed would help mentally ill (or nervous) patients to recover their sanity.[25]

Forty-three regulations, signed by Flick and Stockdale in 1904, explicitly defined such a disciplined scheme of life. A rising bell awakened the patients early in the morning. They sponged their upper bodies in cold water, dressed, and then had their temperatures taken for the first time on a twice-daily schedule. Bells called the men to meals at 7:00 A.M., noon, and 6:00 P.M., as well as to extra eggs and milk in mid-morning, mid-afternoon, and at 8:00 P.M. The women ate separately on a slightly later schedule. "All must report promptly. Patients must not take less than three quarts of milk and six raw eggs a day." Indeed, breakfast and supper were limited to milk and eggs until patients progressed to four hours of daily work. A little vinegar added to a broken egg in a glass disguised the "mawkish raw taste," according to Neale, and with patience, care, and encouragement, he noted, everyone could take the diet. "Food should be taken as a duty," read one of the regulations, "even when there is no desire to eat."[26]

After the beds were made in the morning, no patient could enter the sleeping quarters until he or she went to bed. No loitering there was permitted. All but those on the sick list and those assigned to work were to take their cure at a kiosk. A rule required them to do not less than twelve hours of cure a day in summer and eight hours in winter. Any writing a patient might wish to do should be done there. Although life in a kiosk lent itself to friendly interaction, limited of course to people of one's own sex, a regulation banned one topic from discussion: "Conversation between patients regarding their symptoms, or any subject relating to their illness is prohibited." All patients were to be in bed, with lights out, at 9:00 P.M.[27]

Institutional order required a number of other restrictions—none of them unusual in comparable hospitals or sanatoriums. Drinking alcohol was not allowed, and all packages were to be inspected by the authorities. Except for fresh fruit, all food and drink were to be returned to the senders. Profane or obscene language was not to be tolerated, obnoxious conduct was punishable by dismissal, and patients could not "congregate in mass meeting" without prior permission from the superintendent. Sunday was to be observed as a quiet day, with no games or other weekday sports. All whose condition allowed it could apply to the superintendent for permission to go to church, but they had to go and return in a group, "under a Lieutenant." They could not otherwise leave the premises without special permission. And always, wherever the patients might be, they had to take special precautions with their sputum. Posted around the property were signs reading " 'If you spit on the ground, you will be discharged.' " Because the institution had relatively few employees, Flick explained, it had to enforce its regulations "with military rigidity. For breach of certain rules, there is expulsion without appeal."[28]

The growing complexity of the organization and the larger numbers of resident and visiting physicians created issues that related increasingly to medical authority and responsibility. Stockdale, caught in the middle and holding views of his own on most matters, strove to make rules, set standards, and bring some uniformity to everyday decisions. He raised questions of policy and tried to get Flick to give answers that would systematize the administration and be fair to the patients. When a visiting physician found that a patient was unsuitable, for example, who should send the patient away, he or the resident physician? Should the patients of just one visiting physician be allowed special dietary privileges? The resident, James H. Heller, had told him that Dr. Walsh wanted the milk increased for all of his men, but "if Dr. Walsh's men are given 4 qts. the balance will set up a large howl." Stockdale recommended a rule that patients could be discharged only after they could work eight hours daily; Dr. Neale's dismissals, which Stockdale considered premature, had instigated this suggestion. And could there not be clear definitions of "disease arrested," "improved," and "much improved"? The doctors differed in their usages. Discouraged by the quality of the sanatorium's work and by his own receding authority, Stockdale offered his resignation on August 22, 1904. The board of the Free Hospital accepted it, and appointed the resident physician Heller in his place.[29]

Successes and Costs

The atmosphere of the changing sanatorium drew praise from its visitors. In *The Era Magazine*, Edward Nocton wrote of the "sunlit kiosks snug against a mountain" where groups of hatless men sat, "talkative and cheerful in their idleness, like men to whom life is all that is kind. Off from the left comes the babble of romping children," a small number of whom were admitted to the sanatorium. During the warmer months, patients rested in the orchard or gathered fruit. "With a willingness pathetically eager, the afflicted persons, with few exceptions, obey the rules, anxious to do anything within their power that will restore them to health." As the weeks went by, they saw their bodies once again filling out, their weight increasing, Nocton continued. Work helped to restore their muscular vigor, and dejection turned gradually to optimism and hope. "Outsiders expect to see a lot of pale, cadaverous inmates sitting about coughing, spitting, and swapping symptoms," observed George G. Kalb, a resident physician in 1904, "when in fact one sees a crowd of happy, redfaced men, women and children working, attending school or sitting in the Kiosks. They sing by the hour, usually the popular airs."[30]

Lawrason Brown, an experienced physician from Saranac Lake, praised the sanatorium after visiting there in 1905. "I had heard so much about the 'Barn' that I expected to see a rough place with very few modern conveniences," he wrote to Flick; "I cannot tell you how surprised and

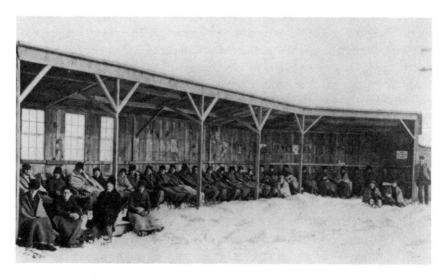

Figure 13. "Doing Cure in Kiosk 16° Below Zero," White Haven Sanatorium. From the *Annual Report of the Free Hospital for Poor Consumptives* 6 (February 1904). Historical Collections, College of Physicians of Philadelphia.

delighted I was to find such a modern plant." In February 1905, William H. Allen, general agent for the New York Association for Improving the Condition of the Poor, paid a visit to White Haven. "I hope Dr. Heller has told you of our listening to summer songs out in a kiosk," he reported to Flick, "with the stars as big as plates and the thermometer three below zero,—a bit of romance which we had hardly anticipated. What has impressed me more than anything else that I have ever seen within an institution is the pulsating missionary spirit that testifies to frequent visits on your part." The institution is "an object lesson of economy and intelligent cooperation with patients."[31]

Patients expressed their own appreciation. F. A. Craven, for whom Dr. Neale had secured employment after his discharge, noted in 1903 that both Dr. Flick and Mr. Stockdale had made the sanatorium as pleasant as possible for him. "It has been for me the means of saving my life and I shall always feel the deepest gratitude." Mrs. Fred G. Day echoed these feelings in a letter to Flick in 1905. "My friends consider my case wonderful and my physician is much gratified as to the result of your treatment. I know how much you have done for me and am grateful beyond expression."[32]

Statistics of the maturing institution document an increasing satisfaction among its patients. Of the men and women who left the sanatorium, those who did so within one month of admission fell steadily—from 70 percent during the first seven months of its existence to 15 percent by the year ending early in 1905. The proportion of patients who stayed for more than three months rose from 5 percent to 64 percent during the same period. At the same time, the sanatorium maintained the rapid turnover that Flick desired. Although the average length of stay did increase significantly over this period—from eight weeks to thirteen weeks—the latter figure marked a peak that was not exceeded until early 1919.[33]

Reported results, moreover, remained favorable, and costs per capita low. Of the 646 patients discharged between early 1903 and early 1905, after staying for more than one week, the annual reports classified 67 percent as being improved or much improved and another 23 percent as having had their disease arrested. The average patient gained 13.44 pounds. These results were roughly similar to those achieved in previous years. Although the weekly cost of maintaining a patient in the sanatorium rose with a change in bookkeeping practices, it still remained in a satisfactory range: $5.76 as reported in February 1904 and $6.49 in the following year. In 1904, by comparison, the Rush Hospital for Consumption and Allied Diseases reported an average weekly maintenance cost of $9.13; St. Agnes' Hospital, $11.69; St. Mary's, $9.10; and the Home for Consumptives at Chestnut Hill, $7.00.[34]

Despite Flick's and Stockdale's efforts to economize, however, the costs of the expanding sanatorium exceeded expectations and exhausted the resources of the Free Hospital. In the fall of 1904, the society found it necessary to mortgage the sanatorium for twenty-five thousand dollars; it could not otherwise pay for its current expenses. Although the society managed to pay off most of the mortgage by 1906, it continued to borrow, and remained in varying degrees of debt for years afterward.[35]

Expansion at White Haven incurred an additional cost: the Free Hospital stopped its care of advanced and dying consumptives in Philadelphia. During the year ending early in 1904, it paid for the maintenance of forty-six such patients in the city, but these were the last. When St. Agnes' and St. Mary's Hospitals lost the Free Hospital's subsidy, the numbers of consumptives treated there fell precipitously. The proportion of medical patients who were classified at St. Agnes' as having phthisis ranged between 13 and 16 percent between 1899 and 1902, but dropped to 4 percent in 1903 and then to 1 percent in both 1904 and 1905. At St. Mary's, 8 percent of its medical patients had phthisis in 1903 but less than 1 percent did in 1904.

Although the Free Hospital had opened a new asylum for poor consumptives at White Haven, other doors that Flick had pried open for them for a few years fell quietly shut again.[36]

Other institutions, to be sure, still accepted poor consumptives without charging them a fee. These included the Phipps Institute, the Philadelphia Hospital (renamed the Philadelphia General Hospital), and the City Mission's two facilities, the House of Mercy and the Home at Chestnut Hill. In addition, the Jewish Hospital in Philadelphia had taken up the work. In 1890 it created segregated wards for consumptives, and in 1900 it opened the Lucien Moss Home for Incurables of the Jewish faith. Although this Home also accepted men and women with other kinds of diagnoses, more than half of its patients in the early 1900s were listed as having phthisis.[37]

The Continuing Problem of Advanced Cases

Although the Free Hospital needed to economize in every way possible, it could not control its selection of patients. Despite all attempts to choose suitable applicants, men and women with advanced tuberculosis slipped through the screening process and entered the sanatorium. Between early 1902 and early 1905, the sanatorium's statistics show a gradual trend toward more advanced cases. The proportion of patients with the least-advanced tuberculosis declined, while those with clinically detectable cavities in their lungs—the worst category—increased from 5 to 9 percent.[38]

Screening undoubtedly excluded many acutely ill or dying patients, but some of the examining physicians lacked the skills to make the desired judgments. Others found it personally and professionally difficult to reject unqualified applicants. Dr. W. J. Ashenfelter recommended Mrs. Redinger for admission, even though he did not think she would benefit. Both she and her husband were so very anxious to have her go to the sanatorium, he explained, that he sent her "with the hope that I might be mistaken." Dr. Robert S. Maison knew that he had sent an unsuitable boy, but was hoping that Flick's "personal decision will prevent any hard feeling toward me by the family and a certain physician of Chester." "I have cases here that have been on rest list for months and months and will never get off it," Stockdale complained in 1904. "The cases we are sent are altogether unsuitable but Dr. Neale would not reject a case Dr. Gayley sent, and so it goes."[39]

Unsuitable patients such as these upset the economy of the sanatorium. Unlike the patients with early disease for whom the institution had been designed, they needed nursing care, close medical attendance, and proper domestic help. They needed rest and could not contribute their work, thus adding doubly to the expense of their care. "Half of our people here are practically dead wood," Stockdale grumbled in May 1903. They "not only cannot wait on themselves, but take up the other men's time to wait on them." Twenty-three of the men should be resting completely, he noted. They should not even "wash dishes or make sputum cups"—tasks for which he had always depended on patients. "Such work as scrubbing and sweeping, making sputum cups, waiting on the table, washing and drying the dishes, picking up papers from around the grounds . . . is work that must be done every day." With twenty-three men out, the rest of the men would have to do these jobs, and who would work about the premises to improve the property?[40]

Dependency on patients' labor sometimes slipped insidiously into exploitation. In "Number One Cottage the women all with one exception lost weight last week from picking stone which was the[i]r occupation for the week," reported Stockdale in 1903. Similar problems recurred in 1904. "I simply cannot get the every day work done," he complained, "and think you know that I can manage as well as most people. The place is simply a Hospital, and the depending on our patients is really getting to be a farce. I am simply compelled to put persons on 'rest' at light duties to keep things going." Men and women who should have been resting were "working at the wash tub, which is all wrong." To make matters worse, Dr. Neale was discharging patients capable of working; he had just sent two of the good cases home. "Neither wanted to go, one of them only here 106 days. He simply will not wait until they get to eight hours work, and then the public wonder why they go to pieces."[41]

Patients unsuitable because of advanced disease affected more than the economy and the work force of the sanatorium; according to Flick, they also disrupted morale and discipline. "Stationary and retrogressive cases" had a depressing effect on all the others, he observed, and mixing the classes of patients "leads to dissension and breach of discipline." "Those who can work," he noted, "will not want to work, because of the example of those who cannot work."[42]

If the institution was to function as its leaders intended, it had to dismiss its unsuitable cases. Most of the men and women who were asked to leave had been in the sanatorium for six months or more, but others, whose disease was clearly too advanced to improve in the allotted time, may have been sent away after a shorter course of observation and treatment. Dismissals caused resentment, and in November 1903 Stockdale warned of retaliation. After "making some quiet inquiries," he had learned that some men who had been compelled to leave were threatening "to do all manner of things to me among which was to all make complaints etc." "Quite naturally," read the annual report in 1904, "the relatives and friends of such persons are disappointed, and are disposed to find fault." In March 1904, Flick received an anonymous letter from the cousin of a patient who, after seven months, had been turned out of White Haven as unsuitable. The patient, unable to get a job, had had to depend on his family, could not afford the necessary diet, and had finally died. Before his death, however, he had carefully compiled a book that listed fifty-eight White Haven patients who had died, almost all of them after discharge. Although the letter writer had not been able to find his cousin's book, he himself had laboriously traced a number of ex-patients, and he now submitted a bitter list of forty-two names—all "<u>cured</u> (under the ground)."[43]

The annual reports of 1904 and 1905 took cognizance of such results but blamed them on conditions outside the sanatorium. "Many of the people whom we restore to physical health relapse within a year or two because they are unable to obtain employment immediately upon their discharge from the sanatorium," read the 1905 report. "They have to undergo a life of semi-starvation while seeking employment and are unfit for occupation when the occupation comes. Fifty percent of the work which we are doing is lost on account of this practical difficulty."[44]

Such disappointments, however, did not diminish Flick's support of institutions. He suggested instead that the sanatorium be supplemented by a convalescent farm, where patients could go after discharge, and by hospital care of the dying. In the future, perhaps, the Free Hospital could raise the funds for these two purposes. Institutions had preventive as well as curative value; removing consumptives from their homes prevented the spread of disease and thus saved lives.[45]

The future proved different from what Flick was anticipating. He and his colleagues had helped to stimulate a demand for sanatorium care that exceeded the capacities of an organization dependent on charity and careful economy. To meet these rising expectations, the Free Hospital needed governmental help. In 1905, however, it began to lose some of its state funding, and two years later the state government entered the field itself. These changes were to alter the nature and even the goals of the sanatorium.

9. Economy, Charity, and the State

Until 1905, the financial stability of the Free Hospital and its sanatorium depended on state funding, charitable contributions, the work of its patients, and managerial efforts to limit expenditures. The sanatorium tried to select patients with early disease and cure them, if possible, while at the same time preventing the spread of infection. Early in 1905, however, the Free Hospital's fragile foundation began to tremble. Flick had not been willing to appease the politicians, and state aid diminished. In 1907, a newly organized state health department opened its own free sanatorium. To compensate for the loss of state assistance, the Free Hospital made a series of decisions that transformed its sanatorium from a state-supported, charitable institution for poor consumptives to a semi-charitable institution in which most of the patients paid.

When patients paid for most or all of their care, their relations to the sanatorium changed. Those with advanced disease became more acceptable, payment by work disappeared, and special facilities were built for the dying. Sicker patients, however, increased the labor problem at the sanatorium and raised the costs of care. In response, a training school for consumptive women was started in 1907.

In 1910, Flick challenged the state health department in an ideological debate that pitted his frugal, privately managed charity against the centralized, liberally financed system controlled by the government. By this time, however, he had lost his fight. Although the White Haven Sanatorium had found a lasting place among Pennsylvania's institutions, the leadership of the tuberculosis movement, as measured in beds, services, and public recognition, had passed to the government. The methods of twentieth-century Progressivism had won over Flick's conservative, voluntaristic approach. Across the nation, other governments were involving themselves in the work. By 1916, thirty states had opened their own sanatoriums, and counties had also established institutions. The task exceeded the capacities of private citizens.[1]

The State and Tuberculosis

The government of Pennsylvania first took on the care of consumptives through its forestry department. During the latter decades of the nineteenth century, loggers had destroyed much of the forest in the state, leaving the land eroded, susceptible to fire, and almost devoid of wildlife. Joseph T. Rothrock, a botanist and physician, led a campaign to conserve and replenish the woodlands, and in 1895 he became the state's first commissioner of forestry. Rothrock set out to buy devastated land for the commonwealth, protect it from fire and vandalism, and plant seedling trees. Forests had multiple uses, he claimed, appealing to several different interests. They offered hunting, fishing, and recreation; they cleansed the air, reduced flooding, improved the drinking water, and provided timber. Forests were also health-giving, he asserted, especially to those with consumption. In 1873, he had observed convincing evidence that open-air life in the Rocky Mountains often cured consumption. Why not try the mountains of Pennsylvania?[2]

Rothrock, described as a political master of the fait accompli, established a sanatorium for consumptives by first starting a camp and then asking for legislative support. His camp began in the summer of 1902 with a single small cabin in the state forest preserve near Mont Alto, a sparsely populated region in south-central Pennsylvania where South Mountain rises from the eastern lowlands. Voluntary contributions paid for additional cabins, and the camp provided fuel, water, medicines, and weekly visits by a physician. Initially, consumptives and their families had to supply their own food and all other necessities. Despite the primitive conditions, every cabin was occupied and, as Rothrock reported, "results were astonishing." Some of the patients, thought hopeless, recovered. "Public attention was attracted. The thing was spoken about and written about," just as Rothrock had intended, and in 1903 the legislature appropriated eight thousand dollars to enlarge the work. In 1905, it increased its aid to fifteen thousand dollars.[3]

Rothrock's project was to continue for another two years, but in the spring of 1905 a change in the state government altered the camp's future: the old board of health gave way to a new, stronger, and much better-financed department. In matters of public health, Pennsylvania had not been keeping up with states such as New York and Massachusetts. Its vital statistics did not meet federal standards, and recent epidemics of smallpox

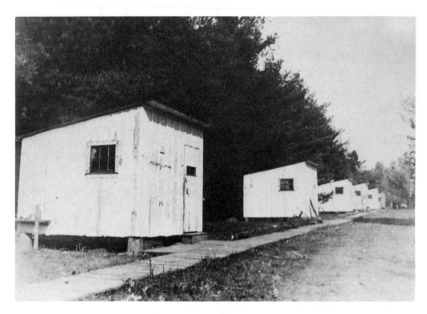

Figure 14. The Rothrock camp near Mont Alto in 1903. Courtesy of the South Mountain Restoration Center, South Mountain, Pennsylvania.

and typhoid fever had helped to make clear that the board could not adequately cope with its tasks. Charles B. Penrose, a Philadelphia physician who had helped to reorganize the city's health department,* went to Harrisburg, drafted a bill for the state's new department, and then lobbied for it. He had more than ordinary influence. His brother, Boies Penrose, was a United States senator from Pennsylvania and head of the Republican state machine. The bill became law late in April 1905.[4]

Appointment to state office in Pennsylvania was usually highly politicized and often corrupt but, in choosing the man to run the new department of health, Governor Samuel W. Pennypacker seems to have made an exception. On June 6, 1905, Samuel G. Dixon, a Philadelphia physician whom Charles Penrose had recommended, became commissioner of health; he was to serve under four governors until his death in 1918.[5]

Both the time and the man augured success. Across the United States, Progressive reformers were looking to government to solve some of the

---

*For the agency responsible for health affairs in Philadelphia, which had several different names, I will use the term city health department.

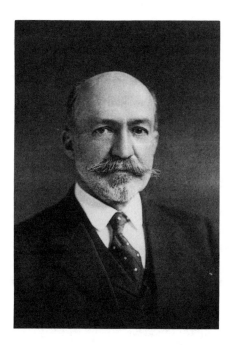

Figure 15. Samuel G. Dixon.
Historical Collections, College of
Physicians of Philadelphia.

nation's problems, and experts trained in public health seemed to have the
knowledge and tools to create a healthier, more prosperous society. Dixon
had both the social and the intellectual credentials for the job. He was born
in Philadelphia of old Quaker stock, trained in law, and in 1886 graduated
with honors from the University of Pennsylvania's medical school. He later
studied in London and in Max von Pettenkofer's laboratory of hygiene in
Munich. In London, he discovered a misshapen form of the tubercle
bacillus, and in 1889 he reported that inoculation with these bacilli increased
the resistance of experimental animals to further injections. This report, he
liked to point out, antedated Koch's description of tuberculin. After holding professorships in hygiene and in sanitary engineering at the University
of Pennsylvania, Dixon became curator and then president of Philadelphia's
Academy of Natural Sciences. By 1905, he had a well-established reputation
as a research worker, sanitarian, and organizer. He and four other officials,
Governor Pennypacker recalled, "were referred to as the influx of gentlemen into the political life of the state."[6]

Dixon moved quickly to build his new department. Among his first
achievements was the organization of a Bureau of Vital Statistics, which
collected data on births, deaths, the causes of death, and the incidence of

certain diseases. The department needed such information in order to identify the state's problems and measure the results of its work. Statistics were useful also in attracting support for programs. For 1906, the registrar of vital statistics reported 9,258 deaths from pulmonary tuberculosis. "Is it not appalling," asked the commissioner's first annual report, "to think that nearly ten thousand human lives should be swept away . . . by a disease now known to be preventable." It was an unnecessary and "lamentable sacrifice," which the department of health felt duty-bound to diminish.[7]

In the spring of 1906, the state's Republican party had committed itself to "the establishment and support of dispensaries, hospitals and sanatoriums for the treatment of the consumptive poor," and in 1907 the legislature passed two impressive bills to combat tuberculosis. In addition to $1,100,600 for its new health department, it voted $600,000 for one or more sanatoriums and another $400,000 for dispensaries wherever in the state they might be needed. These monies were to be spread over a two-year period and administered by the commissioner of health. Governor Edwin S. Stuart, who had given Dixon his prior approval for the plan, signed the bills on May 14, 1907.[8]

Although Dixon deserves the credit for this achievement, the new state plan for tuberculosis also marked the culmination of other efforts. Flick had campaigned for a state sanatorium in the 1890s, before he started the Free Hospital, and the Pennsylvania Society for the Prevention of Tuberculosis, of which Dixon was a charter member, had been lobbying intermittently for it ever since. Popular demand for sanatorium treatment, moreover, probably helped to convince Pennsylvania's legislators that a state system of care was good politics. If they could not get their needy constituents into the White Haven Sanatorium, perhaps the state's own institutions would be more responsive.[9]

The government's action also meant success for Rothrock. In 1907, his camp at Mont Alto was transferred to the health department and became the nucleus for the state's first sanatorium. Rothrock had never wanted to lead the tuberculosis work, and the camp's transfer assured its continuity. He also probably made a profit from related transactions. In 1904 and 1905 he had bought some land and water rights adjacent to the camp at Mont Alto, and in 1905 he opened a private sanatorium there. He spent $1,120 for the property, improved it with one building and seven cabins, and in August 1907 sold it to the state for part of its new Mont Alto sanatorium. The state paid him $27,550.[10]

Dixon's strategy to combat tuberculosis was organizationally and po-

litically masterful. Through its sanatoriums, the state offered both treatment for patients with early tuberculosis and care for those with advanced
disease. By rapidly escalating the number of beds available, it held out hope
to those on waiting lists. Dispensaries—established in every county—
evaluated patients, funneled some into the institutions, and distributed
milk and eggs to others. By limiting dispensary services to those unable to
pay for private care, Dixon tried to avoid competing with local physicians.
Dispensary nurses, like those at the Phipps Institute, carried instructions
into patients' homes and tried to identify additional cases. The dispensaries
also offered part-time paying jobs to physicians. A new state laboratory,
based at the University of Pennsylvania, did free diagnostic tests for the
commonwealth's doctors, and Dixon developed a research program that
included the manufacture of his own tuberculin-like fluid. "Dixon's fluid"
became available at the state sanatorium in 1907 and in the dispensaries in
1909. Like Flick and Ravenel, Dixon was pursuing the elusive goal, a cure
for consumption.[11]

Toward Paying Patients at the Free Hospital

As the state was formulating its plans, the Free Hospital for Poor Consumptives was struggling to free itself from debt and complete its ambitious
building program at White Haven. Its prospects in 1905 seemed dim.
Charitable contributions had leveled off, the sanatorium was economizing
as strictly as it could, and its chances of getting assistance from the state
seemed small. The Free Hospital was asking for a biennial appropriation of
three hundred thousand dollars, but its political support had soured since
1903. It was to get but a fraction of its request—seventy thousand dollars—
much less than two years earlier.[12]

The Free Hospital, anticipating the fiscal squeeze, decided to charge
the patients for part of their care. Early in April 1905, it established a sliding
scale that determined the schedule of payment. For roughly the first two to
four weeks, when the patients were housed in one of the new infirmaries,
they paid seven dollars a week. As their condition improved and allowed
them to work, the charge diminished progressively. When patients could
work for a full eight hours, they paid nothing. If they could not pay all or
part of the charges, the board of management tried to make up the difference.[13]

Within less than a year, the sanatorium tightened this policy. A four-week stay in the infirmary became a more strictly enforced maximum, and then physicians assigned patients to one of two groups. Those who were well enough entered the graduated work program in Department No. 1, and those whose disease was "a little more advanced" entered Department No. 2, where they continued to pay seven dollars weekly. Patients unable to work or pay were discharged as unsuitable.[14]

Annual reports acknowledged the economic necessity of the new policy, but justified it as socially and morally sound. It countered the two evils—dependency and idleness—that nineteenth-century charity workers had found so abhorrent. Some of the applicants to the sanatorium could well pay part of the charge, observed the reports, but instead they "throw themselves upon the Society as objects of charity." If they would only carry part of the burden, they could "maintain their sense of independence" and "avoid the stigma of pauperization." Families should not be entirely relieved of paying for their sick, nor the individual from struggling against disease. It was better philanthropy "to help carry the burden than to lift it." Flick at this time was starting to use similar rhetoric in criticizing the Phipps dispensary.[15]

Patients' work, so important to the economy of the sanatorium, became an expedient part of the medical treatment—a necessary step in their rehabilitation. As Joseph Walsh explained in 1906, work prepared the patients to resume their regular employment after discharge. "The sanatorium would be remiss in its duty if it sent them home without showing them the amount of work they can do without harm to themselves. This can only be learned by having them work at the sanatorium and gradually increasing their work till they do as many hours as their occupation demands."[16]

Some prospective patients looked upon this arrangement as an acceptable way to pay for their board and treatment. "I have sold my household and gathered up $28," reported Rubin Krasnopolsky in 1905. "I will try and pay for 1 mounth [*sic*] and if you can give me some work for the other mounth I will be greatful." Others worried about their abilities to do the required tasks. "I am willing to do any work that I am able to do," wrote Mrs. Thomas J. Clark, "but . . . my trouble has been greatly aggravated by over work. . . . Would a patient who does not do heavy work at home, such as washing, ironing, etc. be required to do it there?" Still others gambled on feeling better, but lost the four-week bet. Mr. Dotts had been at the Sanatorium for one month, wrote his wife in 1906. "The money was given to him for the first 4 weeks payment of $7.00 [weekly] and then we thought it would come down to $5.00." Mr. Dotts still had a fever, however, and needed another fourteen dollars for two more weeks. His wife, unable to find the money, hoped he could stay on as a free patient. "I have two very small children to support and myself," she explained, and "my wages are but 5.00 a week."[17]

Between 1905 and early 1907 the patients' work and their payments helped to finance the expansion of the sanatorium. Although the payments did not fully compensate for the drop in state assistance, they reached $21,474 by the year ending early in 1907. By building additional shacks, the sanatorium increased its bed capacity to 196. It reserved 100 of these beds for free patients. Improvements kept pace with enlarging capacity: a new reservoir, a new ice house, and a beautification program. With the help of the patients, who did much of the landscape gardening, the grounds were transformed by flowerbeds, macadamized roads, and paths. A chicken-house and a piggery were established, and an enlarged staff of employees was organized into four departments: engineer, farm, chicken, and construction and repair. By early 1907, moreover, the Free Hospital had reduced its debt to fourteen hundred dollars.[18]

The new system of payment also affected the kinds of patients admitted. Within these two years, the men and women with clinically detectable cavities in their lungs rose from 9 to 28 percent. By paying fees, even a patient with far-advanced disease could now enter the sanatorium with full approval.[19]

The spring of 1907—another year for the biennial appropriation—found the ambitions of Flick and his colleagues even greater than before. In addition to further expansion at White Haven, the men wanted to start a second sanatorium closer to Philadelphia. Their request for three hundred thousand dollars had little chance in the legislature. Flick's relations with the politicians had not improved, and Dixon's health department was soon to open it first sanatorium. The situation called for a new tactic. After Flick learned that the House Appropriations Committee had approved only thirty thousand dollars, he sent a threatening letter to Governor Stuart. The Free Hospital, he declared, would decline the appropriation, put the sanatorium on an all-pay basis, discharge the free patients, and refer them to the state health department.[20]

With the help of Chester D. Potter, a reporter for the *Pittsburg Dispatch* who covered the capitol, Flick followed the threat with action designed to force the issue. The patients were pawns in the subsequent fight. On May 14—the very day that the governor approved the bill for the state sanatorium system—Potter wired Flick from Harrisburg that the Senate had finally passed the Free Hospital's bill at one hundred thousand dollars. If Flick would come to the capitol the following day, he thought they could get the House to concur. Additional pressure on the politicians was necessary. "Patients at White Haven ordered to leave June 1," Potter concluded, "have started trouble." June 1 was a carefully chosen date: it marked the beginning of fiscal support for the state sanatorium. Soon Dixon began to receive "a great many letters from patients at White Haven saying that they are to be turned out on the 1st of June." Flick acknowledged to Dixon his role in initiating the letter-writing campaign, although he was acting, he said, out of necessity and "a spirit of kindness." He had told the patients that, if the state did not grant the requested appropriation for White Haven, "they would have to provide for themselves elsewhere unless they could pay for the cost of their maintenance. . . . I advised those who could not provide for themselves to write to you and to the institutions which received State aid in order that they might not be turned out helplessly."[21]

Dixon, outmaneuvering Flick, won the skirmish. He did not respond to the flurry of letters until May 31, thus making the patients face the full threat of expulsion and testing the will of the Free Hospital. Dr. Harry Z. O'Brien, now superintendent at White Haven, described the uncomfortable situation on May 29: "None of the patients have received answers to their letters to Dr. Dixon. Twelve have reported that they expect to be able to pay $7.00 per week. Most of them are discouraged . . . and will only write to their representatives after a great deal of urging. Almost all say that if they are unable to stay here they will go home." Flick's colleagues, meanwhile, urged him to take a less confrontational approach. The executive committee wanted the free patients whose outlook was good to complete their cures, and the board of directors did not believe that it could raise enough money from donors to make up for the state's aid.[22]

A compromise brought the sanatorium a little closer to an all-pay institution, but some of the change was temporary. Again, the Free Hospital raised its charges. Early in June 1907, it abolished its sliding scale for working patients and began to charge seven dollars a week in Department No. 1 and nine dollars in Department No. 2. For almost three months in the summer of 1907, the Free Hospital did limit its new admissions to paying patients, and it tried to pressure some of its free patients to scrape together the weekly fees. It did not, however, take harsher measures. The state and the Free Hospital settled on seventy thousand dollars, and by late August the sanatorium could again accept new patients who were unable to pay. The number of free beds rose to 120 by the end of the fiscal year. Public criticism of the pay requirements, however, persuaded the society to change

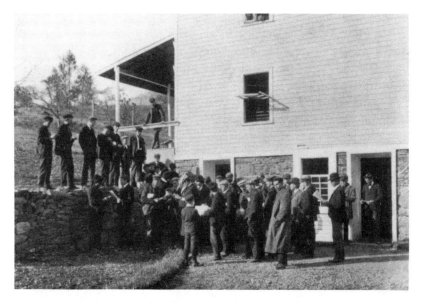

Figure 16. "Arrival of the Mail," White Haven Sanatorium. From the *Annual Report of the Free Hospital for Poor Consumptives* 9 (February 1907). Historical Collections, College of Physicians of Philadelphia.

its name to the Free Hospital for Poor Consumptives and the White Haven Sanatorium Association.[23]

The episode in May and the increased charges that followed unsettled the patients and worsened the labor problems at the sanatorium. Many of the free patients—especially those who felt least sick and were already working for their maintenance—left the institution. Although the sanatorium was usually filled to its capacity of 196, O'Brien reported only 161 patients on July 23. Of these, only 40 were on the free list. "There are 42 patients in bed," he noted, "72 on rest and 47 on work. Of the latter, 7 are children." In all areas of domestic work, the sanatorium was short-handed. To make up for the lost labor, Flick suggested employing some cured ex-patients, and for ten dollars each per month O'Brien managed to find seven willing to take the jobs. He was still, however, in critical need of workers.[24]

Work and a Training School for Nurses

Lack of nursing care also proved serious. "We have no one to take charge of the Women's Shacks, in which there are a number of quite sick patients who need considerable intelligent care," O'Brien reported on June 27. "We also need a nurse for the sick male patients, who can no longer be kept in the Men's Infirmary without overcrowding." He had written to the graduates of the training school at the Phipps Institute and offered them jobs, but only two replied. Both nurses declined.[25]

In response, Flick turned to the same source of labor that had succeeded at the Institute: consumptive women at the sanatorium. "I think it might be well for your Committee today to take up the question of establishing a training school . . . and employing a head nurse," he wrote to Joseph Walsh on July 25. "We will have to do something to get more nurses." In August 1907, the Free Hospital appointed Mrs. M. Elizabeth Hoffman, an early graduate of the Phipps Institute Training School, as the head nurse. Others who had done the nursing at the sanatorium would have to leave. "I was able to discharge one of our $40.00 nurses without putting anyone in her place," wrote Dr. Walter F. Wood, who had now replaced the ailing O'Brien as superintendent. Flick was pleased. With the school established, he responded on August 26, "we will get over the nursing difficulty. We will complete this training school on our return from Europe. Meanwhile do the best you can with it." Over the next few months, pupil nurses replaced ten of the eleven matrons and orderlies at the sanatorium.[26]

All recruits for the training school came from among the patients at White Haven—by policy, if not always in practice, those who were in good physical condition and had been working an eight-hour day. The first class of five nurses completed their two-year program and graduated in 1909. Three more graduated in 1910, seven in 1911, and twelve in 1912. Although the quality of the nursing care did not meet medical standards consistently, Flick and his colleagues considered the school a success. The Free Hospital increased the numbers of people who provided nursing care at the sanatorium and gave the pupils training in a field that physicians considered peculiarly suitable for those with arrested or cured disease. According to the annual report in 1910, the nurses had excellent job opportunities after graduation. They had "gone out into useful lives" and had "become missionaries in the crusade against tuberculosis."[27]

Furthermore, the school proved sound economically. Expenditures for nursing salaries continued to rise during this period, but roughly in proportion to the growing numbers of patients. Because the patients were sicker than before, the services were almost certainly greater. In addition to board and lodging, the Free Hospital paid its head nurse seventy-five dollars a month and its students ten dollars a month. If only salaries are counted, expenditures for nursing care of each patient stayed reasonably stable, averaging about twenty cents per patient per week. Of the sanatorium's total expenditures for patient maintenance, the proportion spent on nursing salaries ranged from 2.5 to 3.0 percent.[28]

Expectations of work applied to men and women other than the pupil nurses. The sanatorium continued to require work of the patients in Department No. 1, even when they paid seven dollars a week. At the discretion of the visiting physicians, patients in Department No. 2 were also asked to participate. "It is explained to the patients that the work is part of the treatment and that it is necessary for a proper restoration to a life of usefulness," Flick wrote to an inquiring physician in 1908. "This I think goes a long way towards reconciling them."[29]

Some patients, to be sure, complained about their work or thought that it made them worse, and some visiting physicians tried to keep their patients at rest for longer than the rules prescribed. As Dr. William B. Stanton observed, however, other patients saw their increasing capacity to work as a sign of improvement. Hindsight suggests that this kind of improvement sometimes reflected healing tuberculosis but could also be due to physical conditioning, which, along with the weight gain achieved by the diet, could give an impression of returning health. Whatever the effects of work on tuberculosis (they are still unclear), Flick and his colleagues judged the program satisfactory. At the 1909 meeting of the National Association, Flick described White Haven's work program and listened to the report of a similar system at the Massachusetts State Sanatorium. Comments, though cautious, showed no major dissent. In another decade or so, U.S. physicians began to favor a longer, more strictly enforced rest treatment for tuberculosis, and the work imposed by some institutions came to be seen as scandalous. Meanwhile, patients' labor was clearly advantageous to the sanatoriums. Flick estimated that their work at White Haven was roughly equivalent to the services of twenty-eight paid employees.[30]

An All-Pay Institution

Savings from patients' labor could not balance the sanatorium's budget, however, and in 1909 the Free Hospital took its final step in becoming an all-pay institution. Once more it asked the state for three hundred thousand dollars, but late in January it found the request stalled at the first step in the appropriations process. The State Board of Public Charities recommended only eighty thousand. Flick, charging constant political discrimination, announced that the White Haven Sanatorium would soon be financed entirely by private subscriptions; free beds would be abolished on the first of June.[31]

In the annual report of February 1909, Flick again justified a pay institution on social and moral grounds. Most people with early tuberculosis were not yet pauperized, he argued; they were still trying to help themselves and had not yet become dependent. Assistance by friends and employers served to maintain their social connections and ensure a permanent cure. Tuberculosis placed a heavy burden on both the family and the community, and "we should not use the measures at our command to pauperize and debase. We should give aid where aid is needed . . . but not indiscriminately throw open free institutions to everyone who has tuberculosis, whether he is able to help himself or not."[32]

In his reference to "free institutions," Flick was attacking the state's tuberculosis program. Dixon's health department had "established 600 free beds at Mont Alto" and was contemplating "many more in different parts of the state. Millions of dollars have been set aside for this free work," Flick noted, "and there is some danger of converting a great philanthropic movement into a demoralizing influence upon our people. Indiscriminate charity works for degeneracy rather than upbuilding." The man who had led the fight against tuberculosis for almost twenty years, now on the defensive, was deprecating the large amount of money that had entered the campaign.[33]

The Free Hospital proceeded with its plan to require all of its patients to pay. Fees from patients would not entirely cover the cost of care and the Free Hospital would continue to make up the difference. Flick asked the visiting physicians to "make it plain" to all of their free patients "that it will not be possible to continue at White Haven Sanatorium after 1 June, unless they can find some way to pay the cost of maintenance." Flick also recommended that all examining physicians for White Haven be allowed to charge two dollars for evaluating a prospective patient. Such a fee, he suggested, would make them "more loyal agents to the sanatorium." The board of managers concurred and the plan was implemented. The institution that had once tried to limit its numbers of patients was now trying to increase them.[34]

When the new charging system started on schedule in June, "the number of patients immediately dropped to nearly one-half of the capacity of the sanatorium." The drop resulted in "an abrupt reduction in the working resources from patients, those on longest hours going out first and making a higher ratio of employees to patients necessary." Edward Baker left after having worked eight hours for only one day. "He said if he could work eight hours, he might as well go home and work." In January 1910, the sanatorium was still "running at about one half full." Most of the patients had far-advanced disease. For the year ending early in 1910, 65 percent of the patients had clinically detectable cavities. The reduced occupancy and the rising proportion of sicker patients further increased the maintenance costs per capita. Expenditures per patient per week for nursing salaries rose 43 percent, from twenty-one to thirty cents.[35]

Nevertheless, the institution survived the transition and gradually found a niche for itself between the growing number of small, more expensive, private sanatoriums and the large, free, public institutions that were financed by government. Payments for patients' board increasingly covered the costs of maintenance, and charitable contributions took care of any deficit. Contributors also paid for further construction. Mrs. Henry Phipps gave the money to build a sixteen-bed brick cottage for female patients, and Mrs. Eckley B. Coxe, the early friend and benefactor of the sanatorium, gave generous support. By rejecting state assistance, the Free Hospital could now admit previously prohibited out-of-state patients, and early in 1910 Walsh and his medical administration committee began to recruit out-of-state examining physicians to help attract additional applicants. Although the annual patient weeks did not surpass the level reported early in 1909 for almost two more decades, they gradually, if haltingly, increased.[36]

Care of the very sick and dying became an increasingly important part of the sanatorium's work. Mrs. Coxe had first suggested this change in 1909. Some of the very ill patients whose board she had been paying at White Haven had been "obliged to leave, as having reached a stage where no improvement could be expected. In all of these cases," Coxe observed, "there was no alternative but our County Poor House, already over-crowded, or homes where the risks to others would be great." She offered to pay for a four-bed shack for such patients, along with a nurse to provide the care. In 1910, the Free Hospital accordingly opened a Department No. 3 for apparently incurable or dying patients at a charge of ten dollars a week. The department soon had a waiting list.[37]

The payment of fees altered relations between the sanatorium and its

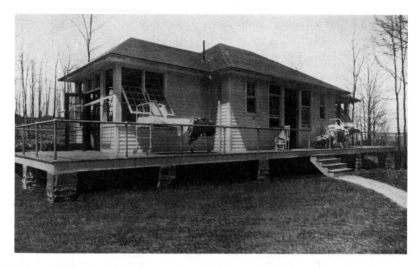

Figure 17. "Shack 1, Department No. 3," for very sick or dying patients, White Haven Sanatorium. From the *Annual Report of the Free Hospital for Poor Consumptives* 13 (February 1911). Historical Collections, College of Physicians of Philadelphia.

clientele. For some men and women, it guaranteed that care would continue until they died. Between the years ending in early 1909 and in early 1916, the proportion of patients who died at the sanatorium rose steadily, from less than 2 percent to more than 18 percent. The payment of fees also gradually excused patients from having to work. This change did not occur because the sanatorium's patients were sicker. Department No. 3 was kept modest in size, and the sanatorium actually succeeded in attracting larger numbers of less-advanced cases.[38] The change resulted instead from a more honest classification of patients. "Many of the patients in Department No. 2 were really No. 3 cases," Flick acknowledged in 1912, "and many of the patients in Department No. 1 were No. 2 cases." Slowly, patients' assignments shifted out of Department No. 1, where work was expected, into the other departments, where patients paid more but did not work. Those with cavities shifted first, and then the others, and by 1916 Department No. 1 had almost disappeared. Work, according to Frank A. Craig, in his account of White Haven, "was largely discontinued when the patients began to pay." The ideology that had justified patients' labor faded away when institutional survival no longer required it.[39]

Charity Versus the State

While the White Haven Sanatorium settled into its reasonably stable position, the state was rapidly expanding its facilities and services. In 1909, the legislature was so impressed with the results, according to Dixon, that "without any per[s]onal effort on my part, the appropriation to the [Health] Department was increased to $3,000,000; of which . . . $2,000,000 [was] for the eradication of tuberculosis." The little camp at Mont Alto, which had accommodated only 28 patients when the health department took it over in 1907, grew to an average of 730 patients by 1910. By this time, Andrew Carnegie had offered the state a tract of land near Cresson, once a health resort, where a second sanatorium was to open in 1913. The state had also bought some land near the town of Hamburg for a third sanatorium. These two additional institutions were to serve western and eastern Pennsylvania respectively, thus supplementing the more central Mont Alto. By 1910, moreover, the number of state dispensaries had reached 115.[40]

Flick, having reached the limit of what he could accomplish with frugality and charity, attacked the state's efforts as wasteful, immoral, and medically incompetent. After first expressing his disgust to Dixon himself, Flick took the debate to the public by delivering an acrimonious speech to the state medical society in 1910. He disparaged the trifling accomplishments that the state could show for its three million dollars, and attacked its methods of preventing tuberculosis. The state had barred expert physicians from employment unless they gave up their connections to private organizations, he asserted, and it had retarded the development of local institutions for tuberculous patients. To man the dispensaries, it had hired physicians for political reasons, not for their experience; these doctors knew nothing about tuberculosis and could not educate others. The "Mont Alto Camp" was "a huge joke." Its large size precluded efficient management, and the "absolute discipline . . . essential to good work . . . cannot be maintained in large, poorly equipped institutions." Most of the patients at Mont Alto, Flick declared, were "only mildly contagious or not contagious at all," and the preventive value of segregating them was "exceedingly small." Instead, the intensely contagious patients with advanced disease should be institutionalized, but for this purpose Mont Alto was ill-equipped, inaccessible, and too far from the patients' homes.[41]

Flick contrasted these activities with the accomplishments of privately

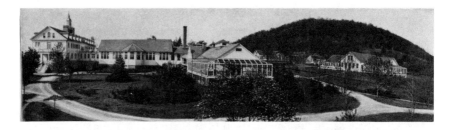

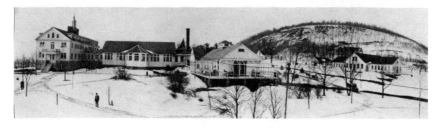

Figure 18. White Haven Sanatorium in summer and winter. The three intercon-
nected buildings, from left to right, are the administration building, the dining hall,
and the men's infirmary. From the *Annual Report of the Free Hospital for Poor
Consumptives* 18 (February 1916). Historical Collections, College of Physicians of
Philadelphia.

sponsored organizations in Pennsylvania. He estimated that the latter had
given to the crusade $1,500,000, to which the state had added $500,000 of
assistance. On his list of private achievements was first the "public enlight-
enment on the subject of tuberculosis"; then the White Haven Sanatorium;
the Henry Phipps Institute; "the idea of making tuberculosis nurses out of
cured consumptive girls; the idea of making useful work part of the scientific treatment of tuberculosis in working people; the practical demonstration that tuberculosis can be cured in any climate and in any place; and the
tuberculosis dispensary as it is operated throughout the United States at the
present day." While all these benefits resulted entirely from the efforts of
private organizations, Flick continued, others stemmed partly from them:
the National Association for the Study and Prevention of Tuberculosis, the
International Congress on Tuberculosis, trained medical experts, private
sanatoriums, the advancement of knowledge, and, "as the cap-sheaf of all
this work, nearly fifty per cent. reduction in the death-rate from tuberculosis in Pennsylvania." Thus the bitter, scarred, but still combative vet-
eran tallied up the victories, as he saw them, in his own crusade.[42]

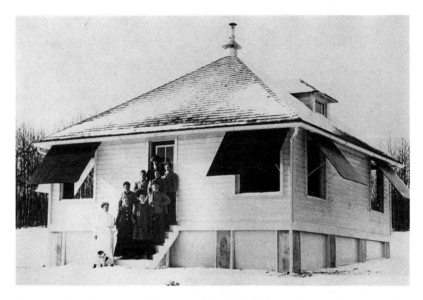

Figure 19. A "Dixon Cottage" at Mont Alto, with eight patients and a nurse, winter 1907–08. This was the typical accommodation, designed by Dixon himself. Courtesy of the South Mountain Restoration Center, South Mountain, Pennsylvania.

Flick's allegations against the state are difficult to assess. The health department did not report its costs during the early years; Dixon was careful to cover his fiscal tracks. As the health department's reports acknowledged, the care at early Mont Alto did suffer from overcrowding and lack of facilities. Initially, there were no infirmaries; patients lived in tents and cottages and had to walk to both the bathroom and the dining room even during the winter. Nevertheless, applicants were plentiful.[43]

To what extent political pressures influenced appointments to dispensary posts remains unclear, but they undoubtedly had an effect. Such charges, however, were inextricably mixed with medical self-interest. When the York County Medical Society met in 1909 to debate the worth of the dispensaries, for example, physicians alleged political appointments and unethical behaviors, but at the same time they were complaining about competition that they considered unfair. Dispensary physicians, they claimed, saw paying as well as indigent patients, they took the paying patients into their own offices, and for a ten-dollar fee they wanted to remove those patients' adenoids. Advertisements for the dispensary listed its physicians as tuberculosis specialists, the complainers continued, thus

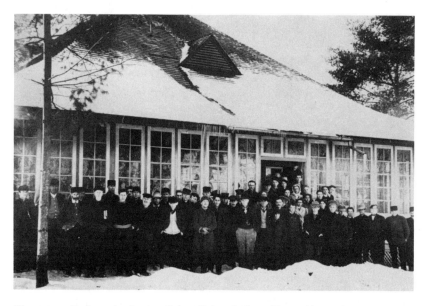

Figure 20. Patients in front of the dining hall at Mont Alto, winter 1907–08. Courtesy of the South Mountain Restoration Center, South Mountain, Pennsylvania.

giving them undeserved prominence by unethical methods. The dispensaries, in short, were encroaching on private practice. "The dispensary is welcome to my poor [patients]," concluded one of the physicians, "but not to my rich patients."[44]

For the next few years, the public debate continued over the proper approach to controlling tuberculosis in Pennsylvania and helped to clarify the two competing strategies. Flick argued for a medical staff with special scientific training, while Dixon chose to involve a fairly large number of general practitioners and educate them in the process. Flick, reiterating the infectious hazards of dying consumptives, urged their institutionalization during the last few months of life. The department of health, while acknowledging some value in this approach, emphasized the dangers represented by ambulatory patients early in their disease. Flick continued to favor a decentralized system of small, local institutions that would be responsive to their communities and supported by private philanthropy, with additional aid from the state. But the tuberculosis problem was "too great for philanthropy alone," Dixon asserted; "the State must lead, erect, assume and supervise the chief burden of this greatest menace to its citizens.

It would be irrational to throw the burden . . . upon a few earnest and struggling bands of patriots while the trained forces of the Government sat inactive." Most local communities, added Albert P. Francine, now chief of a state dispensary in Philadelphia, had "neither the means nor the awakened interest" to establish their own institutions. He argued instead for a few large institutions with their efficiencies of scale, state financing, and centralized control.[45]

The argument between Flick and the state health department exemplified two competing approaches to the care of the poor. Flick's position was rooted in nineteenth-century ideas of voluntarism, frugality, fears of creating or perpetuating dependency by giving away aid and services, and a profound suspicion of government and the corrupting effects of politics. If Flick had not always had these beliefs, his observations of the state's activities and the threat they posed to his own organizations undoubtedly helped to convince him. Dixon, on the other hand, argued that only the state government had the capacity to protect the public's health. He used the political process skillfully to gain support for his program. If politics tainted appointments or admissions, it expanded the care system to an extent that charity could not achieve. It was a major step in Progressive reform. The state system also had a result that even Dixon may not have intended. While giving medical treatment and protecting the public—its overt functions—it also expanded the welfare system under the guise of medical care.

While the differences in program and philosophy sharply divided the debaters, the state sanatoriums resembled the one at White Haven in many ways. With minor exceptions, the therapeutic regimens were much the same—fresh air, proper diet, and suitable proportions of rest and exercise, all under the supervision of physicians and nurses. Admittedly, state physicians preferred a balanced diet over a rigorous milk-and-eggs program, and the state used only "Dixon's fluid" while Flick and his colleagues favored tuberculin. But patients who could worked in the state sanatoriums, as they did at White Haven, and state physicians too emphasized the value of institutional routine. "The nearer to strict military discipline," noted William G. Turnbull, medical director of the sanatorium at Cresson, "the better [the] results."[46]

Patients who entered Mont Alto closely resembled those at White Haven. Around 1909, approximately a third of each group had been born abroad. Only 2 to 3 percent were black. Both the Free Hospital and the state screened their applicants with means tests, and those accepted by both sanatoriums came chiefly from the working classes. About 60 percent of them were between the ages of twenty-one and forty. Most of the patients in both systems of care entered a sanatorium only after their disease had progressed beyond the early stages. Despite the state's interests in segregating those with incipient tuberculosis, it could so classify only 13 percent of the patients discharged from its sanatoriums between 1907 and 1913.[47]

The systems of care developed by both charity and the state centered on specialized institutions, characteristicaly located in mountainous or other rural areas. While echoes of climatological thinking lingered in the rationales for selecting these locations, it was there that land was both available and cheap. As a result, the distance of sanatoriums from major cities intensified the isolation of patients, some of whom were shunned already because of their disease.[48]

For very-advanced and dying patients, Flick tried to establish an alternative system closer to their homes. General hospitals in Pennsylvania, he argued in 1909, had twelve hundred vacant beds; if only the state would pay hospitals a dollar a day for the care of these consumptives, tuberculosis could probably be wiped out in fifteen years. When a bill for this purpose failed in the legislature, Henry Phipps offered ten thousand dollars to reimburse any of the voluntary hospitals in Philadelphia that would accept dying consumptives on similar terms. All the hospitals declined.[49]

While the White Haven Sanatorium and the developing state system accepted tuberculous patients of limited means, the more affluent had to make other arrangements. Early in the twentieth century, resorts and a change of climate still beckoned to some of them, while others preferred to manage at home. Starting in 1901, a third alternative developed in Pennsylvania. By establishing private sanatoriums, men and women found that they could render needed services in return for a weekly fee.

10. The Private Sanatoriums

A sanatorium could be a charity, a semi-charity, a public enterprise, or a private business, depending upon its auspices and the means of the patients served. As physicians began to promote the idea that tuberculosis could be treated and cured in Pennsylvania, a number of men and women saw opportunities in running a private sanatorium. A large vacant house or a farm in attractive surroundings could be turned into a business—much like a boarding house or small hotel but one that was dedicated to the care of tuberculous patients. A cluster of such establishments first appeared near White Haven, where both the healthful reputation of the area and access to experienced caretakers were valuable assets; others started closer to Philadelphia. The private sanatoriums attracted some of the more affluent patients out of resort hotels and lodgings and out of their homes into this new environment. Managing such an enterprise, with all its fiscal, domestic, and medical problems, proved to be a highly competitive business, in which profits were possible but the risk of failure was high.

The Proprietors and Their Sanatoriums

Elwell Stockdale and his parents started the first private sanatorium in Pennsylvania in 1901, not far from the primitive camp that he managed for the Free Hospital. "[Your letter] is awfully encouraging and hope it all comes out right," wrote Stockdale to Flick on November 20 of that year. "It will be a God send for my folks. You can count on us being ready about Nov. 30th I think. ready cash is of course the stumbling block but think all will be well." Sunnyrest Sanatorium opened on schedule, with a capacity of twelve beds. In February 1902 Stockdale reported only two vacancies, and the family was starting to think of expansion. Two maids, who waited on table, a cook, and a woman to help with the cleaning constituted their staff, and Miss Elizabeth Burns served as the nurse. Stockdale, who felt too busy at the White Haven Sanatorium to bother with details at Sunnyrest, had

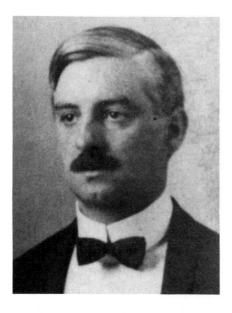

Figure 21. Elwell Stockdale.
Courtesy of Edward M. Keck.

organized it into three departments: medical, under Miss Burns; business, under his father; and housekeeping, under his mother. "Each ones duties are carefully defined and arranged," he reported, "so that Miss Burns is the only one who ever comes in contact with the patients except on Saturdays from 11 to 1 when all bills are payable to my father. Complaints or requests . . . must be made through Miss Burns."[1]

The new sanatorium consisted of a large house and cottage on the eastern side of the Lehigh River in East Side Borough—an easy walk across the bridge from White Haven's two railroad depots. While patients later complained occasionally of the smoke and noise from passing steam engines, all who could walk a few hundred yards had ready access to transportation and to shops. Between 1902 and 1907, a series of Stockdale purchases, worth about $7,720, enlarged the property into a substantial tract of land that fronted on South River Street and extended two blocks rearward up the eastern slope of the Lehigh Valley. There, with the help of several mortgages, Stockdale and his wife, Elizabeth, whom he married in 1903, built a central dining room, added cottages and bungalows, and increased the sanatorium's capacity to about fifty beds. In summertime, they expanded to seventy-five by pitching tents.[2]

That the care of consumptives might be good business occurred to several observers of White Haven, among them Margaret McDonald, a

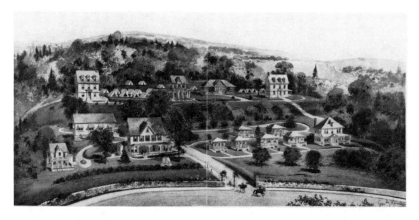

Figure 22. Artist's rendition of Sunnyrest Sanatorium. From *Sunnyrest Sanatorium, White Haven, Pa., for the Diseases of the Lungs and Throat* (ca. 1909–1912). Pamphlet in the Historical Collections, College of Physicians of Philadelphia.

single woman aged about forty-nine, whose mother and father, both born in Ireland, had died in 1901 and 1903, respectively. Margaret, now the owner of the family farmhouse just beyond the northern boundary of White Haven, decided to put the land to a new use. In April 1904, Flick learned from his old friend, Father Michael Bergrath, pastor of White Haven's St. Patrick's Church, that McDonald and her family were planning to start a sanatorium. Flick promised to help in every way possible, and Stockdale thought that Sunnyrest could send them some patients. By early May, Margaret McDonald, helped by her brothers and sisters, had opened her sanatorium, soon to be named Fern Cliff, and Flick had sent them a patient. The early months were probably chaotic. When Miss Mary Mahony, an experienced nurse, reported to Flick that Miss McDonald had hired her to start early in August, Flick was very pleased. "I trust," he wrote to Mahony, "you will be able to restore order there."[3]

Connections in the town through work, family, and the church undoubtedly helped to build a clientele. Both Elwell Stockdale and the McDonalds were Roman Catholic, and Fr. Bergrath was interested in the success of his parishioners. Stockdale's wife, like the McDonalds, came from a White Haven family. The physicians who served at the Free Hospital's sanatorium, moreover, knew both Stockdale and the nurses, Burns and Mahony, and would have felt comfortable with sending them patients.

The women who next ventured into the tuberculosis business lacked

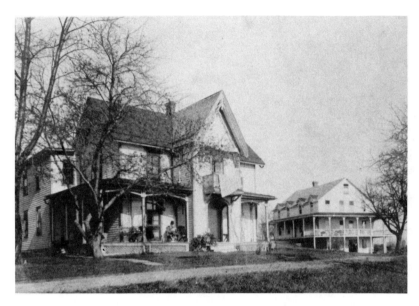

Figure 23. Fern Cliff Sanatorium, White Haven, Pennsylvania. Courtesy of Mr. and Mrs. Albert Maier.

these advantages. In 1905, two trained nurses from Philadelphia entered the increasingly competitive field. One was Miss Mary Irene Wightman, a forty-eight-year-old woman who had graduated from the training school at the Philadelphia Hospital in 1888 and had served as head nurse of the Visiting Nurse Society of Philadelphia from about 1893 to February 1905. The second was Miss Amy E. Potts, who had worked intermittently for the Visiting Nurse Society since at least 1893 and who had served as Wightman's assistant there. Potts, now aged forty-six, had been born in England, came to the United States in 1889, and trained at the Massachusetts General Hospital in Boston. For reasons that are unclear, the Board of Managers of the Visiting Nurse Society had asked Wightman to leave her post as head nurse, and Potts resigned at the same time.[4]

In March 1905, the two nurses purchased for $1,400 a 12.72-acre tract of land a little north of Sunnyrest and farther up the hill. This property became the Orchards Sanatorium. In the latter part of 1906, the nurses paid another $1,000 for almost an acre of additional land and, at the same time, mortgaged all their properties for $3,000. Although Flick later added the Orchards to his list of recommended sanatoriums, his response to the first inquiry about the place was at best cool. "I do not know anything about the

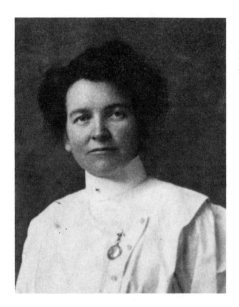

Figure 24. Agnes E. Moss.
Courtesy of Mary S. Bracken.

Orchards," he wrote to Mrs. Helen Mauck in August 1905. "I have received a circular saying that the place is conducted by two nurses."[5]

In contrast to Wightman and Potts, Miss Agnes E. Moss was well acquainted with the town and with the visiting physicians at White Haven. She had gained this advantage from having been a patient and then a working, though still tuberculous, nurse at the sanatorium. Moss came to the U.S. in 1897 at the age of about eighteen. She was born in Omagh, County Tyrone, Ulster, and at the time of her emigration had just graduated from the two-year nursing school at the county's hospital. Moss worked for a time at Municipal Hospital, Philadelphia's institution for contagious diseases. When she became ill from tuberculosis in 1902, Joseph Walsh sent her to the White Haven Sanatorium for treatment. She was no stranger to the disease. Her father and both paternal grandparents had died of it, as had four of her sisters.[6]

Like many of the early patients at White Haven, Moss survived some strenuous times. She lived in a tent for some of her stay, and during the winter months she and other patients tucked newspapers under their mattresses and between their blankets to shield themselves from the cold. In May 1903, Stockdale identified her as "just the nurse" for the infirmary and, toward the end of August, recommended her for a salary. With the title of matron, she worked for about two years, but in August 1905 and again in

January 1906 she coughed up blood and had to return to bed. Late in January 1906, Flick found her a job at the Philadelphia General Hospital, hoping, as he explained, that the lower altitude might help her, but Moss declined the offer. "As I expect I should have to do a nurses duty . . . And as I have still considerable pain in my right side, Just at present I know I would not be able for it," she responded. "I fully intend to get as well as I did 3 years ago, as I am going to fight the battle to the finish."[7]

By July 1906, Moss felt well enough to accept a position as nurse at Fern Cliff, and in the spring of 1908 she was ready to enter the business herself. "I am about to rent the late Mrs. McFadden's house and will open April 1st," she reported to Flick. "I intend to board tuberculosis patients; and if you could recommend any patients who are awaiting their turn to get into the Sanatorium it would help me in my new work." Moss's ambitions went further than her rented quarters in central White Haven. In June 1909, Fr. Bergrath lent her money for a down payment, and for $1,100 she bought a house and lot on the corner of Church and Wilkes-Barre streets. Within another two years, she acquired two adjacent lots for $100 each.[8]

People who wanted to see the sanatoriums in the area during the summer of 1909 could find them all in roughly a two-mile walk. Starting at the White Haven Sanatorium, part way up Green Mountain on the south side of the town, they would descend the hill to the road, cross the creek, pass the cemetery, and head north along the fairly level Church Street. Then they had to climb again, up the hill rising to the north, where the road passed Hill Crest, as Moss named her new sanatorium, and on another quarter mile or so and up another rise to Margaret McDonald's Fern Cliff. A stroll back to town and across the bridge over the Lehigh River would take them to Sunnyrest and the Orchards.

Three other private sanatoriums opened in or near Philadelphia. Miss Margaret G. O'Hara started the first and most successful of these in 1903. O'Hara was born of Irish parents in 1866 in Ontario, Canada, and graduated from the nursing school of the Philadelphia Polyclinic Hospital in 1897. A charming, vivacious, and enterprising woman who was fond of music and the arts, she too had had tuberculosis, probably in the late 1890s. She apparently studied hydrotherapy in New York City with its leading proponent, Dr. Simon Baruch, and then came to the White Haven Sanatorium for the summer of 1902. There, as described in Chapter 5, she supervised the new women's department and ruffled the discipline that Stockdale was trying to establish. Like most trained nurses of her day, she had also cared for private patients in their homes, but in the spring of 1903 O'Hara, now thirty-six, embarked on work of a larger scope.[9]

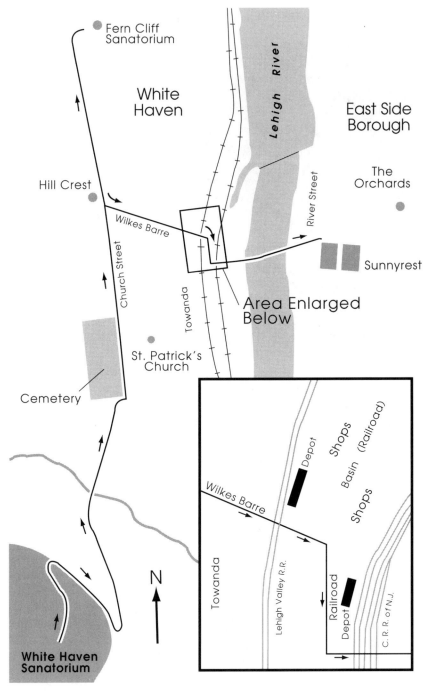

Figure 25. A tour of the sanatoriums in the White Haven area, 1909. Map by Yvonne Keck Holman, Alternative Productions.

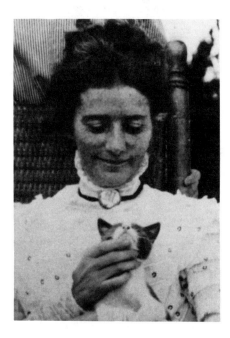

Figure 26. Margaret G. O'Hara.
Courtesy of Kathryn Riordan.

"At the suggestion of a number of physicians for whom I have done nursing," read her handwritten announcement to Flick, "I have opened a private rest-cure house in Mt Airy Philadelphia. The location is an excellent one, the house which is of stone, stands on a hill and is surrounded by two acres of well wooded lawn. . . . Patients will receive the best attention and every thing will be done to make their surroundings pleasant and agreeable." By 1904, her Dermady Sanatorium with its house and annex could accommodate twenty-five patients.[10]

O'Hara was popular with the physicians with whom she worked, but her sanatorium did not find favor with the community. Fears of contagion and neighbors' anxieties about falling property values faced many tuberculosis sanatoriums, and within a few years O'Hara had to move. In January 1906, she purchased 64.5 acres of land in Springfield Township, mortgaged it for fifteen thousand dollars, payable in seven years at 5 percent interest, and by April of that year moved her patients to her new location. On the property were two barns and a three-story farmhouse that served as both nurses' quarters and administration building. Tents of O'Hara's design were pitched in a field north of the house and gradually, as her resources permitted, she converted them into small wooden cottages.[11]

To reach the new Dermady Cottage Sanatorium, patients and their

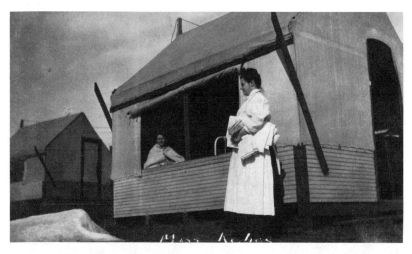

Figure 27. A patient in one of the tents at the Dermady Sanatorium, with the nurse Miss Kehoe. Note the snow drift. Courtesy of Kathryn Riordan.

families could take the Pennsylvania Railroad from Philadelphia's Broad Street Station to Morton Station, ten miles to the southwest, where Dermady's driver met them with horse and buggy. From there they travelled north and west about 1.4 miles through rolling farmlands, and then turned left between two stone posts into the sanatorium grounds. If alert, they might have noticed a discreet sign near the entrance: "PERSONS WITH COLDS WILL KINDLY NOT ENTER THE DERMADY SANATORIUM." To the left of the driveway lay the square house, with a spacious verandah wrapped around two sides. Ahead was the larger barn, but the patient's destination lay to the right, in one of the tents or cottages that clustered on that side of the driveway and spread back from the road and up toward the crest of a gentle slope. Within several years, O'Hara built on this higher ground a dining room with its own kitchen, a recreation hall with a library, and one cottage large enough to accommodate eight patients, each in a private room. Behind the main house she added her own bungalow, which she called with heartfelt Irish conviction Sinn Fein—Ourselves Alone.[12]

A few miles from Mt. Airy, where O'Hara started her work, Mrs. Mary M. Wilson, a Quaker woman, began to think of entering the same business. She was not a trained nurse but had had experience with tuberculosis: both her husband and her daughter suffered from the disease. Mr. Wilson had

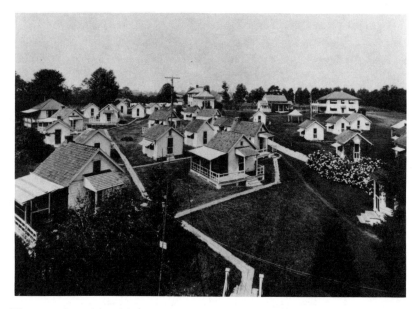

Figure 28. Overview of the Dermady Sanatorium. Small cottages have replaced the tents. Courtesy of Kathryn Riordan.

"grown stout" under Flick's care. On September 13, 1904, Mrs. Wilson visited Flick to get his advice about setting up a sanatorium, and within ten days she found a suitable house in Glenside, just north of Philadelphia and nicely situated near the railroad. She inspected the house carefully and felt satisfied with its elevation, view, and surroundings, and with its windows and ventilation. "I shall be prepared to receive paitents [*sic*] by Oct. 6. [19]04," she reported to Flick, "and will install a nurse as soon as I have two or three paitents."[13]

Meanwhile, uncertainties troubled her. "I have thy book, Consumption, a Curable and Preventable Disease. Now can thee spare me a few moments to go into the question of diet restrictions . . . more fully. Do all thy paitents have the same diet that Mr Wilson has had?" In mid-October, as Wilson anticipated the arrival of George E. Macklin, one of Flick's wealthier patients, she queried again. "Will thee please let me know if I am to furnish paper napkins and bags, that is if they are included in the board or if I shall furnish them and charge for them. . . . Thee knows there is much for me to learn in this." Flick apparently referred her to Margaret O'Hara, and a week later Wilson reported that she had seen Miss O'Hara at Dermady and "found her most kind and courteous," the visit "very instructive." In terms of sanitation and exposure, she added, lacking a bit in tact, "I find my rooms, and house is superior to hers."[14]

While most of the private sanatoriums in eastern Pennsylvania were started by one or two people, or at most by a family, one began as a group investment. In 1905, Flick received a fourteen-page pamphlet announcing elaborate plans for the new Radnor-Wayne Sanatorium for Consumptives, to be built on sixty-seven acres of land thirty minutes by rail to the west of Philadelphia. A "number of public spirited citizens, of Philadelphia and New York, who are equipped with ample capital" had authorized the venture, aiming to make it the largest and best-equipped sanatorium in the world. The plan indeed had need of capital. In November 1904, Maxwell J. Stevenson, Jr., a young Philadelphia banker, had bought for $5,000 a lovely piece of farmland in Tredyffrin Township, in northeastern Chester County. The purchase was subject to a five-year mortgage for $60,698—a sum presumably intended to develop the property along the grandiose lines described in the pamphlet. When the sanatorium opened in 1905, it looked much more modest and conventional than the initial architectural drawings had suggested. A frame farmhouse served as an administration building, a two and one-half story cottage housed the patients, and "Adirondack tents" spread down the slope behind the cottage, promising "absolute privacy" and "abundant air and sunshine."[15]

Promoting the Private Sanatoriums

Promotional materials of all these sanatoriums echoed the themes of the older resorts with which they were now competing. Brochures and advertisements lauded the altitude, climate, and beautiful scenery, the cold and bracing air of the mountains, the pure spring water, the fresh milk and eggs, the large airy rooms, the convenient railroad connections, and the homelike comforts of house, tent, or cottage. As Stockdale and O'Hara developed the two larger sanatoriums, they added recreation to their lists of assets. Sunnyrest, for example, provided a music room and also "a smoking room with an open fire place for such patients who are permitted to smoke," along with "a pool and billiard table for which no charge is made." Patients in suitable condition might motor through the scenic countryside or take sleigh rides in the winter, while their families could enjoy the local hunting and fishing. For its thirty to forty patients, Dermady boasted a "cheerful well heated Recreation Hall, with toilets, writing rooms, fireplace, large library and piano," which added greatly to a patient's comfort while taking the cure.[16]

Two additional themes that appeared in these publications tried to distinguish sanatoriums from mere resorts: the availability of medical specialists and the attention of trained nurses. Stockdale and O'Hara typically listed the physicians who attended their establishments. McDonald noted that Fern Cliff was "visited by the leading tuberculosis specialists of Philadelphia," and the Orchards and Hill Crest made similar claims. Although the Radnor-Wayne Sanatorium made no such assertion, its 1905 brochure noted that the program there was based chiefly on the work of Dr. Edward L. Trudeau at Saranac Lake. To look to the Adirondacks for medical luster may have been a poor tactic for a place so close to the specialists in Philadelphia.[17]

Virtually every sanatorium also advertised its nursing care although not necessarily in every notice or in much detail. The Radnor-Wayne Sanatorium emphasized the value of Miss Mahony, who had left Fern Cliff to become the head nurse of the new establishment. "One of the most essential attributes to the successful operation of a Sanatorium is the selection of a chief nurse," claimed a later brochure, "for it is the chief nurse who is largely responsible for all which appertains to the comfort of the guests." Mahony's skill and experience, well-recognized by the medical profession, it added, made her thoroughly competent to fill this important post. "Five nurses including a night nurse are in attendance," read a Sunnyrest pamphlet, "and patients are given the attention received in a private room of a modern hospital." For patients awakened by cough, pain, sweats, or unfamiliar sounds near their tents, assurance of nighttime nursing must have been very important. The Orchards and Dermady also specified this service. Electric call bells linked each tent and cottage to the main building at Dermady, and the night nurse, "bundled up to her eyes in woolen garments" during the winter, picked her way along the plank walkways to answer the patients' calls.[18]

Discriminating readers of the advertisements might also discern some differences among the sanatoriums that revealed the individual characteristics of the establishments and also, no doubt, the personalities of those who ran them. Stockdale alone mentioned the discipline. "Doing the proper things to cure Tuberculosis means doing many things that one would not do at home," warned a Sunnyrest pamphlet. "Thus a Sanatorium with discipline is necessary and all are expected to conform to the rules. It is seldom that patients fail to do this and when they do they are promptly sent home." O'Hara, in contrast, never referring to discipline, asserted that "nothing which sympathy and conscientious duty can do to further the efforts of the physician is left undone." Moss, who ran the smallest sanatorium, made an asset of its size, stating that Hill Crest was "more homelike than is possible" in larger institutions, while McDonald, subtly criticizing Sunnyrest, found advantage in Fern Cliff's half-mile distance from the railroads. The location, she noted, obviated "any disturbance by whistles, steam escaping from engine safety valves, or running of trains."[19]

Although differing in some ways, the sanatoriums shared a common mission: the active implementation of a regimen to cure tuberculosis. The environment, the diet, the treatments, and staff were all directed toward this goal. In 1905 the editor of the *Journal of the Outdoor Life*, a magazine for laypersons and patients published at Saranac Lake, commented on an important change in terminology that underlined this single objective. "Until comparatively recently the terms 'sanatorium' and 'sanitarium' were used synonymously," the editor explained. "Now 'sanatorium' in connection with institutions for the treatment of persons suffering from tuberculosis is regarded as not only preferable, but also etymologically correct. 'Sanatorium' is from sanare, to heel [*sic*]; a place in which to be treated. 'Sanitarium' is from sanitas, health, and is usually applied to a healthful place, a resort for convalescents, and not for the special treatment of disease." Although many persons with tuberculosis still camped out, went west, and stayed at resorts in both the United States and Europe, the medical cure was becoming ascendant.[20]

The Business

Running a private sanatorium proved to be a tough, laborious, and risky business that demanded a wide variety of skills. If an establishment was to survive, it had to attract and please patients, satisfy their families, maintain a roster of visiting physicians, and furnish the care and supervision that all of them expected. The sanatorium was doing part of the doctor's job, just as it was substituting in part for the patient's family.

Nurses or other members of a sanatorium's staff took over the many clinical tasks and judgments that relatives or perhaps the physician would otherwise have had to perform. They counted pulse rates, took temperatures, kept records, and saw that the patients received their prescribed diets

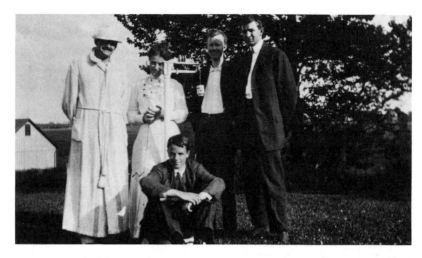

Figure 29. Margaret G. O'Hara and four patients, with scales that typically helped to define a patient's weekly progress (or lack of it). Courtesy of Kathryn Riordan.

and treatments. They gave injections of tuberculin or other substances, applied blisters, cupped their patients' chests, rubbed the europhen-in-oil into the patients' skin, and fumigated each room after it was vacated. Because physicians usually visited a sanatorium only once every two weeks, clinical judgments during the intervals fell to the sanatorium's staff—how to maintain the proper discipline, for example, whether to alter a patient's regimen when symptoms changed, and when to call a local physician to evaluate an urgent case.[21]

A sanatorium also had to create an environment where patients could feel secure and contented and where family members could be satisfied with an appropriate mix of attention, pleasure, treatment, and discipline. The patients were paying for their care and, in contrast to those at the Free Hospital, could often make other arrangements if they felt dissatisfied. In addition to taking their diets and treatments, private patients could enjoy the countryside near Sunnyrest, ramble through the woodlands or lounge in the fields of daisies at Dermady, or rest in the quiet atmosphere at the Orchards. The reputation of a sanatorium depended in part on other patients, and a congenial group helped to attract additional business. Each establishment developed its own particular clientele. A "great many sisters and priests" went to Fern Cliff, where Mass was said daily, while Dermady, also popular among Roman Catholics, became known for its "very fine class of people."[22]

The variegated assortments of men and women who collected in the sanatoriums created some thorny sets of problems with which those who managed and worked there had to contend as best they could. Mrs. Thompson, for example, in egregious disregard of the rules at Sunnyrest, absolutely refused to use her spit cup. In turn, she was terribly upset by Mr. Melvin, who sat next to her "discussing his symptoms and explaining how his 'vomit looks.'" Mrs. Berger was so fearful of contagion that she threatened to leave when she learned that one of the kitchen maids had been treated for tuberculosis, and Stockdale, angered by the whole affair, felt obligated to fire the unfortunate employee. At Dermady, one young patient gushed infectious sputum from her mouth whenever she turned onto her right side, and others lost control of their bowels or bladder. And late one evening, Mr. J. V. Walsh was shocked to see his intoxicated brother, a Dermady patient, making his way through the Philadelphia railroad station as he tried to get back to the sanatorium. Somehow the proprietors had to adapt to such problems without alienating their patients or the doctors who attended them.[23]

They also had to juggle their income and expenses so that they made a profit without pricing themselves out of business. Income came from the patients' weekly payments. Both Sunnyrest and Dermady charged between twelve and twenty-five dollars a week during their earlier years, depending on the type of accommodations. By 1911 or so, Dermady was charging fifteen to thirty-five dollars, while in 1914 Sunnyrest charged from twenty to forty dollars. The smaller sanatoriums charged less, roughly twelve to fifteen dollars a week. In addition, some of the sanatoriums offered board and lodging to other than regular patients. Sunnyrest, for example, quoted a daily rate of $2.50 for guests and visitors, while Dermady boarded out-of-town patients for a night or more to lessen the strain of a long trip between home and Flick's office.[24]

From a patient's viewpoint, these weekly expenses could become quite onerous, and they were not the only costs. The weekly charge did not cover medicines, which Flick estimated at $1.50 a week, nor did it usually pay for personal laundry. Finally, physicians made their own separate charges for their biweekly visits. The younger men with whom Flick was associated charged ten dollars for their first visit and five dollars for each subsequent visit, but Flick, the leading specialist, charged twenty-five dollars and ten, respectively.[25]

While patients often fretted over their expenses, the owners of the sanatoriums had their own fiscal concerns. First, they had to raise the capital, and some who considered going into the business never could make the initial investment. Frances A. Eastlake, from Paoli, Pennsylvania, for example, had thought of opening her home to tuberculous patients, but after talking with Flick about it she had found the project beyond her resources. "I could not furnish a 'Capital of one thousand dollars,'" wrote Eastlake in 1904, "could not, at the start, 'employ a trained nurse,' could not 'make the stipulated sanitary improvements in my house' + c. + c." Even the limited dreams of Ella Hackenburg must have been blighted from the start. "The reason i write [is] i want you to get me a couple of boarders that is in search of health," she wrote to Flick from New Jersey in 1909. "We have a Wonderful Well of water for health and Mountain air," she continued, reflecting some familiar themes, "and any one in Search of health would do well to grasp the oppertunity to come instead of going to Ocean Grove . . . how much beter it would be to come and rome the woods for health . . . and be rugged   get some of the weelthy to try it." Hackenburg was desperate: "i am poor," she concluded, "and my aged Mother is with me   we are alone and i cant do nothing else for a living."[26]

Once the capital was raised and the quarters were made suitable, those who ran the sanatoriums continued to incur expenses. They had to buy the food or try their skills at raising chickens, keeping cows, and growing and preserving vegetables and fruits. They had to maintain the grounds and purchase supplies such as fuel, disinfectants, disposable tissues, and sputum cups, and they had to provide the necessary transportation to take the patients, and sometimes the physicians, to and from the depots. They also had to find and hire an appropriate staff, pay their wages, and often provide them with room and board.

The size and nature of a sanatorium's staff depended in part on the number of patients. In 1910, for example, Margaret G. O'Hara had ten employees who lived at Dermady: two hired men, one cook, one dish-washer, one servant, one nurse, and four servants who worked as nurses but presumably lacked formal training. O'Hara also hired day help, such as the tray boys who carried milk to the patients. Sunnyrest's staff seems to have been larger. Out of the forty-three households in East Side Borough listed in the 1910 Census, three men and ten women worked in a hospital, probably Sunnyrest. These included four nurses, two servants, two cleaners, one laundress, one waitress, one driver, and a chef and chef's assistant. Stockdale, moreover, had hired the widow of Dr. James Heller as the stenographer for Sunnyrest. She boarded in town with Dr. and Mrs. Shoemaker.[27]

Margaret McDonald had a smaller staff for Fern Cliff's thirty patients, and half of them were members of her family, all single. Her younger sister, Sarah, the Census reported, acted as superintendent along with Margaret, while another sister, Catherine, served as matron, and two brothers, John and Thomas, worked as laborers. In addition, the McDonalds employed a cook, a waitress, and two nurses, one a graduate of the training school at White Haven. At Hill Crest, where the 1910 Census listed five patients, Agnes Moss established the necessary discipline and provided all the nursing care herself. Sustained by a personal optimism and a bright sense of humor, she loved nursing and was determined to get her patients well. Moss also served the meals, helped with the laundry, and planned most of the menus, while her younger sister Teresa, who had come to the United States in 1902, ordered the food and cooked.[28]

Most of the sanatoriums had to meet monthly payrolls. The salaries they paid probably resembled those at the Free Hospital. In 1906, for example, Stockdale offered Clara C. Waugh, a recent graduate of the training school at the Phipps Institute, "a position at Sunnyrest at $38 per month clear of all expenses"—a salary she wished to accept. At about this time, the Free Hospital paid its nurses $40 a month, the chef $60, the assistant cook $30, the housekeeper $20, the matrons $15, and the waitresses $10, in addition to room and board. To pay their employees and meet the installments due on their properties, those who managed the private sanatoriums had to keep them as full as possible. "Wish you would scare me up 1/2 Dozen patients—especially one or two for my shack," wrote Elwell Stockdale to Flick in 1906. "I hate to see $325⁰⁰ wasted."[29]

When patients wrote to Flick inquiring about suitable accommodations, he usually responded with a list of sanatoriums but left the selection up to the patients and their families. Although physicians could influence these choices, sanatoriums depended importantly on the favorable opinions of other patients. Amy Potts, for example, observed that "more patients come to us through patients who have been at the Orchards themselves than directly from the Drs," and some invalids weighed with care the relative advantages of Dermady and Sunnyrest.[30]

No sanatorium could escape criticism, and patients as well as their families complained. "Last week at Mt. Airy during that heavy rain," wrote Daisy W. Laidley, "it poured through my tent . . . until the floor was wet all over," and the following afternoon, when she developed chest pain, "there wasn't a nurse to do anything." Mr. Pollard, whose son was at Fern Cliff, reported that "Richard's room and tent had not been taken care of at half past Twelve" and the food there was still poor. Too, some of the patients had "migrated to the village and procured 'Ham and Egg' breakfast"—an escapade of which he disapproved—and neither "Miss McDonald or any of her assistants seem inclined to write and give us any information" as to Richard's progress. Much of the grumbling doubtless reflected the actualities of sanatorium life, but both human perversities and reactions to illness probably twisted and embellished some of the observations. "I regret to advise you that we were compelled to ask Miss Moore to leave," wrote Stockdale to Flick in 1906. "She was upsetting every one in the place and is simply a trouble breeder. When she gave such outrageous reports of Miss O'Hara we felt sure we would come in for the same thing."[31]

Success of a sanatorium depended on many factors, probably first among them the attributes of those who ran them. Pleasing the patients, attracting physicians, and making a profit out of the venture required capital, energy, experience, personality, connections, and a sound sense of business. Proximity to White Haven clearly offered advantages, and it was no accident that sanatoriums clustered there. Patients with limited resources often entered them temporarily while awaiting admission to the White Haven Sanatorium, and the region still benefited from its healthful reputation. For medical and nursing services, moreover, the charitable and private institutions were mutually supportive. The sanatoriums could rightfully claim the attentions of an unusually experienced medical staff while at the same time, by offering opportunities for private practice, they helped to reward the physicians for staffing the Free Hospital. In addition, the private institutions offered employment to graduates of the nursing school at White Haven, and in turn they advertised the nurses' special training. Stockdale, Moss, and O'Hara drew on their Free Hospital connections to establish their reputations and attract referrals. The proprietors, the physicians, and the nurses all lived in a small world, interrelated at many levels. Joseph Walsh, for example, served as visiting physician to the Free Hospital and attended his private patients at the local sanatoriums. He also shared dinners and stimulating conversations with Margaret G. O'Hara and her friends at Dermady, and when Agnes Moss married and had a daughter in 1913 he became the child's godfather.[32]

Failures and Benefits

Not everyone who opened a sanatorium succeeded. Although Mrs. Wilson's establishment in Glenside made a promising start in 1904 and George

Macklin praised it to Flick as "without question the Best you have," even Macklin saw signs of trouble. From "a Business Point of View," he observed, "I am afraid she cant keep this up unless you send her two or three more Patients." In December, difficulties of another sort came to Flick's attention. "Now all is not o.k. at Glenside," wrote Louis Woelfel, rector of St. Martin's Church in Pittsburgh. "Mr. Kossler complains about how Mrs. Wilson is overcharging him above what she promised to do for the money. He sees no fruit and no nuts and is very much put out at what he calls leg-pulling. He wants to leave."[33]

In February 1905, Mrs. Wilson's troubles deepened. She had to vacate her rented house in Glenside and, although she promptly found new and satisfactory quarters in Penllyn, six or seven miles farther out from Philadelphia, the added distance made it more difficult to attract business. When Flick had to travel very far to see an individual patient, he charged twenty-five dollars an hour. In contrast, when he had a cluster of patients in one place, he charged his usual twenty-five or ten dollars. Now that his traveling distance to Mrs. Wilson's had increased, he told her that he could not send her patients unless they could come to his office or were willing to pay his special fee. "I am very much worried because of my financial condition," wrote Wilson on March 22, 1905. "I put every dollar I posessed [sic] in the Sanatorium and have now reached the end of my resources. I have been using princapal since January." Flick expressed his regret and agreed to refer cases to her, but added that he could not go to Penllyn unless enough patients warranted the trip. His economic interests conflicted with those of the beleaguered proprietor.[34]

Mrs. Wilson's fortunes continued to spiral downward. By May 1905, she found it necessary to send her "help away because of the expence" but wanted a woman to assist with house work—preferably at ten dollars a month "if I can possibly get some one for that." By summertime, she had to move even farther from Philadelphia, this time to Gwynedd, and her patients, citing a host of complaints, were in an uproar. Mrs. Mervine, who left the sanatorium before she had intended, explained that "conditions about me are wholly responsible," while Mr. Griesmann smuggled a letter out of the house to Margaret G. O'Hara through Richard Field, a fellow patient, so that he might safely arrange to move. Field, distraught with the whole mess, accused Wilson of overcharging, extravagance, insulting behavior, and personal vulgarity. Whatever the truth of the allegations, Wilson, with only one patient left by September 12, 1905, appealed to Flick for the last time to send her some patients. "I am sorry that you are in such a predicament and shall be glad to help you if I can," Flick responded, but then, dashing any hope that he might have given her, he added: "From the cases which you have had you could have had many returns, and the fault undoubtedly must be your own. . . . Some of the patients whom you have had have sent a large number of cases to other places so that you evidently have not pleased them."[35]

Mrs. Wilson was not alone in her failure. The Radnor-Wayne Sanatorium faded from Flick's list of recommendations after 1906, and never appeared on national listings of sanatoriums. The reasons for its lack of success we can only surmise. Its mortgage was unusually large, and its lack of medical connections, along with its geographic isolation, may have prevented it from attracting a clientele. In December 1909, John Henry, the prior owner of the land, successfully sued for the return of his farm, and in January 1910 the Chester County sheriff sold it back to him for five thousand dollars. By late 1909, Potts and Wightman had closed the Orchards after having made "a very strenuous effort to succeed," as Flick described it. Potts returned to the Visiting Nurse Society of Philadelphia, and Wightman, living near White Haven in 1910, worked as a special nurse.[36]

Others, however, continued to try their luck in the business. Between 1910 and 1912, a series of women, all previously connected with the White Haven Sanatorium, ran the new Clair Mont Sanatorium north of town, and in 1911 two men opened the Brookhurst Sanitorium south of Sunnyrest. Neither establishment survived for long. In 1912, J. J. Best, one of the men who had started Brookhurst, asked Flick to explain his sanatorium's inability to attract patients. "Tuberculosis is decreasing very rapidly," Flick replied, "and a great many sanatoria have sprung up in the last few years. Some have been compelled to close for want of support. I do not believe that any of the private sanatoria have been very prosperous in the last year or two and it is quite possible that your failure is due to the fact that you were the last to come into the work."[37]

Subsequent developments confirmed Flick's explanation but with one exception. Miss Sarah E. Pollack, a 1911 graduate of White Haven's training school who had managed Clair Mont and then worked at Brookhurst, later succeeded in a new effort. In 1918, she and her husband, Thomas M. Bleuit, bought the previous Orchards Sanatorium from Mary I. Wightman and changed its name to Clair Mont. Mrs. Sarah E. (Pollack) Blueit continued as superintendent of the new Clair Mont at least through 1934.[38]

Meanwhile Flick, who was no longer associated with the Phipps Institute and was undoubtedly faced with competition that came partly from men he had helped to train, was finding his own private practice dwindling. "I have personally not been busy for a very long while," he confided to Dr. F. N. Yeager in April 1913, after the latter complained of dull times in his own practice; "[I] can duplicate your experience in every detail."[39]

Despite the diminishing number of patients seeking his care, or perhaps because of it, Flick himself plunged into the sanatorium business. Late in March 1913, he opened a six-bed sanatorium at the corner of Eighth and Pine streets, just above his office in downtown Philadelphia. He had carefully furnished his upstairs rooms and persuaded Mary Mahony (then head nurse of the Eagleville Sanatorium) to become his nurse in charge. Late in April he sent out a large number of letters to physicians and others, announcing his new venture. By having his own sanatorium, Flick emphasized in these announcements, he could provide advanced scientific treatment and could also exert closer personal supervision and greater control over the patients than he could in other establishments. Since late February, he had been writing to some of his patients along similar lines. For treatment at the new sanatorium, together with room, board, medicines, and all medical fees except his initial charge of twenty-five dollars, Flick asked thirty to fifty dollars a week. Some of the patients responded positively to Flick's letters, including at least three from Dermady, where Margaret O'Hara was now ill and conditions seem to have deteriorated for a time, and Flick began to implement his characteristically meticulous regimen.[40]

The ingredients of his "advanced scientific treatment" differed little from the regimen he had promulgated for years. Admittedly, he had abandoned creosote as a routine treatment, had adopted tuberculin for selected patients, and was now exploring the usefulness of pneumothorax—the purposeful partial collapse of a lung by injecting gas into the pleural space. For the most part, however, he still depended on diet, europhen-in-oil, and supervised rest and exercise. It was the rigor with which he could now impose his therapy that he hoped would distinguish his new sanatorium. He carefully specified the quantity and timing of every part of the treatment, and his staff, at least for a time, weighed the dishes before and after each feeding and recorded the ounces of fish, potatoes, beans, or whatever else the patients had actually eaten. By gradually increasing the activity of certain patients who had grown dependent and timid during the course of their disease and by manipulating the amount of nursing attention that they received, Flick hoped to train them back to activity and self-reliance.[41]

Through the intensity of his efforts, Flick was probably able to regulate each detail of his patients' regimen, but he could not control everything. One of the problems beyond his reach was the noise of a big city. "Among the unnecessary noises, I class boisterous conduct on the streets during the night," he complained to Director Porter at City Hall on April 1, 1913. "There is scarcely a night that I am not awakened by shouting, boisterous singing, loud talking, or noise of such a character which means nothing to anyone and is absolutely unnecessary." Flick thought that a "dance hall in Eighth Street below Lombard" was probably responsible, but that was not all. He had improved his property by installing a good cement pavement, and now "the children from all the little streets in the neighborhood use it as a skating rink with all the noises that go with such recreation." Some of the street cars at night, moreover, went too fast over the crossings and around switches. The clatter "awakens a person with fright. Without exaggeration, it shakes our buildings and rattles our chandeliers." The city's responses had no lasting effects.[42]

More serious than noise was the inexorable nature of some of the patients' diseases. George Hiestand, whom Flick was trying to wean from dependence during April and May, died at home in August, and Judge Baker, another patient whom Flick was training in self-reliance, hemorrhaged toward the end of June. Flick had been planning to close his sanatorium during the hot Philadelphia summer and go with Baker to the Jersey shore on vacation. Baker's illness, however, interrupted these plans, as Flick reported to Margaret O'Hara, and he kept the sanatorium open at least until July 28, when Baker died.[43]

In a rare interchange that revealed the strains of running a sanatorium, O'Hara responded to Flick's loss. "I realize very fully what you went through with Judge Bakers serious and fatal illness," she wrote sympathetically. "It does make it harder for you when you are right there and again when the patient is in your home. It is different. The association is closer." "If you do go back to Morton," Flick replied to O'Hara, who was recuperating in Canada, "you ought to be extremely careful about coming in close contact with the worriments of the Sanatorium." In a blunter letter to William J. Clark, a patient at the White Haven Sanatorium who wanted the superintendent's job there, Flick elaborated on this theme a year later. "The management of a sanatorium for tuberculous people is very trying, on the physical condition of the individual and requires rare executive ability, and some experience. Physically you would not hold out three months. I say this advisedly, because I have seen others try it and break down."[44]

Flick by this time, feeling his age at fifty-seven, had brought his venture to a halt. Early in 1914, he had not felt well, he reported to his sister; therefore, "I have closed out my little private sanatorium at the end of the first year. I find that I am not quite as pliable and cannot stand as much as I could some years ago and so have decided to take things a little easier." Flick mentioned no other reasons for his action, but possibly he could not attract sufficient business. His papers contain few references to the sanatorium through the fall and winter of 1913–14, and his admiring biographers, a daughter and a niece, were silent about it.[45]

Despite the several failures, private sanatoriums continued to function; they filled a need and provided benefits. Patients who could afford to pay the charges enjoyed a greater degree of privacy than others could find at the White Haven Sanatorium or in public institutions. They also found a wider range of choices among physicians and treatments. They could enter and leave a sanatorium with greater freedom, perhaps share a suite with husband or wife, and arrange for the special attention of a private nurse if they could afford the extra expense. They probably found an atmosphere more congenial to their tastes, and despite the recurring complaints they probably savored a better selection of food. And naturally, as persons of means, they were not required to work.

Well-to-do patients were also beginning to find their alternatives restricted. As fears of infection grew, stimulated by the propaganda of the antituberculosis forces, health resorts both in Europe and the United States began to exclude consumptives. "I have kept a resort here for seventeen years," wrote Mary M. Gally from Nordhoff, California, in 1903, "and until the last five years had more or less consumptives, but public opinion compels me to close my doors to them if I wished to keep the tourist trade." In 1907, the editor of the *Journal of the Outdoor Life* deplored the growing restrictions, noting that tuberculous invalids now had only three choices: to stay at home, to lie about the nature of their disease, or to go to "one of a few resorts where tuberculosis is openly acknowledged and willingly and sympathetically received."[46]

While patients found in the private sanatoriums an environment where they could get the desired attention without prejudice or subterfuge, some of those who managed the institutions also reaped rewards. Stockdale, O'Hara, Moss, and the McDonalds all created successful enterprises. Their patients often felt better; many went home to their families and some resumed their work. Tuberculosis, the common enemy, seemed to yield a bit to the proprietors' energies, giving them personal satisfaction as well as monetary gain—doubly gratifying to a man or woman who started the work with limited means and precarious health.

Other persons who were affected by the growth of sanatoriums were the nurses who took care of the patients in these and other settings. As the fears of infection grew, a history of having had tuberculosis increasingly handicapped a person's chance of finding employment. In caring for tuberculous patients, however, apparent recovery from the disease could be an asset, not a liability. A group of nurses who specialized in tuberculosis emerged out of the need for services on the one hand and the need for work on the other.

11. Attention, Care, and Doctor's Orders: Tuberculosis Nursing

Nursing was chiefly women's work. Although male attendants had served in the military and in early U.S. hospitals, and although a few men entered the new training schools, nursing had long been an integral part of a woman's domestic duties, part of her care of the family. As nursing emerged as a paid occupation during the nineteenth century, the prevailing ideals of middle-class womanhood helped to legitimate the new role. The kind, gentle, nurturing, conscientious woman, honed by the training school into a dutiful, informed, and disciplined worker, was seen as the natural moth-erlike figure to serve in the sickroom at home and perhaps in the hospital. This image, however, like the culture from which it emerged, also restricted the nurse's development. It limited her autonomy and helped to make her subservient to the usually male physician.[1]

Available work in turn-of-the-century society affected a woman's deci-sion to enter nursing. Farm work, teaching, clerking in shops, domestic service, working in mills and factories, and the newer white-collar jobs such as stenography all offered alternatives, but they paid poorly, some had a questionable reputation, and most demanded long hours of labor. As hospitals multiplied in the late nineteenth and early twentieth centuries, the training they offered and the subsequent opportunities that the experience promised seemed to some like a reasonable bargain. The women needed work, the training school provided a protected transition from home to the world outside, and nursing offered a single or widowed woman a respect-able way to support herself.

The life of a nurse was hard, but not without rewards. The care of her patients, tedious and exhausting as it sometimes became, helped others and also helped the physicians with whom she worked. She drew satisfaction from a job well done, from accomplishing something worthwhile. The skills acquired through her training and experience, along with her own personal qualities, usually enabled her to improve her financial position. She climbed a rung or two up the social and economic ladder. But hers was a woman's ladder; it did not extend very far.

The Nurses and Their Training

In February 1906, the Sunday edition of Philadelphia's *North American* celebrated the first graduation of nurses from the Henry Phipps Institute with a long, generously illustrated article. In language rich in religious metaphor, it praised the devotion and self-abnegation of the new nurses. "With hearts aflame with love for fellow-beings and minds humbly subjected to a discipline of self-sacrifice," six women had "entered their life work." The writer acknowledged that most of the women in the training school needed to work for their living, but still marveled that consumptives who had been restored to health—"literally born into a new life"—might choose to remain in "that valley of the shadow" to care for others. "None who lacks experience with tuberculosis victims can begin to realize the self-sacrifice of devoting one's life to nursing them. It means almost forsaking the world, just as if a nurse shut herself up in a convent." Yet the six young women had "chosen this path of charity, through gloom and despair. Who shall say that the spirit of the martyrs is dead? The work of these nurses is a sermon in itself."[2]

Whatever the extent to which her five classmates accepted this selfless and womanly image of their role, Mary Cornell expressed herself in much the same way. Perhaps the image gave her a sense of worth. Of the six graduates, Cornell had been "nearest to death," and she considered her cure the "most remarkable." In July 1902, several physicians had regarded her case as hopeless, she reported. Determined to take the treatment, however, she had cleared a third-story room of all its furniture except for a large chair, and there she had sat all day, with windows open "even after zero weather came." At first she could hardly walk because of weakness, but she persisted with the regimen: three quarts of milk and six eggs daily, with one meal at midday. By January 1903, she had gained seventeen pounds. Her turn then came to enter the White Haven Sanatorium, where she gained another nineteen pounds in one month. "It is purely through a desire to help suffering humanity," Cornell concluded, "that I have taken up the work of nursing consumptives."[3]

More practical considerations must also have shaped the nurses' decisions. Of the eighty-one who graduated from the training schools at the Phipps Institute and at White Haven between 1905 and 1913, eighty were women, most of them single and a few widowed. When they had become ill, well over 90 percent of them were working—almost a fourth in factories, roughly a fourth in households, and about one-fifth in clerical or similar positions. The rest included saleswomen, milliners, school teachers, and a few who were already trained or partly trained as nurses. They must have weighed the prospects of tuberculosis nursing against the long hours, low wages, oppressive conditions, and uncertainties that characterized their previous occupations. A change itself seemed advantageous. As Mary E. Lee explained to Flick, "I dread going back to the school room having taught ten years, thereby losing my health."[4]

To enter one of the two training schools, a woman was supposed to have had a common-school education and she had to be fit to work an eight-hour day. Flick preferred candidates who were accustomed to hard work. If a woman had had an easy life, it would "make the hardships of a training school seem severe and undesirable to her. This may give rise to complaints and dissatisfaction." Some of the pupils undoubtedly had active tuberculosis. In 1908, Joseph Walsh reported that a majority of the thirty-five pupils admitted to the Phipps training school had moderately advanced disease, a "small number were early cases, and a few far advanced." One pupil in the last category had "a cavity at the top of each lung" and "moist rales all over both lungs."[5]

Opportunities in the field appealed to the women, but there were drawbacks and anxieties. Miss Steinberg had worked as an unpaid employee under Agnes Moss at White Haven, but was afraid to risk the training school at Phipps. Mary McNamee entered the school, but only after bargaining hard to protect her health. She insisted that she be allowed to keep up her treatment strictly, report to a doctor every week, and return immediately to White Haven should she become sick again. Other women, once in training, failed to complete the program. In 1907 five probationers—16 percent of all students then in the two-year school at Phipps—"lost courage" and left during their first month. Of all the students listed during the first two years of the school at White Haven, 67 percent never graduated.[6]

Active recruitment of pupils was necessary, and superintendents at White Haven, staff physicians at the two institutions, and head nurses, all of whom had an interest in full cadres of pupils, assisted in attracting them. A certificate that documented a graduate's accomplishments, while not worth as much as a diploma from a general hospital, helped to entice prospective students into the field. Anna G. Murphy, a valued matron at White Haven between 1902 and 1905, for example, twice consulted Flick about the relative merits of entering the Phipps training school or taking a position as a nurse in a private sanatorium. Flick advised her to get a certificate and Murphy, "anxious to make a real success of this work," took the counsel and graduated in 1907.[7]

During their twenty-two months of training, successive groups of millhands, saleswomen, stenographers, domestics, and school teachers, all convalescing from tuberculosis, worked to become specialized trained nurses. Physicians lectured on medical subjects, and the head nurse gave textbook and practical bedside instruction. The pupils learned to "keep an accurate and methodical record of temperature, pulse, respiration, and other clinical details of their patients." They learned to handle soiled clothing, bedding, bandages, and evacuations. They were expected to carry out the doctors' orders "strictly and literally," and staff physicians tested them with questions such as, How much strychnine is in a teaspoonful if a six ounce mixture contains two grains? How would you treat a pulmonary hemorrhage? And, what is the best method of taking care of a patient's knives and forks? The pupil nurses gave medicines, applied remedies, and ministered to the comfort and welfare of their patients. They were to treat all patients "with the utmost gentleness, and under no consideration [were they] to engage in any argument or dispute." Each nurse was responsible for the discipline and condition of her ward and was to tolerate neither profanity nor disrespect. In turn, she was expected to give "prompt and respectful obedience" to the superintending nurse and to remain standing whenever a doctor was present. In short, the trained nurse was to be knowledgeable about disease and its treatment, reliable in her performance, efficient and competent in her skills, gentle and kind yet firm with her patients, and obedient to her superiors.[8]

Starting in 1905, a new group of nurses trained in tuberculosis joined the work force every year. Although most graduates from the schools in general hospitals went into private-duty nursing, those who trained at Phipps and White Haven were different. Roughly two-thirds of these women took positions in sanatoriums or hospitals, while less than a tenth took private cases. Flick usually gave them preference when hiring or recommending nurses, but they competed with others in both settings. Although healthy nurses often avoided tuberculosis work, some were either unafraid or pressed by need to take whatever job they could find.[9]

Expectations of the Nurse

To a busy physician with a large practice—especially one whose patients were widely scattered in homes and sanatoriums, hours away by train—few aids could have been more valuable than a competent nurse. She mailed him regular reports about his patient, and he altered his management according to her observations. She initiated treatments for both minor complaints and medical emergencies, and even reminded the doctor to bring a scalpel on his next visit to drain his patient's abscess. Specialized training facilitated this working relationship. The nurse who understood the doctor's expectations could anticipate his decisions, manage the details of the patient's regimen with little medical explanation, and save the doctor's time.[10]

Physicians also expected the nurse to help them control their patients, to establish the discipline that they thought so essential to healing. To the institutions she should bring order, and in patients' homes she should impose the regimen, thus protecting the sick from their weaknesses and from the temptations of families and friends. Charles J. Hatfield, when a staff physician at Phipps and at White Haven, praised such a nurse in 1907. "In private practice," he declared, "with a patient who insists upon being treated in his own home—surrounded perhaps by forbidden luxuries, surrounded usually by a devoted family, always ready to help him break through prescribed lines—she is beyond price."[11]

Peter Dettweiler, the German director of the sanatorium at Falkenstein, had emphasized the importance of medical control, and after 1900 his ideas had been gaining favor among tuberculosis specialists in the United States. According to Dettweiler, "the smallest details of the patient's life are controlled by the supervising physician, and nothing of any importance is left to his or her judgment." The patient and doctor should relate to each other as student and teacher, penitent and priest, in an atmosphere that nurtured "implicit confidence" and "strict obedience." Flick began to express himself in similar terms about 1902, and he expected a nurse to facilitate this kind of relationship.[12]

In the idealized views of contemporary society, women seemed particularly able to guide and take care of the sick, and physicians frequently preached and praised their virtuous qualifications. "A loyal, devoted and high-minded nurse," Hatfield observed, "represents to many minds the highest development of womanhood." Frank A. Craig, then another staff physician, echoed this theme in his 1911 commencement address at White Haven. "The work is better done by women than men," he explained, "since the instinct of motherhood which is strong in every woman will guide those on the road to health and set the steps of those scarcely [able] to walk in this new path of life."[13]

Some patients had expectations of their nurses that matched exactly those of their physicians. They wanted the nurse to make the needed observations, implement the medical orders, and make them obey, even against their own wishes. Anxious over deteriorating health, peevish with illness, and often made tense, depressed, or lonely by family frictions, they asked for control and complained of its absence. Mrs. Thompson tried to make sure that her new nurse would do just as Flick commanded. "I am going to ask you to make an appointment with her," wrote Thompson, "so that she may understand thoroughly just what rules I am to follow—to lead as far as possible a Sanitorium life here—which I am almost positive I can do—if you will impress it upon her to be very firm."14

Family members, unable or unwilling to help the patients with treatment or to impose it upon them, expected the nurse to do it instead. With the proper medical instructions, the nurse was supposed to substitute for the patient's willpower and for family persuasion and discipline. Mr. Levis thought that his wife needed a strong person to see that she took her diet. "A weak character is apt to be guided by Mrs. Levis's impulse," he explained. "Anyone who has been sick as long as she has, can hardly be depended upon to keep up her proper treatment in the face of her very discouraging times."15

While patients and their families asked for control and discipline, they also yearned for a nurse who was kind, companionable, personally attentive, and emotionally satisfying—someone who could adapt to the household or bring a semblance of family warmth to a sanatorium. Mrs. Killip's relatives, for example, were hoping to find "a bright cheerful private nurse (almost a companion) to lead her to forget her loneliness." Absence of family, conflicting responsibilities of related caretakers, and marital discord all increased the need for finding a stranger to help with an invalid's care.16

Diverse desires such as these sometimes tugged a nurse in one direction and then another; so did her dual responsibilities to physician and patient. It was the physician who gave her orders, often recommended her for a position, and may have taught her in school. He usually had additional authority derived from education, class, and gender. It was the patient or the patient's family, on the other hand, who employed her, whom she was duty-bound to serve, and with whom she had to live. Tensions and conflicts were almost inevitable. Although they must have been felt in any setting where nurses worked, they are most evident where relationships were most intense—in private-duty nursing.

Intimate Needs, Intimate Conflicts

When the care of a patient shifted from family to nurse, results were unpredictable. In some instances, the nurse brought great relief and comfort. The stranger became a friend, supplementing a family's care or, if family was lacking, substituting for it entirely. As a nurse moved into the intimate family circle, however, she sometimes disrupted relationships and tried to take more control than either the patient or the family wanted to grant. The extent to which she succeeded in meeting competing expectations depended in part on her own skills, but it also depended on the patient, the relatives, the physician, and the regimen for which she had taken responsibility. Four examples illustrate the range of these relationships and the nature of a nurse's work.

Richard Field had lost his nurse, and his desperate plea to replace her makes clear her value to him and the anguished dependency of a sick man. In 1905 Field had entered Mrs. Wilson's sanatorium. The proprietor had objected to his lack of discipline (he ate Bologna sausage in his room) and had also accused him of intimacy with Miss Brown, a nurse whom Field had brought with him from Arizona. In response, Brown had departed. After Field too had left the sanatorium, he had tried to make other arrangements, without success. Defending himself against Mrs. Wilson's allegations, he appealed to Flick for assistance:

> As I am still unable to walk 100 yds. or get up and down stairs without help a nurse is absolutely necessary. I have not walked 5 minutes a day in the last five months. The truth is I am perfectly helpless. I have not been sensually passionate in months and have no desire that way. I have just broken my engagement because I cannot marry nor do I ever hope to. I am so fearfully weak I must have a nurse and I suffer so with my brain, that at times gets into a whirl, I must have some quiet, attentive person with me. I should think the fact that at Mrs. Wilsons the only gains I made were while I had a nurse would disprove her charges. I gained every week my nurse was with me simply because I was quiet and contented. When she left four months ago I lost and have lost every week since with but one exception. . . . I want a nurse who is cultured, quiet, and who can, in a decent way, make a fellow swallow lots of milk. I am worried as I seem to have lost my fighting spirit and I have fought tooth and nail for 15 months.[17]

Desire for a woman's care and attention was not limited to single and perhaps isolated patients such as Field. Happily married persons, even men's wives, often welcomed a nurse into the intimate sphere of family life.

The nurse took over the work required by the regimen and also gave the family some respite from the emotional and social demands of caring for an invalid. George Hiestand had been ill for more than six years when, on Flick's recommendation, he and his family hired Miss Rebecca McCabe. Her work pleased everyone and, when Flick admitted Hiestand to his private sanatorium four months later, McCabe accompanied her patient. When Hiestand insisted on having the nurse's cot moved into his sanatorium bedroom, Flick objected. The patient was "coddled too much," he wrote to Mrs. Hiestand; he was growing too dependent and would make better progress if he could learn "some self-reliance and self-confidence." Mrs. Hiestand, however, supported her husband's wishes. "It is a great relief to me to know he has a <u>nurse</u> he <u>likes</u> right near him," she replied. "She gives him a better bath and rub than he ever had before. However she is not only a nurse[,] she entertains him and you'd find he would get very nervous shut up in four walls with nothing to do."[18]

Combining care and companionship with a strict medical regimen tested and sometimes exceeded a nurse's abilities. Nurse, physician, and patient could get locked in a grim, tedious battle as the patient, wracked by progressive disease and glutted with milk and eggs, resisted continuing treatment. In the spring of 1911, Miss Lillian Ried had returned from the Dermady Sanatorium to her home in New Jersey, where two successive nurses, Miss L. M. Hall and Miss Sue Earley, took care of her until she died on October 12. The nurses' twice-weekly reports detailed the gain of a quarter pound or the loss of a half pound; a brighter facial expression but cough, fever, weakness, and palpitations; watery stools from the purgative powders; and the insufferable heat of the Jersey summer. Through the long, worrisome months, however, one persisting theme dominated their correspondence with Flick—the struggle over the patient's diet.

> *Flick, May 17:* Tell Miss Ried for me to keep up her courage as I think she is doing very well. The little vomiting will not do her any harm.
> *Hall, May 23:* The emesis still persists as you will see by the chart.
> *Flick, May 24:* It might be well for you to give her a dose of castor oil as it may stop the vomiting. See that she takes her full diet every day.
> *Hall, June 20:* Her morning lunch she vomited immediately after taking. Gave her three more eggs and two glasses of milk which she retained. It was a hard fight all day.
> *Hall, [late June]:* Could you kindly let me have relief as soon as possible. . . . I feel that I need rest badly, before I break down.
> *Flick, July 5:* I expect Miss Earley, one of the nurses from White Haven, to relieve you on next Saturday and I trust you may be able to hold out until then.

Earley, July 26: I cannot force her to take more Diet.

Flick, August 2: Tell Lillian that I would like very much if she would take a little more milk. Give her . . . the whites of as many eggs as she can take.

Earley, August 23: Lillian is not feeling any better   I cannot force any more food or milk.

Flick to Lillian Ried, August 29: You have been improving lately and I want you to try very hard to get well.

Earley, September 15: Lillian . . . is not trying to take any more diet I am sure she could if she wanted too.

Flick, September 18: If she would only take more milk and eggs, I am sure she would improve a great deal. Tell her that she must try and increase the number of glasses of milk and that she must again try and take more eggs. Use all the persuasion you have to get her to do this.

Earley, October 5: I cannot get her to drink any milk   she is not bothered about her condition   she does not care.

Two convictions drove Flick's therapeutic persistence. By controlling the patient, he believed, he could often control the patient's disease. In terms of priority, moreover, the alleviation of suffering was far less important than cure. These convictions pitted the physician's authority against that of the family, sometimes leaving the nurse caught awkwardly in between. Miss Anna Walsh, a 1910 graduate of the training school at the Philadelphia General Hospital, had been caring for Chester Bobb for about six weeks when the conflict reached a crisis. Like Lillian Ried, Chester had been a patient at Dermady, but his parents, whose only other child had died four years earlier, wanted to continue the treatment at home. Following Flick's suggestions, the Bobbs built Chester a shack in the yard, bought a goat for its presumably more digestible milk, and hired "a good trusty nurse" to supervise the regimen.[19]

Neither the first nurse nor Walsh, who succeeded her, found the case easy. Although the eighteen-year-old Chester usually tried to take his treatment, he was easily annoyed, "spoiled," and "inclined to be stubborn" regarding his diet. He was "cross" when awakened for milk at six in the morning, and wanted "to sleep in the house when he takes a notion," rather than staying in his shack throughout the night. His mother sided with her son. "His mamma is very nervous and afraid it might be too damp out in the shack," Walsh reported, "and she is afraid of the wind blowing on him, and if he is left out in the shack when we go to bed she is most likely to have him back in his bed-room by morning." When Flick suggested that Chester return to a sanatorium, both parents refused.[20]

Paid caretakers—physicians or nurses—had limited ways of asserting authority. When a patient improved, the very recovery attested to the caretaker's wisdom and skill, but without such evidence other methods had to be used: persuasion, command, dire prognostication, and finally, the cessation of services. This last method acted as both a threat to enhance compliance and a peaceful way of resolving incompatible expectations. After visiting Chester in October 1911, Flick sent Mr. Bobb a stern letter. His visit had convinced him that Chester "has broken loose from discipline"; Flick had "dismal forebodings of what may come in the future." Because Chester's mode of life and treatment would largely determine the outcome, he warned, "his exercise should be under strict control and not taken at random or to suit his whims. . . . He must be carefully fed and . . . kept in the open air continuously." Chester himself "must not be permitted to judge what is best for him either in the way of exercise, diet, or medical treatment and these things must not be under the control or subject to the wishes of those who are tied to him closely by bonds of relationship. He should be subject entirely to the directions of his physician in every detail under a competent nurse and no one else should have any voice in the interpretation and execution of the physician's directions."[21]

Flick assured Mr. Bobb that he would gladly continue to treat Chester, but only if every detail was followed and he was kept fully informed; otherwise, the Bobbs should find another physician. On November 20, Walsh made a comparable suggestion. No matter how hard she had tried, she could not persuade Chester to take his diet. Perhaps Flick knew of a more capable nurse with whom he would feel more satisfied. Each caretaker had sensed correctly that a change was desirable, and on December 3 Mr. Bobb graciously dismissed them both.[22]

The Strains and Rewards of Nursing

Emotionally and physically, nursing demanded much from those who practiced it. Private duty often placed the nurse in a distraught household, where she had to give of herself to the patient and adapt to the ways of the family. Even a happy home taxed her resources. "Being with the family so much," one experienced nurse observed, "has been hard for both the patient and the nurse." Long hours that often included twenty-four-hour responsibilities, uncertainties about the length of a case, and, probably worse, uncertainties about getting a case at all disrupted a nurse's life. While time between cases gave her some much-needed rest, waiting for the next call and being prepared for it must have created suspenseful anxieties. All the necessary personal belongings and perhaps some equipment for the care of the patient had to be ready. "I am going to try private work," and would appreciate a case, wrote Stella M. Brown, a Phipps graduate of 1911; "just send me a telegram and I will be ready to come on the next train."[23]

Conditions of the work and hopes of improving them sent many of the nurses on a restless search from one job to another, from institution to private cases, and back again. A rare nurse such as Margaret G. O'Hara broke free from a hired position to become an employer who managed her own enterprise yet maintained the individual contact that was central to nursing. The careers of most nurses, however, moved sideways, not upward. Miss Edith Metzler, for example, who graduated from White Haven in 1911, worked on the women's tuberculosis ward of the Philadelphia General Hospital, tried to get a private case, and then found herself a job at Bellevue Hospital in New York City, all in the course of a few months. Metzler had not liked the "disposition to domineer" that her work at the General Hospital seemed to cultivate. She was also looking for better pay.[24]

In their efforts to better themselves, nurses weighed income against the continuity of the work. Sanatoriums and hospitals offered more steady employment than many nurses could find in private duty, but they paid considerably less. In addition to the board and lodging that the nurse could usually find in either situation, institutions paid about thirty to forty dollars a month. When a private nurse was actually working, in contrast, she earned at least twice as much: fifteen to twenty-five dollars a week. Only an administrative position, for which relatively few nurses qualified, could match the income of private duty.[25]

By the time Metzler was looking for work in 1911, competition was intensifying. Overproduction of nurses for private duty had started as early as the 1890s, as increasing numbers of hospitals used pupils to work and then graduated them to fend for themselves in the labor market. In comparison with general hospitals, tuberculosis institutions did not depend so much on pupils, but by the 1910s increasing numbers of these too were beginning to open schools. Opportunities for nurses to work in such sanatoriums thus diminished, as they had at White Haven after the school started. Private sanatoriums, moreover, competed with nurses for patients. Although they hired some nurses, they also attracted affluent patients who individually might have employed a private attendant instead. Tuberculous patients in need of a private nurse were thus becoming scarce. "A short while ago when I needed nurses very badly, I could not get them," Flick replied to Metzler when she asked about a private case, "and now that nurses are available, I have no call for them."[26]

Untrained women, especially those who had had tuberculosis themselves, competed for the work. They felt qualified by their own illnesses, by the experience some had gained at a sanatorium, or by the care they had given an ill or dying relative. "While I have no real training," wrote Nellie K. Smith, who had been a patient at both White Haven and the Rush Hospital, "I taught myself a great deal at the Hospital and am fully capable of following a doctors orders." Such workers were in some demand. Potential employers did not always consider it necessary to have a trained nurse; they needed a person to help with the household chores in addition to caring for the patient, or they hoped to spend less money than a trained nurse expected to get. For the care of one young patient, for example, Mrs. P. White asked Flick if he knew of "a woman in need of employment, who would be able to attend the patient at her home? Someone whose case is not too far advanced to admit of her nursing another; and, who would be glad of a good home with slight recompense."[27]

Medical practice was also highly competitive, and physicians too wanted the work. "As my wife is unfortunate to have contracted tuberculosis," wrote Dr. M. B. Holzman to Flick in 1908, "and as my means do not allow me to have her away in a suitable clime, I have decided to . . . ask you if you know of any tubercular person that I could accompany in the capacity of nurse and physician." Thus, he explained, "I could also keep my wife in a suitable climate. Mrs Holzman is of a very nervous disposition and it is impossible to send her to a san[a]torium."[28]

Despite the competitive pressures, the stress, and the uncertainties of their work, nurses preferred it to their alternatives. They had learned a skill that raised them a notch or two above their previous jobs. According to available records, not one of the graduates from Phipps or White Haven returned to her previous line of work. The women had increased their earning capacities substantially, according to Joseph Walsh, and "almost all . . . improved their station in life." The graduates' salaries ranged from fifteen to thirty dollars a week, he reported in 1915, and averaged seventeen dollars. Although these weekly figures overestimated the nurses' income over the course of a full year because they did not allow for rest time or lack of employment, they were still probably better than the nurses' prior earnings. In their previous occupations, which also carried a risk of unemployment, the women's wages had ranged from seven to fifteen dollars a week and had averaged nine.[29]

Upward mobility meant more than simply money; it meant status and satisfaction. In 1915, Walsh gave six examples of special success among the graduates of the Phipps Institute and the White Haven Sanatorium: one owned and managed a sanatorium, one was a superintendent, and four were directresses of nurses. Anna Murphy, the White Haven matron who had sought Flick's advice about entering the Phipps training school, took a position in Louisville, Kentucky, in 1908. "You will be glad to know that the work in this little Sanatorium has been a pronounced success," she wrote, "and that it is one of the pupils of White Haven and of your Training School who has worked hard with Dr. Rembert to make it such."[30]

Both Flick and Walsh asserted that better health also rewarded the nurses. In terms of mortality rates, Walsh observed in 1923, nurses did 39 percent better than consumptives who entered other careers. Both physicians, however, observed these rates only after the nurses' graduation, not at the time that they entered the schools. Their two-year training, with its high attrition, had undoubtedly winnowed out many of the less hardy women—before they were counted—and the mortality rates for the pupils cannot be determined."[31]

The Life and Work of Mary Mahony

In the life and career of Mary Mahony may be glimpsed the value of a nurse's work, its hardships, and its satisfactions. Mahony was born in Pennsylvania in 1870, the second of six children. Her parents had come to the United States from Ireland in the 1860s, and by 1880 the family had settled near Easton, Pennsylvania, where her father worked at an iron furnace. Mahony entered the two-year training school of the Philadelphia Hospital early in January 1894, nine years after the school had opened. This was a time of change at the old municipal institution, and the new school, founded in the tradition of Florence Nightingale, was reforming the care of patients. Mahony graduated in 1895 and worked there for several years afterward.[32]

Between 1895, when she was a senior student, and 1899, when the records cease, Mahony made brief evaluations of students in the training school. The words that she used most often described a good worker: willing, thorough, industrious, conscientious, reliable, careful, quiet, and neat. Students had to learn their appropriate place and behavior in the hierarchy, and Mahony commended them for being obedient and respectful. In relations with patients, she approved their being kind, thoughtful, good-tempered, and gentle. Occasionally, she praised a student as observant and intelligent or criticized one as quick-tempered, nervous, or slow. These comments sketched the turn-of-the-century nursing ideal.[33]

In 1902, two physicians wrote to Flick about a nurse at the Philadelphia Hospital who, during the winter, had been found to have tuberculosis; after a period of treatment at Saranac Lake she had returned to Philadelphia and wanted to enter the White Haven Sanatorium. Although this nurse's identity is not established, she fits no one in the Flick correspondence other than Mary Mahony, who went as a patient to White Haven in 1902. By January 1903, Elwell Stockdale had recognized her value. He had her in mind as the nurse for Sunnyrest, should Miss Burns leave there, but also saw her as just the person to fill a vacancy on White Haven's staff. She and Miss Murphy between them, he thought, could cover the three cottages. "Think $25[00] [a month] would hold her," he wrote to Flick, "as she is anxious to continue her cure."[34]

Mahony stayed at the sanatorium through the middle of February, but she soon had better opportunities. First she moved to Sunnyrest, and late in November 1903 Flick offered her the superintendent's position at the Henry Phipps Institute at seventy-five dollars a month. "I think you could fill this position consistently with the maintenance of your health," he advised, "as you would have practically no nursing to do but merely . . . superintend the institution." "Will be most pleased to accept the offer as soon as I can be relieved from duty at Sunnyrest," Mahony responded. "I shall endeavor with God's holy help to show my appreciation by conscientious performance of duties and trust I will be able to fill the position." Mahony moved back to Philadelphia in mid-December, but during the winter her health faltered. She developed a bad cold and, "owing to her rather severe duties," as Flick later explained to George E. Gordon, "has not recovered from it." Early in April 1904, he recommended a trip to the seashore, and after a short stay in Atlantic City Mahony went home for a rest. In June, she resigned from the Institute. Early in August, she became the superintendent at the Fern Cliff Sanatorium, where she stayed for at least a year. Then, for an unknown length of time, she served as the head nurse of the Radnor-Wayne Sanatorium west of Philadelphia.[35]

By April 1908, she was ready for private duty. From May to July, she worked on a case in Belle Vernon, Pennsylvania, probably leaving after the family had learned the routines of treatment. In November, she nursed a man in Moorestown, New Jersey, but he soon found it necessary to reduce his expenses and manage his own recovery. In January 1909, when Flick wanted her for a case in Mauch Chunk, Pennsylvania, she was already caring for one of Dr. Walsh's patients in Wilmington, Delaware. She stayed in Wilmington at least until March 1909, when Flick recommended her highly to Dr. Marvel for one of his patients. This time, the family refused to hire her. "The woman," Mahony explained, "felt I was not strong enough to do the nursing she required." On March 31, Mahony went to another patient in Slatington, Pennsylvania, and stayed until he died late in May. By then, she "was quite fatigued" and went home to rest.[36]

Between 1909 and 1912, Mahony returned to institutional work, this time at the Jewish Sanatorium for Consumptives at Eagleville, Pennsylvania, but she also took private cases in both homes and institutions. In January 1911, she reported to Flick on Mrs. Sharples, a patient whom even Mahony was finding "very difficult to manage." Mrs. Sharples and her husband objected to some of Flick's treatments, wanted to try something different, and suspected Mahony of withholding information from them. "These things are not pleasant to bear," Mahony wrote to Flick, "but those two are not accustomed to obey orders other than their own." Mahony, however, won them over. Although she had to leave them when her younger sister Catherine died during the winter, the family welcomed her back in March. She stayed with them through early July when, after several weeks of great suffering, Mrs. Sharples died. "Miss Mahoney [*sic*] was to us like one of the family," Mr. Sharples reported to Flick, "and we shall never forget her kindness and care." Later, he sent Mahony a gift of seventy-five dollars, with a letter of thanks.[37]

Soon after leaving the Sharples family, Mahony took over the care of Father Kelly, a patient of Dr. Walsh's at Fern Cliff. When in July Flick wanted her to replace the nurse who was caring for Chester Bobb, Mahony could not accept the position. Father Kelly was extremely ill, and it "would be very disturbing for me to leave him," she replied to Flick; "he will not allow me out of the room. . . . I am sorry to not be able to accommodate you . . . but Father Kelly is the dearest friend I have and this little comfort he has in my presence is the last act I can do for him   he has always been my sweet consoler." Mahony suggested that she might be able to take Chester's case a little later; and early in August, when the priest seemed better, she finally felt that she could leave him. "On informing Fr Kelly that I had to leave to day," however, she wrote to Flick, "he became very upset and cried Dr. Walsh talked the matter over with him and decided I had better remain two weeks longer." The weeks stretched out, and Mahony stayed at Fern

Cliff for another four months. "Father Kelly still needs me but is willing to have me take your case," she reported at last to Flick on December 2. "He does not improve poor creature   is so dreadfully nervous and lonely   I never before realized how dependent one can become when they are weak and sick   he seems to feel so confident when I am here."[38]

On December 6, 1911, Mahony telegraphed Flick that she could go to the Bobbs in three days, but by this time Flick had been dismissed. When Mr. Bobb learned that Mahony was free, however, he must have asked her to come. On the evening of December 7, Mahony arrived at the Bobb home in western Pennsylvania, where Chester was extremely ill. He had had a hemorrhage of nearly two quarts, his pulse was exceedingly rapid, and his breathing was shallow and "very oppressed." Although he was taking a quart of milk daily, she observed, "the act of swallowing causes labored breathing. The parents dont seem to realize his condition." Chester died suddenly on December 21. "Mrs. Bobb is quite prostrated," wrote Mahony from Easton on Christmas Day; "she was so devoted and self-sacrificing the boys death was a great shock to her   they were very sorry to have me leave yesterday but she wanted me to spend Christmas with my mother. . . . I am ready for work   any call from you will be appreciated."[39]

Private cases proved to be scarce and, on April 1, 1912, Mahony went back to Eagleville as the head nurse. "The private work has been so dull lately," Flick wrote to Anna Murphy, "that even Miss Mahony has taken a position in an institution." Mahony stayed at Eagleville for about a year, and late in March 1913 she moved to Philadelphia to work in Flick's new sanatorium. There she functioned as head nurse, but during the summer she also did private duty at the sanatorium. She nursed Judge Baker during his terminal illness, probably until he died on July 28. "I still feel tired," she reported to Flick on August 6, "but am resting quietly at home." "Do not attempt to work until you have fully recovered yourself," Flick warned, "as I fear you are not any too strong, and you might break yourself down seriously by over-working."[40]

On September 7, Mahony reported herself "thoroughly rested" and "ready for work at any time," but Flick had no cases for her. In October, when he asked her to accompany a patient to Florida, she was caring for a little boy whom she could not leave until his parents returned. By the time she was free, Flick's patient had hired another nurse. When Mahony received her next call from Flick in March 1914, she could not accept it. "Sorry unable to take case," she telegraphed from Easton, "sick with cold." Flick wrote to Mahony for the last time on September 30, 1914. He had found "a heavy cape, lined with red," and after more than a year he had finally realized it was probably hers. If so, he would be glad to send it. Miss Jane Mahony responded to the letter. Her sister had no use for the cape, she told Flick; it could be thrown away. Her sister had been ill for months and could not write herself.[41]

Before the year's end, Mary Mahony, whom Flick had once described as "one of the best trained nurses in tuberculosis in this country," died and was buried in St. Joseph's Cemetery, Easton. She was forty-four. Dr. Martin F. Sloan, superintendent of the Eudowood Sanatorium in Towson, Maryland, might well have been delivering her eulogy the year before. When he spoke to the second graduating class of the sanatorium's training school, he commended the women for their achievements and praised their new work. Urging them to be gentle and kind, tidy and neat, cheerful and obedient, he suggested their womanly place in society. "Your work will not be accompanied by the sounding of trumpets or announced in the head-lines of the press, but will likely be done away from the gaze of the crowd," he counseled the new nurses, themselves recovering consumptives. "Your name will [probably] not be recorded in the medical annals of the future, but remember the words of George Eliot, who said 'the growing good of the world is partly dependent on unhistoric acts; that things are not so ill with you and me as they might have been, is half owing to the number who lived faithfully a hidden life, and rest in unvisited tombs.'"[42]

Mary Mahony touched many lives, both in long and intense relation-ships and in transient encounters. Among those she knew briefly was George E. Macklin, a well-to-do man from Pittsburgh. As Macklin tried to follow Flick's regimen while retaining some semblance of a normal life, his experiences illuminate the interactions among patient, family, physician, and nurse early in the twentieth century.

12. The Final Years of George E. Macklin

The care of consumptives did not shift abruptly from home or resort to institutions; it took time to build the sanatoriums and hospitals and to persuade the patients to go there. During the first two decades of the twentieth century, well-to-do patients sampled one method of taking the cure, and then another. They traveled to reputedly healthful climates and they tried the new sanatoriums. They hired servants, nurses, and physicians to take care of them and, if one proved less than satisfactory, they tried another. Their hope and their faith in physicians sustained them, but they also questioned the treatment and tried to negotiate changes. An affluent man such as George E. Macklin had many more choices than Annie E. Hackett or other poor patients, and he was better able to bargain effectively with his physician. Compliance with medical rules was still important, however, and control of the patient was still an issue. Macklin's final years illustrate the experiences of a well-to-do consumptive during a transition period when the "scientific" treatment of tuberculosis was still quite new. His persisting hope and his final dependency, shared by the thousands like him, help to explain the expansion of medical care.

George E. Macklin, the forty-year-old general manager of the Pressed Steel Car Company in Pittsburgh, had been ill since 1901. He had spent two winters in Colorado, but in the spring of 1903 he was not yet well and F. N. Hoffstot, a brother-in-law of Henry Phipps, recommended a consultation with Dr. Flick. "I should like very much to have you look me over and talk over with me in general your views on tuberculosis," wrote Macklin to Flick on April 30. "I presume you can readily understand how a man with the trouble is interested in the advancement of anything that might lead to a cure; and, I am also extremely anxious to have someone look me over who has and is making a study of the disease."[1]

On May 13, after a successful meeting in Philadelphia, Macklin telegraphed his acceptance of Flick's recommendations and asked that all the necessary arrangements be made for him. He would go, as suggested, to the

Sunnyrest Sanatorium at White Haven. In a letter written the same day, he explained his goals for the sojourn. "I want to be made as comfortable as possible up there, but don't expect any frills; and I think it would be a good idea if we had the two tents put up together so we could use [them] . . . any way we want to arrange them. I would not want to be uncomfortable just to prevent a little extra expense. . . . My one point is to get there and be there . . . so that you will be able to tell me just about where I stand, that is the all important question with me just now." He hoped that his stay in the sanatorium would not bar him from work. "Would you have any objection to me having my Secretary come up occasionally, say once a week," Macklin inquired, "so that I could go over some papers that might be of importance, or, would you prefer that I do absolutely nothing while there? Of course, he would only be with me a few hours during one day in the week." By May 25, 1903, Macklin had satisfactorily established his quarters at Sunnyrest. "The Tents are working nicely," he reported, and "I am able to keep up the 16 Glasses of Milk and 12 Eggs per day. and now 24 hours open air."[2]

Macklin's only complaint was hard coughing, which caused pain in his neck muscles and worsened his usual sleeplessness, but complications in the nursing arrangements soon disrupted his stay. Mr. C. J. Hunt, a private nurse whom Flick had sent, arrived ill. Then he developed a sore throat and Macklin sent him to bed. On the night of June 1, Hunt was given a room in the house so that he could be next to the bathroom, but the next day his throat was worse, his temperature rose to 103°, and the local physician suspected diphtheria. "They have put him in Third Story room," wrote Macklin hastily on June 2, "and Doctor has sent for a nurse for him as it would not do for Miss Mahoney [*sic*] to attend him and be about the rest of us if he has anything like Diphtheria and of course, it is very important to keep it from rest of Patients so only the Doctor Miss Mahoney and Mrs Stockdale know of it. The lat[t]er I think is quite worried for fear it will become know[n] . . . and all the Patients get out."[3]

Macklin accepted the conspiratorial silence regarding the dread infection in good humor. "It is suggested that Neither the Telegraph or Telephone be used in referring to what I wrote you about Mr. Hunt," he added in a second letter to Flick the same day. "As it would be all over Town in short order and as I understand it, their Ears are wide open and Lip[s] not sealed." He supposed there was nothing "to do but await developments. It is rather a queer situation for me to be getting a Nurse for a Nurse, and being out of it myself. However Miss Mahoney attends to all my needs and I can get along."[4]

After six weeks or so at Sunnyrest, Macklin had apparently achieved

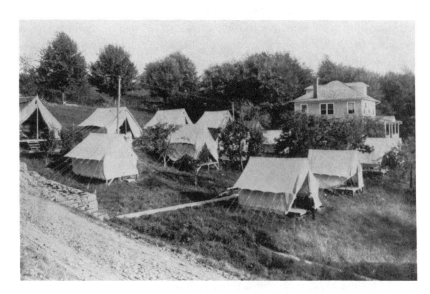

Figure 30. Tents at Sunnyrest Sanatorium. From Guy Hinsdale, *Atmospheric Air in Relation to Tuberculosis* (Washington, D.C.: Smithsonian Institution, 1914) but dated 1904 by its appearance, in part, in *Souvenir of Sunnyrest Sanatorium*, in Flick's Pamphlet Collection.

his main goal, and by late June it was time to move on. He and his wife found a place for the summer about seventy miles east of Pittsburgh—closer to home and closer to work. "We have located at Ebensburg with head quarters at above Hotel," he wrote from Maple Park Springs on July 7; "have tents some distance away from house. and think am going to be comfortable. . . . It certainly is a beautiful place and I think cooler than White Haven." He had "not gained any in weight the last week. probably due to Traveling about so much. but otherwise am feeling all right."[5]

C. J. Hunt, now recovered from his sore throat, accompanied Macklin to Ebensburg. "His stomach is in a fair condition," Hunt reported on July 11, referring to Macklin's difficulty in tolerating his milk and eggs. "Rales are audible 12 inches from his body. . . . He raises a great deal of sputum." On July 7, Hunt had decreased Macklin's exercise because of a rise in temperature, and the next day had advised him to discontinue it altogether. The fever lingered, however, and by July 20 Macklin had developed some soreness in his left chest and a rasping sensation in his throat. Nausea and belching persisted even though he had discontinued his six o'clock eggs.

"What he wants especially is relief for his stomach," wrote Hunt. "I have used salts and it gives us results. Then I should like to be of some use in controlling his temperature. Europhen is rubbed in each morning and night; the right side is dry cupped every other night; the left, twice each week; iodine is used each night."[6]

Over the next two weeks, Macklin began to feel "better and Stronger" and resumed his exercise. At the same time, he dismissed his nurse. "I was getting very little service from him," he explained to Flick; "outside of the rubbing at night and morning I saw very little of him. a little to[o] much Golf, Base Ball, and Girl for the Boy. He is a nice young man and will come out all right, when he gets into the world and has some of the Edges knocked off. But just now I had no time to train anyone." Macklin felt pleased with Hunt's replacement. "I have my Old Valet from Pittsburg who is doing all my rubbing cup[p]ing and everything Hunt did and so much more that I am as comfortable as a fellow could be. away from Business."[7]

Through the late summer and early fall, Macklin's condition improved gradually, and he eased himself back into the business that meant so much to him—a directors' meeting in New York, for example, and occasional trips to Pittsburgh. He faithfully continued his regimen, however, and assured Flick that he was remaining obedient. "I want you to feel that I am ready at all times to do your bidding," he wrote on August 21, "and you only have to say what you think and I will be with you."[8]

By mid-October, Macklin had returned home to Pittsburgh. Although he presumably worked regularly, he kept up his treatment. "I am sleeping out doors, on the porch, and taking the open air as much as possible," he reported on October 19. "When the mornings are foggy . . . I pay no attention to it and go right out into it. . . . I notice no serious results from this excepting when we have had two or three mornings in succession my pipes will play a little tune." As the cold weather intensified, the rigors of sleeping outdoors increased. "These nights are a bit crisp on a fellow's nose," he noted on November 25. "If you know of a good asbestos covering would be glad to have you advise me." By the end of December, Macklin had had enough of the cold. "If you don't mind, I would also like to have an alternative prescription for sleeping out of doors," he requested of Flick. "It is pretty cold out here—snow, and the wind *blows*, and last night the wind blew my slippers away and I had to go into the house through the snow in my bare feet! Do you call this humane treatment? Kindly advise." Flick consented to his sleeping indoors as long as he kept his bedroom windows open.[9]

Early in January 1904, Macklin's temperature rose and a pain appeared in his left side, which he recognized as his "old friend, pleurisy." He painted his side with iodine, and when that failed to help he tried an "anti-flugistine jacket"—a kind of plaster especially fitted for the chest. This "pulled it all out," but his fever continued. Flick assured him that he had "done exactly the right thing" by staying in bed and suggested putting "a fly-blister over the same place because there still may be a little pleurisy there and perhaps some effusion." Flick worried, however, that Macklin was overdoing. "You probably have been a little too active recently because you have felt well," he cautioned, "and it may be that you have started up an activity of your disease by overexertion. It makes me nervous every time I see you go to New York because I realize you are taking a great risk." He recommended that Macklin stay in bed "until the activity that is going on has subsided," even if it took a few weeks. "The little storm will blow over," he added reassuringly, "and you will be none the worse for it."[10]

Flick was correct for a time. By late February, Macklin had improved sufficiently to resume his usual activities and, despite occasional "colds" and other relatively minor flare-ups, felt optimistic. He persisted diligently with his treatment, even increasing the quantities of oil so that he now had it rubbed into his whole body, not just into his armpits and thighs. "It takes a lot of it," he reported resolutely on June 1, "and I have slept in the hot Summer nights with better things than a skin full of grease, but, they tell me that a fellow with a 'busted lung' is up against it and he has either got to knock the lung out or [it] will knock him out, and I think I have got it by the tail and on the run down the hill and I want to keep it on the run."[11]

Even a therapeutic mishap could neither daunt Macklin's spirits nor reduce his confidence in his physician. "I did as I was told, as I usually do, and put on a fly-blister," he related to Flick on June 21; "as a result I am now minus, over the top of my right lung four by five inches of skin, and the surface very much resembles porterhouse steak." Attempting to carry out Flick's directions, Macklin had "left the plaster on about an hour and a half, and then substituted hot towels." Perhaps he had left the plaster or the towels on too long, he acknowledged; "I don't know which,—only I know I got a hole burned in me." Because Flick now wanted him to use a fly-blister once a week, "I would be glad to know where you want to take the next piece of skin off; or, if you can kindly tell me wherein I erred in putting this one on, I will try one more, but, I will promise you if it makes me as sore as this one you will have to change your prescription. Otherwise, I am feeling tip top."[12]

Through the early summer of 1904, Macklin continued to do reason-

ably well and even took a pleasure trip. During the first days of August, however, his temperature rose again, the pain in his side returned, and his sputum doubled in volume to about five ounces a day. Although he had previously traveled to Philadelphia at regular intervals to see Flick in his office,
this time he had a different suggestion. "If you think you should look me
over, and can do so," he wrote, "I should be glad to have you come out."[13]

Flick saw no immediate necessity for such a trip, but thought that he
might need to see Macklin before allowing him to to get up. "I would have
to charge you five hundred dollars to go to Pittsburg," he added, "and
whilst I know that you would not object at all to this fee I do not wish to
put you to this expense unless there is very good reason." Instead, he
enclosed a prescription and offered an explanation for Macklin's symptoms.
"I think you have had a small spot of softening and emptying out," Flick
suggested. "In a way it is a good thing for you because you are thereby
getting rid of microorganisms which are much better out than in." "You are
right in supposing that the Money End would cut no figure," Macklin
replied on August 7. "I depend intirely [*sic*] on you, I have no other Doctor
and it is up to you to come and see me, or have me Come to you whenever
you think best."[14]

Three days later, a new note of urgency appeared in Macklin's correspondence. His temperature had gone "up like a Sky Rocket to 100 $^2/_5$,"
and "I cant understand why I cant get better control of this thing. . . . My
Judgment is you are not going to get me well, until you find something to
shoot into me that will either Kill or Cure." By this time Flick was tenta-
tively planning to "run out during the latter part of this week," and Macklin
closed his letter with directions for the trip. "Phone or wire me . . . so I can
have my Coachman at Station to meet you. Get off train at East Liberty,
and Come to House for Breakfast." Flick visited Macklin as planned,
apparently reinforcing his instructions as to bed rest and intensifying his
effort to keep the patient's bowel movements properly loose through the
use of powders and Epsom salts.[15]

While Macklin coped with the treatment in reasonably good spirits, he
also had to contend with critical commentary from his friends. "I am
enclosing a picture of your friend [Doctor] Anderson at Colorado Springs,
who always take[s] great pleasure in hitting your treatment a rap," he wrote
on August 19, shortly after Flick's visit.

> I had quite an article sent me by one of my friends . . . in which Anderson took
> pleasure in giving you a good roasting. All my friends in the West seem to
> think that this is the sort of information to send to me. I am quite sure they feel
> that I am dying in slow stages in this Eastern country. They all think I ought to

be back in the dry country. I tell them one might as well be dead as to live out in that country, so it doesn't make much difference whether you die a slow death here or live a long time out there. The only thing I kick about is that your rules are so rigid that while I am doing this dying I cannot have a good time. I wish you would hurry up and fix that dose that will kill or cure so that I can once more get out and look around with the boys.[16]

"I am glad Brother Anderson is having some fun at my expense," Flick responded on August 23. "In regard to yourself I think it would be advisable for you to go to a sanatorium. . . . The fatigue which you gave yourself when you made that wonderful trip is going to tell against you for sometime and the quickest way to get over it is to go away from everybody and shut yourself up in retreat." After commenting on Macklin's hard breathing and rapid pulse, Flick returned to this theme. "I think you had better just pack up traps and come East and perhaps go to Miss O'Hara's private sanatorium at Mt. Airy, where I can see you more frequently so that I can have you under both close observation and complete control." When Macklin submitted his next report but failed to mention a sanatorium, Flick pressed his point. "I fear you do not realize how much energy you use up at home because it seems so easy to you to transact your business over the telephone and to pass judgment on various matters," he cautioned. "You must not forget that mental occupation burns up tissue very rapidly and that when you pass judgment even . . . while in bed you are using up energy which had better be saved. I would like you to consider seriously . . . going to a sanatorium."[17]

Macklin, however, had other ideas. "I don't want you to think that I have put your letters aside without thought," he wrote on August 27, "nor to have you think. that I feel that I Know better than you, for such is not the Case." He was feeling "as usual Fine. in every way," even though his evening temperature was still a little elevated. He had given a great deal of thought to the idea of going away for a time and "tried to see everything from all sides." Now he proposed a plan of his own.

You Know men go to war and make themselves liable to come back Dead. they take this chance for their Country   Why should we not take some chances for the future comfort of our Families. If I had no one but myself to consider I would not stop a moment. I hope you understand just what I mean. I will tell you in confidence for my Family do not know, that my aim now is to get my affairs in such shape by next Summer if I live that long. So I can give up all active Business and settle Down quietly. I think I understand my condition. I will never be a strong man again and even if I get comparatively well will always have to exercise care. I am not made up of the stuff to stay in business and not have my hand into everything. I know my failings well. If I went away now to a Sanatorium for a month Say it would only give Temporary relief. If I was to stay longer the worry about how my business was going and not knowing would be worse for me than trying to plug along here   I know myself so well. and I must get out of Business alltogether before [I] can give up thinking about it. and unless you see some real Danger of my going all to Pieces I would like to see if I cant fight it out here a while longer. I only allow the office to call me twice a Day and then only when important and am really not under much Mental Strain. just now. I have written you at length, and trust the Reading of it won't Bore you.[18]

"I appreciate your position and sympathize with you in the attitude which you take," Flick responded on August 30.

If you fully understand matters and are willing to take some risk I can see no reason for my opposing you in the matter. I think I would probably do as you are doing if I were in your place. I do not think that the risk you are taking is very great but nevertheless it is a risk and as your physician it is my duty to warn you against it. So far as I am able to judge I am inclined to think that you will come out all right under existing circumstances if you will persevere in the methods which you are now pursuing. You will appreciate that I cannot be sure of my position here and that if you want to be on the safe side you should do as I suggested in my former letter. However, I am willing to help you as things are and to give you all the protection that I know how.[19]

Flick's letter crossed in the mail with another from Macklin, who was now responding to an earlier request for a urine specimen. "I am sending you By Express today Box Containing Sample you asked for," he wrote; "when you see the size of the Box. Dont think some one has sent you a Baby Grand Piano."[20]

Events in September and early October underlined the uncertainties that Flick had acknowledged, and prompted continuing negotiations between physician and patient. Early in September, Macklin's temperature sailed up to 102 degrees—higher than he could remember. If he were to go to Philadelphia for three or four weeks, he wondered if Flick could "get a line on me" that would help "to pull me out of this knockout." Flick countered by repeating his proposal to go to Mt. Airy, but no action was taken. Later in the month, Macklin made an appointment to see Flick in his office but canceled it two days later when he did not feel up to the travel. By October, discussion focused on a new possibility—a trip to Italy, where Macklin might be treated with Maragliano's new serum. Flick consulted with Dr. Ravenel, who had recently returned from Maragliano's laboratory, and counseled against the journey. "As yet the whole matter is too unsettled to warrant you in making such a trip in your present condition," he wrote to Macklin on October 14. "If you would like to try the treatment I think it would be much wiser for us to give it to you here. A new sanatorium has been opened at Glenside in which there are as yet no patients. It is beautifully situated and would give you pretty nearly as much privacy as your own home." If Macklin would go there, Dr. Ravenel could give the injections and Flick himself would keep "a close watch" on him. "The three months rest which you would have to take in the sanatorium would do you a great deal of good independent of what you might gain from the serum. By this method you would risk nothing and would be certain of gaining a great deal."[21]

Macklin agreed immediately. "Get Juice ready," he wired on October 15; "kindly make necessary arrangements for me at Glenside   will arrive about twenty seventh." Two days later, Macklin confirmed his decision by letter. "I want to get into this thing this time and get the full limit. If there is anything in it I want to know it and I presume you do. Of course I do not want to take any more time than is necessary . . . but whatever it is we will stay to the finish. I am extremely anxious to find out whether I am ever to be a man, three-fourths of a man, one-half a man or one-quarter of a man, and when I do learn this I can lay my plans for the future." Flick, responding to some of Macklin's questions, told him to expect injections "every second or third day or perhaps less frequently according to circumstances." During the three months required for treatment, "you will be expected to keep perfectly quiet at the sanatorium and to be no man at all. Business will be a closed book to you so that it is well for you to make provision for a three month's leave."[22]

Macklin settled into the sanatorium at Glenside, where his initial impressions were highly favorable. He worried about Mrs. Wilson's lack of patients, however, not only because of the implications for the sanatorium's business but also because of what he called his own "Selfish" point of view. "If I have to stay here for two or three months," he explained on November 5, "I want it good. If you could get us about three or four men who are Fairly good Poker Players and with Some Money to loose [sic] I think we can winter it out all right."[23]

Already getting restless, he was pushing to start on ten minutes of daily exercise, but Flick held firm and kept him in bed. Ravenel administered the injections, Macklin's attendant rubbed him and gave him cold showers, and, although the patient's pulse rate stayed troublesomely high, his temperature fell to normal. All this treatment, reported Macklin on December 5, "makes me feel like offering to Fight Corbett." He pressed for permission to go home for Christmas. "I don't want you to misunderstand my Idea," he begged on December 14. "It is not for a good time such as I might have if well. But only to be with my little Family   we have asked no one to be with us this year. and will be very quiet." Macklin outlined his plan for the trip to Pittsburgh. "I have no intention of going to my Office or trying any business whatever," he promised. "Have been in Bed two months and its Hell."[24]

Macklin spent Christmas at home, but returned to Glenside shortly thereafter. Early in January 1905, he developed a discouraging "cold" with fever and foul-tasting sputum, which Flick interpreted as "the breaking down and coughing away" of another nodule, but Macklin's spirits rebounded as his symptoms diminished and the weather improved. He had developed some new ideas about his future. "I really meant what I said the other Day about going South for a month," he wrote from the porch at Glenside, apologizing for the pencil and explaining that ink would freeze. "Should I go to a Place on Sea Coast or keep back from it." He had a second question that he wanted to discuss at Flick's leisure. "Now put yourself in my Place and tell me if you were going to Buy a Farm or Place to settle down in for a couple of years where would you go." Macklin wanted "to get hold of something that would give me something to do. to sit around a Sanatorium or Hotel and do nothing is out of my line. Do you think if I should do something of this kind I could shake my Cough and trouble in a Couple of years and be Something of my old self again." He expected Mrs. Macklin to pass through Philadelphia on the following Sunday, when he would spend a few hours with her at the Bellevue Stratford Hotel, and hoped he could drop into Flick's office on Monday morning.[25]

Whatever the nature of their conversation, Macklin decided to go south and on January 27 he arrived in Camden, a town in the sand hills of South Carolina where the porous subsoil and the surrounding pine trees had been touted for their healthful effects. Macklin found satisfactory quarters on the top floor of the Kirkwood Hotel for both himself and his nurse, Charles Bacher. "I feel first rate," he reported on February 7; "am getting more exercise   have big Porch to take it on about 300 ft. long. Dont think am raising quite so much [sputum]." He was continuing his treatment, including Maragliano's serum. Although the weather had been poor, Macklin thought Camden a good place—"nothing here but good Hotel[,] Pile of Sand. and Pine Trees." He was still thinking of the future.

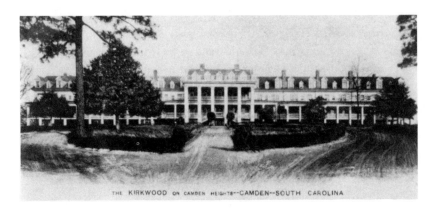

THE KIRKWOOD ON CAMDEN HEIGHTS--CAMDEN--SOUTH CAROLINA

Figure 31. The Kirkwood Hotel, Camden, South Carolina. Macklin's room on the top floor can be identified by the dormer window on the far right of this photo. Courtesy of William Davie Beard.

"I have about made up mind to stay in Country and not go back to work this summer," he noted. "I may go into New England. I wish you would tell me what Altitude I Can stand."[26]

The next report on Macklin's condition came not from the patient but from Charles Bacher. "This afternoon at 5. PM.," he wrote on February 16, "Mr. Macklin was taken with one of his coughing spell[s] . . . this evening he had a hemorrhage of a bright red blood, and was coughed up mouth full at a time, and was somewhat thick and measured about four ounzes." Bacher injected his patient with one hundredth of a grain of nitroglycerine, gave him ice chips to suck, had him "lie flat on his back, and placed a rubber bag of cold water on chest." By 8:00 P.M., Bacher continued, Mr. Macklin was "feeling very good," but at 8:30 P.M. he had another hemorrhage of about six ounces, and Bacher sent for help. Dr. Jno. W. Corbett, a Camden physician, arrived at about 8:45 and left orders for morphine, atropine, ergot, and nitroglycerine should the bleeding recur. "Mr. Macklin said to tell you he is not worried," added Bacher in a postscript, "but is in good spirits."[27]

Flick, reflecting the medical belief that fear itself exacerbated a hemorrhage, responded soothingly to Macklin. "I have Mr. Bacher's letter telling me of your experiences," he wrote on February 18. "The hemorrhage does not mean very much. I would suggest that you remain in bed for a few days and go on a light diet." He suggested stopping the serum injections for a while, and also the creosote. "If the hemorrhage keeps up take the nitro-glycerine but I think perhaps you had better not take the ergot."[28]

A second letter, which Flick started to write on February 20, showed greater concern. "I have been thinking matters over carefully and it seems to me that you had better return North and go back to Glenside or some place near me until your present little upset is over," he suggested. "It is of some importance that you be steered through this difficulty with great care and I am therefore solicitous about you. Evidently there is some softening going on or else you have overexerted yourself and in either event I would like to know exactly what it is."[29]

Meanwhile, anxieties mounted in Camden. On February 19, Macklin asked Bacher to write a second letter to Flick. The patient's temperature had risen that day to 103°, Bacher observed, his pulse to 132. He had had a "nervous attack" with heavy breathing at 2:30 A.M., and then a second in the afternoon. At 4:00 P.M. he had coughed up another five ounces of blood clot. He looked a little cyanosed, as Bacher described his bluish color, and his eyes looked dull. Dr. Corbett had ordered nitroglycerine and ergot to be given every four hours as long as the patient was awake, and if the nervous breathing continued Bacher was to give a quarter grain of mor-phine and $1/150$ grain of atropine "broken in half and given by hypo." Mr. Macklin "just asked me to write you and say he is worried," Bacher con-cluded, "because the blood does not seem to stop. Waiting to hear from you." "Have you received our letter," wired Elizabeth Macklin on February 20, unable to wait another day for a reply; "can you wire advise." Flick responded immediately. Bacher's second letter had arrived before Flick's letter of February 20 could be mailed, and the doctor added a postscript: "have telegraphed to stop atropine, morphine and ergot and to give Epsom Salts. Do not worry about the hemorrhage. You are safer with it going on than with stopping [it] by drugs."[30]

Flick's recommendations as to Macklin's drugs revealed some sharp differences in medical opinion concerning the treatment of pulmonary hemorrhage. He absolutely disagreed with Corbett's therapeutic program. When the physician described his decisions to Flick on February 21, Flick gave him his blunt opinion. "Your treatment is certainly not in line with modern therapeutics of tuberculosis," Flick replied on February 23. "The damaged heart which you speak of is undoubtedly due to the drugs . . . and not to the disease. Calomel, morphia and ergot and even atropia are exceedingly dangerous drugs to use in tuberculosis and should be used only for a most positive indication and with the greatest care." Flick urged that the drugs be discontinued and that "a half dram or even a dram of sulphate of magnesia" be given hourly instead until a "free purging from the bowels" was achieved. This "will relieve the tension on the circulation," Flick explained, "and you will stop both the hemorrhage and the bad heart action." If Mr. Macklin could be "kept quiet and fed properly in the open air with his excretory organs active he may pull through." On the day of his letter to Dr. Corbett, Flick also sent a letter to Mrs. Macklin in which he termed Corbett's treatment "exceedingly old-fashioned" and recommended that she call either of two experts in tuberculosis "even though you have to send quite a distance."[31]

The medical conflict put Mrs. Macklin in a quandary. Mr. Macklin expressed the "utmost faith" in Dr. Corbett, she related on February 26, and to read to her husband Flick's letter was "entirely out of the question, for I cannot agitate him, in any way." To send for a doctor from elsewhere "would be such a surprise to him, and possibly a set back," that she could not think of it. Bacher had told her, moreover, that Dr. Corbett was "gradually doing everything that you have ordered," and Mr. Macklin was "very much improved." Although the climate in Camden was "the most perfect thing you ever beheld," she promised to use her influence to get him north just as soon as it was advisable. "I shall be glad when he is safe back with you," she concluded, "but wish you knew how beautiful this weather is here." Mollified by Macklin's improvement, Flick withdrew his recommendation for a new doctor, and the turmoil quieted down.[32]

On March 12, Macklin began to write again for himself. He puzzled over the reasons for his hemorrhage but could draw no conclusions. He thought that Dr. Corbett had "done what he could in his way for me," but guessed that "I had them all pretty well scared when they could not stop the Bleeding for so long. I hope that when the thing is over you will find that I am better for it and that I have lost a lot of old rotten lung." He was full of questions: "What chance is there for another [hemorrhage?]. What must I look out for? What can [I] do to stop the little leak going on now? Will it hurt me to be up on Porch?" He thought he would stay in Camden until the middle of April.[33]

Despite some continued bleeding, he was feeling "good" on March 15 and "would like to get out in Sun on Porch. . . . My room and Bed are very tiresome." He had also been "planning a little for the Summer," he confided to Flick. "When I get out of this trouble and am in shape. I shall come North probably about last of April or first of May   I have my Eye on 2 Farms one up at Ebensburg and the other up in the Berkshire[s]   I have made up my mind to give up business and am now going to see what [I]

Can do. with no Cares. Fresh Air. and good Food. The Farm I have in Mind has all the Modern Improvements, Bath. and everything and about 1400 ft. Altitude. What do you think of Plan. let me know. I am going to Clean out the Barn and rub down the Horses for a while."[34]

Flick responded carefully to Macklin's concerns. From the charts he had received from Bacher, he thought that Macklin was "doing very well." The hemorrhage would have been less severe if Macklin had been less nervous about it. Should he get another, he should not be frightened by it, nor should he tie up his system with opiates. The blood he was spitting up was probably "mere oozing from an ulceration" and would "no doubt cease in the near future." The quieter Macklin could keep the better, but yes, he could sit on the porch. "As to your going on a farm I think it would be a very good plan. I do not believe that it would make much difference whether you went to Ebensburg or . . . the Berkshires. What you want is an easy quiet life and the place which will give you this is the place which you ought to have."[35]

Macklin was grateful for Flick's attention. "Just staying quiet and letting things take their course," he responded on March 18. "It is now four weeks since I had my first bleeding and over two since the last bad one. still I keep up a Sputum that is over half blood. . . . I must be good and rotten inside   I am getting so tired of the taste of Blood." He felt an increasing urgency about moving north. "This Hotel and in fact the whole Town closes up about the 15th of next month," he explained. "I must be in shape to move by then. I am anxious to hear what you think of my Farm life and if 1400 ft. is to[o] high. I know you are a very busy man. But I am a very lonesome one so write me."[36]

Another hemorrhage shattered the quiet dialogue. Bacher reported it on the very day that Macklin had written his last letter. It was not the hemorrhage that now bothered Bacher; it was who had control of the patient—the nurse or the wife. "It has annoyed me greatly for the last month because there is no sick room rule here," he complained, "and I have no authority but am expected to be under Mrs. Macklin's authority. You have supported me in saying Mr. Macklin must have rest and quiet. But frequently Mrs. M. insists on my leaving the room 'as she knows very well how to care for him.'" Mrs. Macklin, in Bacher's judgment, however, did not behave in her husband's best interests.

When I return I find that she is either in his bed, or demonstrating her affections, and expressing her pity for him, so that he would unconsciously derive some bad effects from it in his present condition. If I suggest anything, then I find myself guilty of making her angry and perhaps find her foot planted heavily on the floor to show what I have done.

On two occasions she was so loud and talkative that Dr. Corbett had to call her attention to it, and mention that the patient must have quiet.

Then again if I must give opiates, I do not want anything preventing quiet and sleep.

Not only is this bad for the patient but an insult to me.[37]

Mrs. Macklin's behavior, according to Bacher, threatened the very core of his obligations as a nurse. "It is my duty to honor, by my management of sick room, the Doctors and Sisters by whom I was trained. And not yield to the authority of a patient's relatives or their kindness. I forgot to say," he added disapprovingly, "that every morning Mrs. Macklin has the patient help her look over advertisements and letters, for a farm. This is a couple hours work." Bacher hoped that somehow Flick could intervene. "It has not been [my] desire to tell family tales," he concluded, "but to know, what is right, for my patient and myself. Hoping that what I have betrayed will bring forth good, and not regret."[38]

At such a distance from the scene, Flick either could not or would not take sides in the conflict. "I would be very glad if you could have Mr. Macklin back to Mrs. Wilson's so that I could have him under my immediate supervision and control," he replied to Bacher on March 20. "As it is I can do nothing but give advice in a very general way." He had just made the same suggestion to Mr. Macklin, he reported, and he thought that the patient would come north as soon as he could. "Meanwhile," Flick noted, "you will have to do the best you can."[39]

For the next ten days, Macklin did fairly well. He had no further bleeding, but when he did raise sputum it tasted "awful" and Mrs. Macklin noted that "the smell was horrible." On the evening of March 29, he experienced "something of a chill" but slept well through most of the night. At 5 A.M. on March 30, however, he coughed "dreadfully" and had a "terrible hemorrhage of sixteen ounces—with syanotic [*sic*] condition." Mrs. Macklin thought he was going to die. By noon, surprisingly, he rallied and asked Mrs. Macklin to tell Flick that he wanted a house near him this summer where Flick could see him each week. Mrs. Macklin realized that her husband's condition was "most grave." She planned to send her little girl and governess back to Pittsburgh that evening, and had asked her brother-in-law to come to Camden. "Now, doctor, can't we arrange, if he rallies from this to bring him north in a private car?" she asked. "Really—I think the personal effect you would have on him, would do him the greatest amount of good." Flick concurred in a letter on April 3. "I have sent an experienced nurse down this afternoon who I think will probably be able to help you quite a good deal," he wrote. "Tell Mr. Macklin to keep up his courage and try hard to get back home."[40]

Dr. Charles L. Minor, a well-known specialist from Asheville, North Carolina, examined Macklin on April 5 and 6. He "found a man of good nourishment, with a lemon anaemic face, slightly bloated, with a respiration of from 30 to 34 and not under 24 for some time; with a pulse of from 140 to 160 and not below 120 for a long time; with a septic temperature and greatly prostrated." The patient was "raising a large quantity (probably 12 ounces a day), of sanguino purulent matter with apparently much pulmonary detritus in it." It was "very offensive." Although the patient's weakness and the risk of recurrent hemorrhage prevented Minor from examining him as completely as he would have liked, he could give a fairly complete report on the chest and abdomen. He found "a large excavation in the middle and lower portions of the posterior part of the left lung," and below this "absolute flatness" which he attributed to the consolidation of pneumonia. There was "much breaking down in the upper anterior portion of the same lung." The front and back of the right lung also showed signs of involvement, with "broncho vesicular breath [sounds] and fine dry crepitations" but no evidence of cavitation. The stomach was "dilated to a fingers length below the umbilicus . . . apparently due to the effects of the morphia." Although Minor considered the outlook "utterly hopeless," he thought the risk of moving the patient was no greater than that of his staying in Camden. He advised Mrs. Macklin "to take him North as soon as she could get a private car."[41]

Mrs. Macklin wired Dr. Minor's recommendations to Flick. Dr. Corbett agreed to accompany the patient to Philadelphia, and Mrs. Macklin requested that, whatever arrangements were made, Mr. Bacher be allowed to continue with her husband. She would leave to Flick the selection of the proper place for care, but she had one suggestion: "that it not be at the Wilson's because Mr. Macklin suffered such depression there. I do not wish in any way to dictate, but where people are suffering and groaning around him, he suffers with them." She herself, she reported, was not losing hope. "I gave Mr. Macklin your message to keep up his courage," she noted in closing, "and when he found he could go—he looked up and said 'Well, I will soon see "papa Flick" won't I?' "[42]

Macklin arrived safely in Philadelphia on April 8. He "is now resting quietly in one of the hospitals here," Flick reported to Dr. Minor two days later, but after the tenth of April the correspondence ceased. On June 26, 1905, George E. Macklin died in St. Joseph's Hospital. In 1887, some lines of William Shakespeare had been quoted at the annual meeting of the American Climatological Association. The two contrasting views that they expressed still had relevance. "The miserable have no other medicine, but only hope," Claudio observed. The duke responded:

> thou are death's fool;
> For him thou labor'st by thy flight to shun,
> And yet run'st toward him still.[43]

Relatively few well-to-do men such as Macklin died of tuberculosis. In 1900, bankers, brokers, and officials of companies as a group had the lowest mortality rate in the United States—92.5 out of 100,000 living persons. Toward the other end of the socioeconomic spectrum, servants, hat and cap makers, clerks, bookkeepers, and nonagricultural laborers died at more than quadruple this rate.[44] For these men and women and others like them, there were no resorts, no private nurses, and no physicians willing to travel long distances to take care of them. During the first decade of the twentieth century, however, visiting nurses began to see a role for themselves in the care of such people. They thought they could help and instruct the consumptive poor and even save some of the sick and their families from death.

13. Into the Homes, Minds, and Lives of the Poor: Visiting Nurses

Throughout the nineteenth century, a number of well-to-do women tried to alleviate the plight of the poor. As individuals or in groups, they sought to guide the less fortunate morally, uplift and teach them, and aid them in material ways. The Visiting Nurse Society of Philadelphia, like similar organizations that began to appear in U.S. cities in the 1880s, was part of this effort. In these societies, the women worked through others—trained nurses who brought comfort, cleanliness, and personal care into the homes of the sick poor and helped them to follow the doctors' advice. During the early twentieth century, the nurses themselves began to emerge from their initial status as mere employees to become the visible leaders of the movement. Among them was Mabel Jacques, the first tuberculosis nurse for the Visiting Nurse Society of Philadelphia.[1]

Comparison of the nurses' work for poor consumptives and the clergymen's work at the Protestant Episcopal City Mission illuminates the changes over the span of a generation. The clergymen of the 1880s were struggling against moral decay and social disorder, the nurses against ignorance and disease. The clergymen preached religious beliefs; the nurses taught how to apply the concepts of science. When the clergymen found consumptives living in destitute environments deemed morally harmful, they arranged for care in an institution where the patients could get both physical necessities and religious guidance. When nurses found their tuberculous patients in hopelessly unsanitary conditions and when the patients did not take the recommended precautions, the nurses urged admission to sanatoriums and hospitals; there, patients could be further instructed and kept safely away from others.

The clergymen and the nurses were also much alike. Although the work was becoming more secular, both groups had moral convictions and goals: they were trying to help the sick poor and improve society at the same time. Both thought their work very important, if exhausting at times as they tramped through the city streets. Both had faith in their guiding principles and both, as they gained experience, increasingly turned to institutions as the way to solve their problems. Mabel Jacques, like the Reverend Durburow before her, found herself holding a minority position. Although preserving families and transforming the homes of the poor into clean, safe, and healthful environments persisted in the goals of the Visiting Nurse Society of Philadelphia, the drive toward institutionalization had greater momentum.

Flick was surely aware of the Visiting Nurse Society's activities. The organization's founder was a charter member of the Pennsylvania Society for the Prevention of Tuberculosis, and articles by or about Mabel Jacques are preserved in his scrapbooks. Visiting nurses, however, rarely appeared in his correspondence or publications, and he gave no apparent support to their tuberculosis work. His lack of interest probably had several explanations. By 1907, when Jacques accepted her new post, Flick was becoming discouraged by what nurses at the Phipps Institute could accomplish in patients' homes. Practicing physicians, moreover, had little organizational contact with visiting nurses. While this very independence from medicine gave nurses room to develop their own role in patient care, it also isolated them from physicians. Visiting nurses, who needed physicians to refer patients to them and to consult with them periodically, sometimes complained of the apathy, uncooperativeness, or frank opposition demonstrated by members of the medical profession. Some physicians, especially those who practiced among the poor and working classes, may have seen the visiting nurse as a competitor. Flick, a busy specialist who saw few poor patients in his office by 1907, would have felt little need for her services. He prided himself on his own teaching abilities, and preferred relationships that he clearly controlled.[2]

Origins of the Visiting Nurse for Tuberculosis

Nine years before Flick and Father Scully formed the Free Hospital for Poor Consumptives, Mrs. William F. Jenks, a young widow from a prominent family in Philadelphia, started her own organization to bring comfort and care to the poor of the city. The concept of organized nursing for the poor in their own homes had originated in England in 1859. In February 1886, Mrs. Jenks heard of the work from an English visitor and felt a "'great enthusiasm at once.'" Familiar with the needs of the poor from her own observations, she turned for help to other philanthropic and well-to-do women, among them the "'rich and generous'" Mrs. Henry C. Lea and several women who were "'intimately connected with the Charity Organization'" and "'deeply interested in public welfare and education.'" With one hundred dollars and a secondhand table that had cost fifty cents, the women opened an office in a back room on Sixth Street on March 1, 1886, and hired a nurse to do the practical work.[3]

The little society had a difficult beginning. It had no official connection with a source of patients, and potential donors balked at the very idea of nursing the poor. "'Why give money to a scheme for over-indulging those who could not possibly continue to pay for the luxury?'" Day after day, however, Mrs. Jenks and a colleague "'trudged about to charitable societies, to doctors, to philanthropic friends,'" and slowly gathered a clientele of patients together with money, supplies, equipment, and nurses to give the care. In 1887, the organization was incorporated as The Visiting Nurse Society of Philadelphia.[4]

By 1895, the Society's staff had grown to eleven nurses, the annual number of nursing visits to 13,748, and the year's expenditures to $8,280. The annual report early that year articulated the goals and methods of the organization. "The Society employs a corps of trained nurses who take care of such patients as absolutely need attention, who are obliged to remain in their homes, and who cannot afford to pay for the full time of a trained nurse." The nurses "visit from house to house (working under any doctor) bathing, bandaging, poulticing, making the patient's bed, taking the temperature, keeping the doctor informed" of the patient's condition. The visits, the women felt sure, were "of inestimable value." They "not only give comfort, often health and life itself to the actual sufferer, but afford to whole families a practical lesson in cleanliness and hygiene." Examples of patients who benefited from these womanly ministrations dotted the annual reports for years.[5]

Numerically, consumptives were not an important part of the nurses' work, nor did their needs warrant particular kinds of attention. Between early 1888 and early 1908, only about 1 to 4 percent of the cases visited had this disease. In the 1890s, the Society classified phthisis among "chronic complaints," along with cancer, rheumatism, old age, and paralysis. A nurse could provide comfort and care for such cases, but there was no special treatment and little hope of recovery. Maternity cases, "sudden and acute illnesses," such as typhoid fever and pneumonia, and "diseases of dirt and neglect," such as bedsores, all competed for her attentions. In 1900, when the city reported that 2,717 persons had died of consumption of the lungs, the Society counted only 50 consumptives among its cases.[6]

A gradual shift in medical thinking changed the relative complacency with which the Society's leaders and nurses viewed the care of consumptives. Flick, arguing for the contagiousness of phthisis as early as 1888, pointed to the house as the source of infection, and by the early 1900s this opinion was gaining support. When William Osler gave his much publicized lecture at the Henry Phipps Institute in 1903, he reemphasized Flick's thesis. "In its most important aspects the problem of tuberculosis is a home problem," he asserted. "In an immense proportion of all cases the scene of the drama is the home; on its stage the acts are played, whether to the happy issue of a recovery, or the dark ending of a tragedy, so commonplace as to have dulled our appreciation of its magnitude." Estimating that fewer than 2 percent of the nation's consumptives could take advantage of sanatorium or climatic treatment, Osler found it inconceivable that society could provide accommodations for all of them. The "battlefield of tuberculosis is not in the hospitals or in the sanitaria," he declared, "but in the homes, where practically the disease is born and bred."[7]

By calling for war in the home—the center of a woman's domain—Osler was sending a challenge to women. Indeed, he had already sent some women medical students from Johns Hopkins into the homes of the poor to scout conditions there and give instruction. In 1900, Adelaide Dutcher, one of these students, identified the enemies that she had found in the slums of Baltimore: crowding, filth, darkness, lack of ventilation, appalling ignorance of the contagiousness of tuberculosis, and carelessness with infectious material. The patients and their families who did view the disease as communicable "live in deadly fear that they [might] transmit or contract [it]. . . . To such the information that elements of contagion are in the sputum, and can be destroyed, is heralded with gladness."[8]

Ruth B. Sherman, a graduate of the Johns Hopkins Training School, quickly saw the implications of Dutcher's report for nursing. "The students' work," she wrote in 1901, "is of most interest to nurses, as being exactly what we ourselves might do, and what we believe many nurses would be glad to do if the opportunity were given them. Such an opportunity . . . exists nowhere at present." While Sherman recognized that visiting nurses functioned to some extent in this way, she envisioned a more focused approach in which nurses could "carry on this special work regularly and systematically."[9]

Sherman's idea was slowly realized. In 1903, after Osler's students discontinued their visits, the Johns Hopkins Dispensary employed its first nurse to visit its tuberculous patients. At about the same time, the Charity

Organization Society and the City Health Department in New York City were also beginning to sponsor tuberculosis nurses. By early 1906, M. Adelaide Nutting, the influential superintendent of nurses and principal of the training school at the Johns Hopkins Hospital, could list at least thirty-two American women in this new field. Of these, two were pupils at the Phipps Institute. In the fervent, authoritarian language commonly used at the time when dealing with the poor, Nutting applauded the valuable work. "There must be a wide-spread, well-directed continuous effort to get into the homes, minds and lives of these people a knowledge of what they must do to be saved," she declared, "and the trained, paid worker is the one force for this purpose at present to be found or depended upon."[10]

In February 1906, the Visiting Nurse Society of Philadelphia reported its own interest in the work. The Phipps Institute reached only the patients from its own dispensary, observed Mrs. L. W. Quintard, head nurse of the Society, thus "leaving the great mass of the city's consumptives without either care or instruction." The Society had been given its first fifty dollars for the purpose, and the *North American* publicized its need for additional funds. "The Visiting Nurse Society aims to reach these neglected ones by going into their homes," reported the paper on July 29, 1906, "isolating them as far as possible from members of their family, supplying the proper diet and insisting on fresh air." Only by education could the spread of contagion be ended. "The Visiting Nurse Society is determined," noted the paper, foreshadowing one of the nurses' future problems, "that the poor shall be safeguarded in spite of themselves."[11]

Mabel Jacques and Her Work

On August 1, 1907, Miss Mabel Jacques started work as the Society's first tuberculosis nurse. Born of American parents in 1880, Jacques had graduated from the training school of the Hospital of the University of Pennsylvania in the class of 1903, and had joined the Visiting Nurse Society of Philadelphia in 1905. Like many others who joined the campaign against tuberculosis, she had had the disease herself. She had taken her treatment at the White Haven Sanatorium.[12]

The role that Jacques developed resembled for the most part the one described by leaders of the Phipps Institute. She and the tuberculosis nurses who followed her taught the precautions, the diet, and the best possible living arrangements; they watched families for symptoms; and they tried to persuade the sick to enter institutions or see their physicians as it seemed necessary. Their services as visiting nurses, however, differed from those of the Institute's pupil nurses in several ways. In keeping with their traditions, they gave personal care when it was needed. Many consumptives, to be sure, needed little actual nursing, and in more than a fourth of the cases the families themselves, once instructed, could assume responsibility, yet the nurses cared for 40 percent of their patients until they died. Many of these men and women had refused to enter institutions, Jacques reported, and could no longer "drag their weary way to a dispensary." The nurses' care was also more frequent than that provided by the Institute. Over the first four years of the work, their annual visits increased from ten to twenty per patient—roughly triple the number made by the pupil nurses. Further, the Society offered assistance to needy patients, and through gifts of its members and a loan closet it might supply clothing, bedding, outdoor shelter, and supplements of milk or food.[13]

Arrangements among various agencies helped to make such assistance possible. The Protestant Episcopal City Mission often provided milk, as did the city health department until around 1910, when it no longer had the money for it. Branches of the Needlework Guild of America contributed clothing; the Octavia Hill Association could sometimes find better housing for a family; convalescent homes for children took the pale, listless, or tubercular little ones for a few weeks at the seashore or in the country; and the health department fumigated dwellings after death. Knowledge of all these agencies and expertise in getting them to cooperate—the social phase of the work—helped to distinguish the visiting nurse from her hospital-based counterparts.[14]

Tuberculosis nursing itself depended in part on a fragile network of cooperating organizations. The Starr Centre Association, a settlement house in a predominantly Italian and black section of Philadelphia, helped to pay for the first few months of the work. In February 1908, Jacques accepted the nursing responsibilities for two tuberculosis classes—one at the Church of the Crucifixion, the congregation of which was black, and one at St. Stephen's Protestant Episcopal Church. The churches provided housing, and the Pennsylvania Society for the Prevention of Tuberculosis supplied physicians to lead the classes.[15]

A tuberculosis class tried to improve upon conventional dispensary treatment by establishing a closer physician-patient relationship; by instructing a relatively small group of patients together and using the interaction among them to facilitate learning, buoy morale, and reinforce discipline; and by supervising the patients' regimen at home more carefully than was otherwise possible. Joseph H. Pratt, a Boston physician, had initiated the method at the Emmanuel Church in Boston in 1905. Through complete bed rest, open-air treatment, careful record-keeping by the patients themselves, and strict obedience, he believed he was achieving a high proportion of cures.[16]

The success of tuberculosis work seemed to depend on the skills and aptitudes of the nurse. In addition to sound training, mental keenness, cheerfulness, and health, Jacques put adaptability, diplomacy, and resourcefulness on her list of qualifications. In homes of the poor, the visiting nurse lacked the equipment provided in hospitals and had to improvise with available materials. As in private duty, she had to adapt herself to patient and family. The visiting nurse also had to deal with immigrants with diverse customs; she had to become familiar with the "queer little ideas about living that are peculiar to the foreign element." She had to know, for example, "that in the orthodox Jewish home there is no fire lighted on the Jewish Sabbath by members of the family, and not [be] . . . surprised or annoyed if she is asked to make a fire herself, provided warm water is required for her work. She must learn to adjust the 'fasch' on the new-born Italian babe, lest the anxious mother worry about the straightness of her baby's arms and legs."[17]

Across the barriers of status, custom, language, and race, the tuberculosis nurse went into the homes of the poor to teach, help, and reorder their lives. The goal was ambitious, courageous, and in hindsight naive. In 1907, more than three thousand people in Philadelphia died of pulmonary tuberculosis, and by contemporary estimates more than nine thousand had the disease. Many of them were poor and foreign-born. These included the Russian Jews and the Italians—the groups who had arrived most recently in Philadelphia and were least accustomed to American ways. They also included the Irish, who among whites had the highest mortality rates from tuberculosis; only the blacks, many of whom had recently arrived from the South, died more frequently from the disease. In addition to the cultural barriers between patient and nurse, care and instruction were typically complicated by low income, crowded living conditions, inadequate ventilation, and insufficient or unwholesome food. It was a daunting task that faced the tiny band of women.[18]

To prevent the spread of tuberculosis and to care for these people, the visiting nurse had little equipment other than her knowledge, determination, caring skills, tact, and persuasion. Her organization was neither rich nor powerful. Her authority depended mainly on what she and her predecessors had earned through kindness, fulfillment of needs, relief of suffering, and efficacy of treatment. Her uniform, together perhaps with an emblem on her sleeve, could convey a sense of authority, but on occasion she found it wise not to display such symbols; they might create fear or betray a confidence. To strengthen her bargaining position with recalcitrant patients, the nurse could withhold services or withdraw material aid, but she usually used these measures as a last resort. They were the final steps in a losing effort to assert control.[19]

The visiting nurse, as Jacques described her work, needed all the skills that she could muster. "Again and again, in making her first visit to a patient, a nurse is received in anything but a friendly manner. . . . The work is usually among the very poorest of the city's poor, a large proportion of whom are foreigners, and these people are full of old superstitions regarding their particular disease, which must be overcome or the desired results cannot be obtained." To gain a patient's confidence, the nurse's approach had to be tactful and indirect: "Through interest in the children and in the little details of the family life the nurse gradually wins her way into the hearts of these poor people. And all the while, little by little, she is working for the ultimate end which she has in view."[20]

One of the cases that Jacques described to illustrate the nurse's methods involved a woman with advanced tuberculosis, referred to the Visiting Nurse Society by a general practitioner. He was "well meaning and kindly disposed," she observed with a touch of condescension or possibly scorn, "but not at all interested or believing in the present ideas of tuberculosis." The patient had a fever, and the doctor suggested that a bath and an alcohol rub might make her more comfortable. The woman lived with her family on a small alley.

> We find her in a stuffy little room, on the first floor of a threestory, threeroomed house, lying on a trundle bed, and despite the warmth of the day piled up with old quilts. On the floor two or three dirty, neglected children are playing with some broken toys. The one window is closed, the shutters barred and the room reeks with the characteristic odor peculiar to the tuberculous. Innumerable pieces of rags containing dried and semidried sputum make a nice camping ground for the flies swarming in through the partly open doorway, only to presently fly out again carrying the destructive germ elsewhere, possibly to some article of food.[21]

"Such conditions, of course, call for action," Jacques observed, and as water was warming for the bath, the nurse went through the house looking for a more suitable room for her patient. "The husband, an Italian laborer of small intelligence, but of good heart, appears to regard the matter rather hopelessly, and truly it is discouraging." The second floor seemed worse than the first, but the top room, even though covered by torn and dirty wallpaper and strewn with old clothes, showed promise. "Quickly we form a plan," Jacques continued, "and partially unfold it to the husband, who nods his head at each remark, with an enthusiastic 'Si, si signorina.' That settled, we turn our attention to the children." The youngest, a baby of six months, "spends most of his time on his mother's bed. This will never do, and we search our minds for a solution." While the nurse bathed her patient, the latter confided in broken English that her husband had been out of work for months and there was little money for food. The nurse departed "with a puzzled but determined mind."[22]

Within a week, the nurse transformed the situation. She persuaded the husband to remove the wallpaper from the top room and whitewash the walls. The floor was scrubbed and a clean bed, two chairs, and a table were installed. With the landlord's permission the windows, which had been nailed shut, were removed and the openings were covered with mosquito netting. The patient's sister-in-law was persuaded to come and stay with the woman, "attending to her nourishment, and giving her all the necessary care under our instruction." The baby was placed in a Roman Catholic home and the other two children were sent to the Children's Seashore House in Atlantic City. After two or three weeks there, they too would be sent to an institution, thus removing them from the danger of infection. Now the patient lay in a "sweet, clean, airy room." Her comfortable bed, positioned close to the window, was "covered with the snowy linen that, she tells you with pride, she brought from Italy many years ago." Next to the bed lay a sanitary sputum cup, and the patient held a paper handkerchief in her hand. "She looks quite happy as she asks about her children in their new home." When the genial general practitioner next visited, Jacques concluded with obvious satisfaction, "he perhaps realized that there were other means of making a patient comfortable in addition to a bath and an alcohol rub."[23]

Jacques's work impressed a reporter from the *North American* who accompanied her in 1909. "To go the rounds with Miss Jacques is to be initiated into the byways of the city, to see the poor in their hand-to-hand battle with poverty and to witness the reviving effect of professional advice and human sympathy upon the man or woman doomed to be a victim of tuberculosis." Among her successes was Joseph, "a cured consumptive"

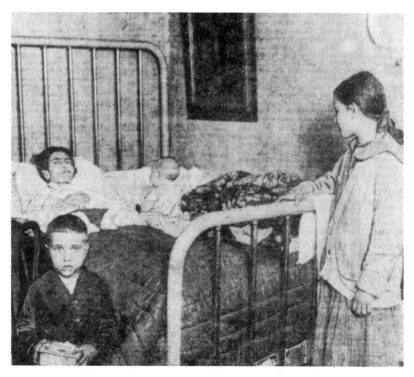

Figure 32. Portrayal of a poor consumptive (left) before and (right) after the ministrations of a visiting nurse. In the second image, the children have been removed from the bedside, the patient has been moved to an open window, and a

who had been pronounced incurable the year before. A tent had been placed in his tiny back yard, the rent paid, his wife and children provided for, and now, able to support himself, Joseph was studying to be a chauffeur.[24]

Once the Society had initiated this special work, the number of tuberculous persons seen by the nurses began to rise. For the year ending early in 1906, the annual report had listed 81 such patients, 3.3 percent of its total caseload; by early 1909, this number had quadrupled to 325, or 11.4 percent of all cases. The number of visiting nurses who specialized in tuberculosis had also increased from one to three. Money contributed in the memory of William Furness Jenks, Mrs. Jenks's husband—a physician who had died of consumption in 1881—supported one of them and funds given in the name of her mother, Maria R. Towne, helped to finance a second.[25]

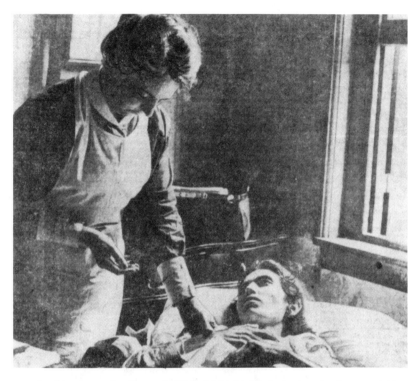

nurse is taking her pulse. From the *Philadelphia Public Ledger*, 26 April 1914. Visiting Nurse Society of Philadelphia Records, Center for the Study of the History of Nursing, University of Pennsylvania.

Tuberculosis nursing was hard, risky, often frustrating, and poorly remunerated. Like other visiting nurses, Jacques and her colleagues rode the sometimes hazardous streetcars to visit their patients in all kinds of weather. They repeatedly climbed up long flights of stairs, worked in badly ventilated dwellings, and took care of advanced and potentially dangerous cases. The patients did not necessarily welcome attention, and the nurses often lacked the authority to do what they thought necessary. Their patients' dwellings were small and unsanitary, and alternative housing was scarce. Funds for food were frequently lacking. Free beds in sanatoriums were hard to find, waiting lists were long, and there were no laws to force careless and uncooperative patients into institutions, even when they were endangering their own children. "Even the strongest women in the service," Jacques observed, "are exhausted when night comes." For such ar-

A GOOD ANGEL TO POOR CONSUMPTIVES

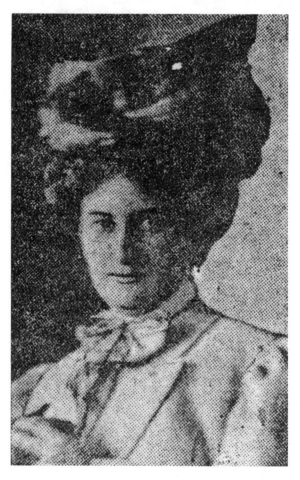

Figure 33. Mabel Jacques, in "A Good Angel to Poor Consumptives," *Philadelphia Press,* 7 October 1907. Visiting Nurse Society of Philadelphia Records, Center for the Study of the History of Nursing, University of Pennsylvania.

duous work, the pay seemed small to the visiting nurses. In 1910, they started out at fifty dollars a month and received increments over their first six months to a maximum salary of seventy dollars. In 1912, this maximum was raised to seventy-five dollars. Because the visiting nurse paid for her board and lodging, her income was roughly the same as that of a nurse in institutional work.[26]

The tuberculosis nurse had her rewards, however, not the least of which was her relationship to patients. As a visiting nurse, unlike her counterpart in private duty, she was not at the beck and call of an affluent patient. In the care of the poor, class relations were reversed. As Jacques portrayed the nurse, she was a resourceful woman of action, an expert, an educator, whose work would benefit the poor of the present and the generations to come. She was a "friend of people of the Ghetto" and "the mother of them all." Once her patients' confidence had been won, she could lead them "like children." She could guide them to health, help to prevent tuberculosis, and eventually, perhaps, even eradicate the disease. Visiting nursing, Jacques observed, with more wishfulness than accuracy, was attracting "many of the most intellectual, wide-thinking, and best trained nurses" of the time.[27]

Public recognition helped to confirm this image of the nurse. Jacques was one of the nurses who spoke at the 1908 International Congress on Tuberculosis in Washington, taking her place among the world's leaders in the crusade against the disease. Her "Educational Leaflet for Mothers" won a silver medal at the Congress, and an exhibit showing two contrasting rooms, before and then after a nurse made it sanitary, won honorable mention. This exhibit, which Jacques demonstrated at the Congress, was cosponsored by the Pennsylvania Society for the Prevention of Tuberculosis and the Visiting Nurse Society of Philadelphia. When the International Exhibition came to Philadelphia, Jacques shared the speakers' platform with leading physicians in the crusade, and the *Philadelphia Inquirer*, printing her picture on its front page, praised the heroism of tuberculosis nurses. These must have been heady times for a woman still in her twenties.[28]

Home Care Versus Institutionalization

During the International Congress, however, just when the outlook for tuberculosis nursing in Philadelphia seemed most propitious, two nurses from Baltimore, Ellen N. La Motte and Mary E. Lent, challenged the worth of instructing the poor in their homes. Both women had graduated from the training school of the Johns Hopkins Hospital. In 1908, Lent was the superintendent of Baltimore's Instructive Visiting Nurse Association, and La Motte was a tuberculosis nurse there—a post she had held since 1905. Early in her work, La Motte had been cautiously hopeful about teaching the poor and changing their lives, but experience had changed her mind.[29]

Blunt, sometimes harsh in her judgments, and showing no sentimentality or romanticism, La Motte pronounced the educational efforts a failure and used her results to prove her case. The lower class, she asserted, "by reason of the very conditions that constitute it a class, is unable to make use of what it learns." There were three reasons, "temperament, environment, and familiarity." Temperamentally, persons of the lower class lacked the moral fiber and the self-control to maintain their struggle for health. Their crowded quarters, small wages, and inadequate food made it impossible to carry out the necessary measures. Finally, because patients saw no quick improvement from treatment and family members saw no ill consequences of relaxing their precautions, they all grew indifferent. La Motte had assessed the preventive efforts of 1,160 patients whom she herself, together with others, had tried repeatedly to teach, and had found the results dismally inadequate: 9 patients careful, 143 fairly careful, 719 careless, and 289 grossly careless. The battle could not be fought successfully in homes, she concluded. When families could no longer take care of their tuberculous relatives satisfactorily, the state should place them in institutions.[30]

Lent supported La Motte's position. In a separate paper at the Congress, she proposed the two true functions of a tuberculosis nurse. By exposing the facts and interpreting them to the public, the nurse should arouse support for the construction of institutions, and she should then persuade the patients to enter them.[31]

In 1909, Jacques challenged these conclusions. Lent's desire to control infection, she asserted, had obscured the values of making the patients happy and preserving their families. Although Jacques agreed that some uncooperative patients—the not-poor as well as the poor—needed to be institutionalized for the sake of the public, others did not need to be and should not be forced to leave their homes. Miss Lent, she suggested, may not have considered the family's happiness. "We know that for years she has been a careful student of the family problem, but has she not possibly through this study become impressed primarily with the squalor, shiftlessness and lack of intelligence and fortitude existing among the people whom she studies, while the question of family happiness becomes a secondary consideration?"[32]

Jacques contended that the nurse must consider this aspect of care if she was to manage the treatment properly. By getting the patient to confide in her, the nurse could learn about the family and determine "what causes her patient worry and what causes happiness." All these factors, Jacques explained, had a "material effect upon the mind of the patient, and necessarily upon his physical condition." Given these data, the nurse's "experienced mind" would know what course to pursue. This might include the placement of children in institutions, as we have seen, and it might involve sending whole families to "work colonies" for consumptives, which she, like some others, considered a good idea.[33]

She drew the line, however, at separating husband and wife. "What effect does the sending of a tuberculous patient to an institution have upon the family . . . ?" she asked in her challenge to Lent. "In nine cases out of ten it means eventually the breaking up of the family." When the breadwinner was institutionalized, the family soon had to apply for charity. An organization then placed the children, while the remaining adult lived "as cheaply as possible, straining every point to pay the children's board and support herself" until she too became ill. If the mother was sent to an institution, the father worked and left the children at home alone or "with an indifferent person hired to care for them. They become unruly, probably live on the streets and are generally neglected; the father loses heart and interest and either places them in an institution, or allows them to go utterly to the bad."[34]

If these people were left alone, Jacques continued, they would certainly become a menace both to themselves and to the world at large, but "under the care and instruction of trained and intelligent people, this should not exist. Who better fitted to do this work than the trained nurse?" Lent had given up too early. "What is the work of six nurses, for four years, to a city of the size and population of Baltimore? . . . The great majority of our patients are among foreigners, or a class of Americans who have lived so crudely for generations, that, in order to accomplish anything in the way of radical change, a complete revolution and reconstruction of the homes must take place." Many patients should go to institutions and many wanted to go, Jacques acknowledged, but as long as they could get the needed care and instruction at home, "the complete segregation of the tuberculous patient seems to me both cruel and unnecessary . . . for it is the home that we must save." Here was a job for the tuberculosis nurse, but "not singly or by twos and threes. . . . Let each city supply itself with . . . fifty or sixty or a hundred if need be, who will give daily instruction to all tuberculous patients, study the home and housing conditions, and give to these poor people who have not been taught to live properly the best of their thought and energy."[35]

At about the time this paper was published, Jacques resigned from the Visiting Nurse Society of Philadelphia. She was interested in becoming the superintendent of the proposed city tuberculosis nurses, but neither the job nor the specialized nurses materialized. Instead of the fifty or more nurses that Jacques had called for in a city's health department, Philadelphia failed to support even one. By 1910, Jacques had moved to New York and had taken charge of a tuberculosis class for the District Nursing Association of Buffalo.[36]

In 1910, the Metropolitan Life Insurance Company started to pay the costs of the nurses' visits to its industrial policyholders. The company's interest was that of a business, not a philanthropy, and it wanted results in the form of reduced mortality. Accumulating data, however, indicated to company officials that nursing visits to tuberculous patients had little, if any, impact on death rates. Statistics in 1914, observed Lee K. Frankel, a Metropolitan official, documented this point. Among the company's tuberculosis patients reported by the nation's six principal visiting nurse societies, Philadelphia had the most visits per case, the lowest rate of transfers to institutions, and the highest death rate. Baltimore, in contrast, had the highest rate of institutionalization and the lowest death rate. Frankel, ignoring the deaths that undoubtedly occurred in Maryland's institutions, concluded that these results partly explained why "tuberculosis nursing did not come within the purview of our work." The company would help its policyholders more if it limited its nursing service "as far as possible to acute diseases where the likelihood of recovery might be influenced."[37]

The Visiting Nurse Society of Philadelphia had different values that included teaching, prevention, comfort, and the preservation of families. In 1912, its board successfully rejected Metropolitan's request to limit the number of visits to tuberculous patients. Company statistics in 1916 showed that, compared to other nursing societies, Philadelphia's nurses still visited such patients more frequently, continued to care for more of them until they died, and transferred fewer to institutions. "The value of this tuberculosis work cannot be over-estimated," observed Katharine Tucker, superintendent of the Society in 1917. The nurses' visits were often "the greatest comfort that these pathetic figures have" and the dangers to others could only cease through constant attention and teaching. Tucker cited the example of Mrs. Smith, who was almost bedridden from advanced tuberculosis after three years of the Society's care. "Through all this long struggle," Mrs. Smith had "followed instructions carefully and in every way tried to protect" her daughter of fifteen from infection. The girl kept their "two small rooms very neat and clean, giving the most thoughtful and tender care to her mother," and the nurse taught her how to keep well. As a result, "though constantly attending the patient, this child is a strong and healthy girl, as well as an excellent nurse." Although the numbers of tuberculous patients had dropped after Jacques's departure, the Society continued to care for about two to three hundred cases per year through the 1920s."[38]

The Diffusion of Tuberculosis Nursing

Meanwhile, tuberculosis nursing was growing in other organizations such as the Kensington Dispensary for the Treatment of Tuberculosis, the Presbyterian Hospital, the Pennsylvania Society for the Prevention of Tuberculosis, and, most important, the state health department. By 1919, sixteen nurses worked at the state's four dispensaries in Philadelphia. Roughly 8 to 10 percent of the first eighty nursing graduates of the Phipps Institute and the White Haven Sanatorium entered this line of work. In 1913 Anna G. Murphy, the valued White Haven matron whom Flick had advised to become a pupil at the Phipps Institute, took a visiting nurse position in New York, and from 1909 to 1912 Mary B. Cornell, the Phipps graduate who had described her marvelous cure to the *North American*, worked in various state dispensaries near Philadelphia.[39]

The state dispensaries helped to shape the nature of the nurses' work. Physicians there, much like Ellen La Motte, were growing skeptical of the value of home care, especially as the first step in management. Sanatorium care should come first, they argued, not so much for its curative worth, which they were also starting to question, but for its educational effects and the value of segregation. The state dispensaries concentrated on casefinding, preventive measures, and followup after discharge. Although their nurses did see patients at home and helped them get assistance from charities or county poor directors, home care of the sick and dying was not part of their mission.[40]

State sponsorship also helped to shape the developing relationships between nurses and physicians. The visiting nurse, as Jacques observed in 1910, was not under the continual guidance of the physician, but of necessity took considerable responsibility. The physician was important to the nurse's work, she acknowledged, but during her visits in patients' homes the decision-making was hers. Although admittedly following medical directions and periodically reporting her observations to physicians, the visiting nurse was reasonably independent; she had her own organization, her own values, and her own services to provide. It was out of visiting nurse societies that Jacques hoped a nursing elite would develop. In contrast, the state dispensary system was explicitly hierarchical; daily authority rested with the medical men. The state-employed nurses in Philadelphia reported for an hour daily at the dispensary, where they talked with the doctors about their cases. The meetings had two advantages, according to Albert P. Francine, director of the first state dispensary in the city: cooperation and supervision. Physicians learned about the patients' home conditions and social problems and could make suggestions. They also checked on the women's work, evaluated their ability to handle the social problems, and judged how well they were keeping up with their visits. As nursing expanded within the state bureaucracy, in short, it did so under the control of medicine.[41]

Regardless of where the nurses worked, the trend toward institutionalization continued. Nurses encouraged patients to enter sanatoriums and hospitals, much as Lent had recommended. If persuasion and reason failed to achieve the desired behaviors, the nurse had a harsher way to compel compliance: threatening to stop the patient's milk, eggs, and other kinds of assistance. Jacques had reservations about this method, but Ellen La Motte found it effective and so did Albert Francine. A few states and a number of cities, furthermore, were starting to legalize compulsory segregation of careless consumptives. In 1911, even Mabel Jacques supported such measures but only to "a certain degree." Absolute segregation, she believed, was "uncalled for, cruel, and, without doubt, impossible." By "impossible," Jacques was referring to wealth and power. "Tuberculosis, although termed a 'poor man's disease,'" she observed, "is found quite frequently among the rich and the powerful. . . . I am sure that they would undoubtedly prove themselves powerful," she noted astutely, "if there should be a movement made for the segregation of all."[42]

Tuberculous men and women of all kinds turned gradually—and with little coercion—to institutions. While wealth certainly influenced their decisions, other circumstances and other forces affected their choices too. Some of the sick responded to public persuasion, and some to personal advice; others acted out of hope, fear, or need. Whatever their reasons for entering hospitals and sanatoriums, their actions helped to keep the institutional system both full and expanding.

14. Persuasion, Choice, and Circumstance

Between 1901, when the White Haven Sanatorium opened, and 1917, when the nation entered the World War, Pennsylvania's consumptives had many alternatives. They could stay at home if they had one, resting or working as much as they could and surrounded by family, friends, and neighbors. They could try the sundry remedies offered in local drugstores or, depending on their circumstances, they could visit private physicians or the increasing number of dispensaries that specialized in their disease. They could ask for a visiting nurse or a nurse might call on them, especially if they had gone to a dispensary. Treatment at home ranged from nothing at all to patent medicines or to various drugs prescribed by a general practitioner or even to elaborate attempts to replicate the open-air life of a sanatorium. Some well-to-do patients, for example, spent twenty-four hours a day on screened, upstairs porches while their less affluent counterparts lived in tents or shacks on the rooftops of buildings or in back courtyards. Others, restless perhaps with life at home, sought a change of air or climate, as so many consumptives had done during the nineteenth century—going to the mountains of Pennsylvania, New York, or North Carolina, for example, or to Colorado and the Southwest. Some boarded out, some stayed at the hotels and resorts that would still accept them, and some, roughing it, camped out in tents or cabins or even made long canoe trips. Gradually, however, increasing numbers of patients chose sanatoriums and hospitals.

A pervasive campaign of public persuasion partly explains the shift from life at home to care in institutions. The Pennsylvania Society for the Prevention of Tuberculosis had led this campaign since the 1890s, and the state health department joined it after 1907. Both organizations tried to shape the system of care and to persuade patients to use it. For the latter purpose, they enlisted the schools, the churches, the press, and other agencies to support their recommendations. At a more personal level, physicians and nurses added their own advice.

Consumptives and their families had their own reasons for choosing

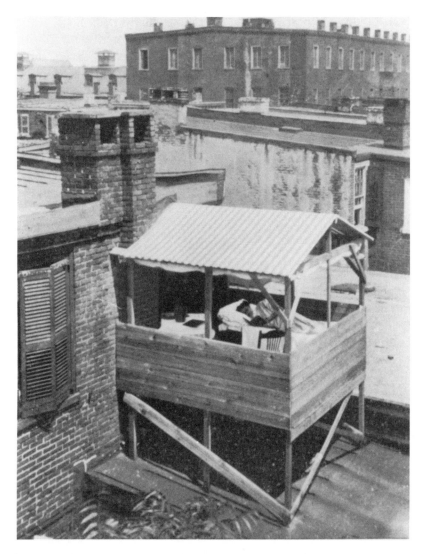

Figure 34. "A Sleeping Porch in a Crowded District of Philadelphia." From Guy Hinsdale, *Atmospheric Air in Relation to Tuberculosis* (Washington, D.C.: Smithsonian Institution, 1914).

sanatoriums and hospitals. The institutions offered them hope, relieved some of their fears, and met some of their basic needs. The advantages of institutional care, however, were partly offset by disadvantages such as loneliness, lack of personal freedom, and loss of privacy. Economic resources, the quality of family relationships, and the stage of a patient's disease each tipped the scale in one direction or the other. The trend in treatment, however, was unmistakable—out of homes and into institutions. Although a few observers questioned the wisdom of this change, they could not stop its momentum; they scarcely tried. There were too many hopes, needs, fears, and convictions wrapped up in the campaign, too many careers involved, too many organizations struggling to survive.

The Pennsylvania Society and the Campaign

The Pennsylvania Society, which initiated the campaign against tuberculosis, was well organized for its purposes. Although physicians held a majority of the positions as its officers and directors, other men and women also served in these capacities. Together they helped to link the Society to Philadelphia's health department, the state health department, the University of Pennsylvania, the Philadelphia Protestant Episcopal City Mission, the Henry Phipps Institute, newspapers, and other organizations. Mrs. William F. Jenks, founder of the Visiting Nurse Society of Philadelphia, for example, served as the Pennsylvania Society's treasurer and a member of its board, and Talcott Williams, editor of the *Philadelphia Press*, served as a vice president through 1913.[1]

Between 1905 and 1917, the previously small, almost impoverished organization, which had usually spent less than one hundred dollars a year, grew impressively in resources. Christmas Seals, which were first sold in December 1907, captured the public's interest, broadened the Society's constituency, and fattened its treasury. Between 1908 and 1911, its income more than doubled, allowing annual expenditures of $9,947 by March 1911. The Society reported that, for the first time, its work was unimpaired by lack of funds. As appeals for support continued, expenditures climbed further, reaching $24,798 by 1917.[2]

The growing income helped to alter the character of the organization's workforce. In 1907, the Society hired its first paid executive officer, and an enlarging cadre of paid employees devoted themselves to the previously all-volunteer organization. Between 1911 and 1917, wages and salaries accounted for about half of the expenditures; they consumed valuable resources, as Flick later complained, but the increased staff helped to raise funds, coordinated and supported the antituberculosis efforts all across the state, and broadened the Society's methods.[3]

Throughout this period, the Society continued to promote the system of care that its members believed would prevent and even cure tuberculosis: sanatoriums, hospitals, and dispensaries. After 1909, it increasingly emphasized the importance of local hospitals for advanced cases. Although the Philadelphia General Hospital, the last resort for the city's indigent consumptives, more than doubled its capacity for such patients between 1904 and 1916, the need for beds persisted.[4] Elsewhere in Pennsylvania, the situation seemed even worse: indigent consumptives might end their days in a county almshouse. In one such place, "ambulant consumptives are entirely free to mingle with the other inmates," the Society complained in its 1911 annual report; "this freedom included the privilege of using the common drinking cup attached to the pump in the yard. If bedfast, the consumptive is committed to the care of the matron, assisted by a feeble-minded inmate." The Society offered to help small communities by surveying their needs and facilities and developing plans for improvement. Providing custodial care for the chronically ill, however, lacked the political appeal of institutions that promised a hope of cure, and fear of infection raised local opposition to building hospitals. The fight was to be a long one, and the gains were to prove modest.[5]

While the Society encouraged communities to create and enlarge tuberculosis institutions, it also worked to eliminate those "heartless, commercialistic triflers" who peddled the fake consumption cures and addictive nostrums that tempted patients away from the "rational regimen and treatment" of scientific medicine. The patent cough medicines, the various vegetable and mineral substances, the serum treatments, the special diets, and the plasters, poultices, and other external applications were all worthless, the Society's magazine asserted in 1911, quoting New York City's health department. Such frauds must be suppressed and the public enlightened by the truth. In this campaign, the Society was a relatively small but active segment of a national drive against quackery, led by the American Medical Association.[6]

The attacks on these treatments rang with scientific conviction and moral righteousness, but the critics were using a biased standard. They assumed the scientific legitimacy of orthodox medicine and did not objectively evaluate its various therapies. While neither the hazards of some of the proprietary "cures" nor the commercial interests of their originators can be questioned, many of the remedies themselves could scarcely be distinguished from approved medical approaches. "Dixon's fluid" was used widely in the state sanatoriums and dispensaries through at least 1916, other physicians administered a variety of anti-bacterial sera, and Flick promoted his special diet, his europhen-in-oil, and his plasters and poultices for years. The physicians, however, repeatedly claimed that their own treatments— unlike those of their commercial competitors—had scientific rationales.[7]

The Pennsylvania Society also continued its educational efforts, teaching people to seek medical attention when symptoms first suggested tuberculosis, to acquiesce in the scientific treatment, to implement preventive measures, and to enter sanatoriums or hospitals when that was medically indicated. People should also live in healthful ways, urged the Society, by being clean, breathing fresh air, eating good food, and adopting regular habits. During its first fifteen years or so, the Society's methods included tracts, exhibits, and public lectures.[8]

The Network of Persuasion

As the organization expanded its paid staff and coordinated its efforts with the National Association for the Study and Prevention of Tuberculosis, however, it developed new or stronger links with three important social institutions—the schools, the churches, and the press—that lent their aura of authority to the Society's propaganda. Work in the schools, which began in 1909, involved a portable exhibit, along with a lecture and discussion by one of the Society's staff. Pupils were sometimes asked to write compositions on what they had learned, and many seemed to have grasped the basic concepts. The children seemed more malleable than adults and quicker to learn and practice the principles of hygiene. The Society, pleased with its results, considered the work unquestionably necessary and worthwhile. Workers seemed relieved, moreover, to shift their efforts into a more hopeful setting. "At best," noted a writer in 1911, "the work with consumptives is discouraging." The program grew steadily; during the year 1916–17 it reached 16,500 children and teachers.[9]

A few churches, as mentioned earlier, supported the care of the tuberculous poor through dispensaries and group classes, and for years clergymen had involved themselves in finding suitable care for their consumptive parishioners. In 1910, the National Association designated a day in April as

"Tuberculosis Sunday," by which it brought a large number of churches into the network of persuasion. During the next few years the Pennsylvania Society, along with its branch organizations, asked local clergy to participate in relaying its message. The tuberculosis societies supplied outlines for a sermon, pamphlets for parishioners, and a Tuberculosis Day Prayer.[10]

The press, like the clergy, had long played a role in the campaign. Flick had used it frequently, Elwell Stockdale had promoted the White Haven Sanatorium through local papers, and the press had covered the 1908 International Exhibition in detail. "The newspapers have done much in the twenty years of the antituberculosis campaign to spread knowledge about consumption," acknowledged the Pennsylvania Society in 1912. "Hitherto, however, publicity work of this kind has been spasmodic. It has lacked the consistent 'pound' that the modern advertiser has used to such good purpose." The Society now tried to correct this deficit by distributing short articles called "health talks," particularly to newspapers in small communities throughout the state. In 1916, the Society sent out more than forty-two hundred press notices, including some from the National Association, to three hundred newspapers on its list. To its own members it sent additional mailings: its annual reports, the *Fresh Air Magazine*, which it published from 1909 through 1911, and then the *Journal of the Outdoor Life*, which the National Association had adopted officially in 1906.[11]

No method of public persuasion reached a greater audience than did the Christmas Seal campaign. In 1911, for example, more than eight hundred businesses—drug stores, cigar stores, department stores, and restaurants—participated in selling the stamps, while nearly every streetcar in Philadelphia carried an advertisement for them. A large banner promoting use of the seals stretched across Chestnut Street near Broad and Fifteenth Streets, and roughly a block away their name shone in lights over the entrances to City Hall. According to Society leaders, the sale of the seals had several advantages. At a price of only a penny per stamp, the seals caught the attention of the poor as well as the rich. By attaching the little stamps to their letters and packages, users learned about the campaign, publicized it, and felt good about helping others, especially at Christmastime. In 1919, Pennsylvanians spent $335,256 on Christmas Seals—3.8 pennies per person.[12]

By finding common cause with other organizations, the Society disseminated its message and its name. With the YMCA, the Boy Scouts, and the Girl Scouts, it promoted good health habits; with labor unions, it advocated better working conditions; with the Octavia Hill Association, it favored better housing; and with the Child Hygiene Committee and Babies' Welfare Association, it cooperated in Baby Saving Shows.[13]

Activities of the state health department resembled those of the Society. In addition to publishing its *Health Bulletins*, the state sponsored exhibits and talks in the schools, promoted Tuberculosis Sunday, and distributed articles on tuberculosis, among other subjects, to newspapers. To encourage use of the state dispensaries, Commissioner Dixon communicated not only with local health officials, county medical societies, and the press but also with employers and, through the clergy, with women's clubs and associations.[14]

Books, magazines, and movies joined in the chorus. In 1903, Flick published his own book for a popular audience, *The Crusade against Tuberculosis. Consumption A Curable and Preventable Disease*, and advertised it in both *Outdoor Life* and *Fresh Air Magazine*. In 1906, he had it distributed to graduates of Philadelphia's Roman Catholic high schools, and Mrs. Charles Hatfield arranged through the Civic Betterment Association to give a copy to all medical students in the city who applied for it. In 1905, Samuel Hopkins Adams, the muckraking journalist, who had first requested an appointment to talk with Flick, published a favorable article on the crusade in *McClure's*. Ten years later, the National Association, in cooperation with the Universal Company, distributed its first movie, "The White Terror." In the same year, the state health department made its own movie, "Pennsylvania's War on Tuberculosis." It featured the sanatorium at Mont Alto, Dixon's "Hillside City of Hope."[15]

Some participants in the campaign worried that people who needed the information most—especially the poor—would not attend lectures or exhibits and did not read newspapers or magazines. It was here that visiting nurses played a special role. In 1909, the Metropolitan Life Insurance Company started its own educational program, taking the message into the homes of its more than four million industrial policyholders across the country. Of all the company's customers, this group had the lowest income, and tuberculosis took a large toll among them. Educating them, observed Philip P. Jacobs, assistant secretary of the National Association, was simply good business. Company agents, who personally collected weekly premiums from these customers, began to take them an illustrated pamphlet, *A War upon Consumption*. In addition to providing information about the disease, the company offered to send upon request a list of sanatoriums, hospitals, dispensaries, and classes, thus encouraging a timely use of approved facilities. Later company pamphlets dealt with "Directions for Living and Sleeping in the Open Air" and "Fake Consumption Cures."[16]

Language of the campaign against tuberculosis expressed the concerns of its leaders as they looked at early-twentieth-century society. Health was wealth, and tuberculosis diminished the nation's wealth by the calculated worth of the lives lost. The disease was a public menace, but chiefly when its victims were unrestricted, unsupervised, and uncontrolled. Then the victims themselves, usually poor as portrayed in this context, threatened the public's welfare. "A very fertile source of infection is the class of vicious or homeless tuberculous indigents who frequently shift habitations," wrote J. Byron Deacon, executive secretary of the Pennsylvania Society in 1911. These should be placed in the General Hospital or its country extension on the city farm at Byberry. "Provision is made for the more intelligent, self-respecting and hopeful type of patient at Byberry," continued Deacon, mixing prognosis with attributes that suggested class, while the "less hopeful cases are sent to the General Hospital."[17]

In metaphors that combined the religious with the military, campaigners preached the gospel of health and hygiene and asked the people to join in the grand crusade. Its army was fighting the deadly enemy, the common foe, the disease known as the white plague. The gospel left little doubt as to leadership and authority: medicine led and controlled while patients submitted, even at the cost of rupturing family ties. The new heroes were those who cheerfully and courageously acquiesced in the treatment. The wise and modern courage, preached an article in the *Fresh Air Magazine* in 1911, was "to give up cherished ambitions, to sit and wait for months and years, to change the whole trend of one's life, to take the cure in honest fashion." The mother who nursed a child through an infectious illness was no longer a heroine, another article noted; the heroine was now the person who supported the hospital and sent the patient there—"to be better cared for than even a mother's love knows how."[18]

Spunk, the patients' magazine at Mont Alto, published "True Heroism" as its lead article in June 1911. To "rally the wavering column," to "risk one's life to save the drowning man," and to "stand by the sinking ship until the last passenger is safely off" were all heroic acts, argued the author, the Rev. George W. Brown, but "the sustained heroism of daily life" was just as exalted.

> Patients . . . at Mont Alto are a living example of this truest heroism, the patient, persistent following . . . of a line of duty self imposed. All men find life under rule an irksome thing at times; some find it painful always. Yet rule is necessary. It guarantees the greatest good for the greatest number. To sink individual preference, to conform to the "crowd" requires courage of a very high[,] order-required[,] heroic character.

To this denial of one's personal preference must be added a renunciation even more difficult, the separation from relatives and friends, the breaking of home ties. . . . Does this require more than ordinary courage? I think it does.[19]

Choice and Circumstance

Although some of Mont Alto's patients may have gained comfort and strength from the praise that Brown said they deserved, decisions to enter institutions and to stay there as long as physicians recommended were not made easily. The promise and reality of life in an institution had to be weighed against the alternatives. Hope, fear, and economic necessity all sent patients to the institutions, while close and supportive relationships, family responsibilities, and dislike of institutional life favored treatment at home.

Sanatoriums, typically promoted for curable cases, offered hope to both consumptives and their families, just as they had for Annie Hackett, Regina O'Leary, and George Macklin, at least for a time. The message that consumption was curable trickled through all levels of society. Many prospective patients and those who spoke for them expressed great confidence in the new scientific treatment, sought it, and even in the face of a bad outcome drew solace from having done everything possible. "I want to save her life if I can doctor," wrote W. S. Ramsey, who wanted the best available treatment for his wife at White Haven, "so at the end, come when it may, there'll be no cause for regret."[20]

Families and friends also hoped that a sanatorium—like a nurse in a patient's home—could impose the necessary treatment on recalcitrant patients, thus restoring them to health despite themselves. Often desperate in their own inabilities to establish control, they proposed a sanatorium instead—for the son who refused to eat the proper foods, for the woman who was too fond of excitement to get sufficient rest, and for the man who drank too much or took cocaine. "I really think he needs a course of compulsory treatment," wrote one distraught mother, and another echoed, "please do not be lenient."[21]

Fear of infection sometimes led to the choice of sanatorium treatment. The Pennsylvania Society continued to preach the dangers of infection, and the state health department added its own dire warnings. Tuberculosis germs poisoned the common drinking cup of country schools and railway trains; infected saliva contaminated paper money, envelopes, and library books; public laundries spread the disease by mixing the clothes of consumptives with those of the healthy; and shoes should be wiped before entering a house. Little wonder that people grew fearful and urged their tuberculous relatives and friends to enter a sanatorium—they were simply protecting themselves and their families. Flick, among others, taught that proper precautions made any but the most advanced and helpless consumptive safe to others, but fear of infection persisted. "I take all the precaution I was learned up there," wrote Mrs. Clara Atherton, who had spent four months at White Haven, "yet I hear my people are afraid of me." Joseph Hayward wanted to go to the sanatorium partly because he feared for the health of his wife and two small daughters. "I know that with the dangers of this disease lurking about me I ought to be away from them."[22]

When family and friends were anxious, a sanatorium could be a haven, and a furlough home fraught with embarrassment and insecurity. "All persons are afraid of him," wrote Elmer McKee in *Spunk*, referring to a young man home on a week's leave from Mont Alto, "for is it not written that 'out of the mouths of babes shall come wisdom and out of the mouths of lungers—bugs?' And are not bugs to be avoided?" Wasn't the young man's cough dangerous, his friends wondered; shouldn't his dishes be sterilized? Could he kiss his best girl friend, worried the patient, and how would she respond? "Do you wonder he is glad to get back to Mont Alto where he can cough without apologizing for it?"[23]

A sanatorium, however, despite its advantages, could be a lonely, depressing, even disgusting place. It meant living with other sick people, being exposed to the sights and sounds of illness, and losing one's privacy. It was more than some could tolerate. Mrs. Levis, who thought that a sanatorium made her morbid, yearned for "the quiet of her own home," and Mr. Rigby complained about White Haven's infirmary where his son was a patient. "To sit at your dinner table and have a call for a bed pan or worse from a near by cot, being compelled to witness the revolting movements incidental to the call is a cruel emitic [*sic*] and far from an appetizer." For some, in retrospect, going to a sanatorium had been a sad mistake. "Rebecca died Sept 2 and regreted having taken the treatment," reported her father, "for when came home was to[o] weak to leave room, where had she stayed home could have driven around and enjoyed life."[24]

Among the circumstances that most affected a person's decision to enter a sanatorium was the nature of family ties. When these were close, many patients and their relatives would not consider a sanatorium. Showing no concern for infection, families insisted on taking care of their own sick members. At White Haven, observed C. W. Gerhart, his wife "would only Pine away after her Children"; he could not send her there. She was "Gritty and active with no give up," and he would do all that he could for her at home. At times, persuaded by Flick or another physician, such patients did enter sanatoriums, but they soon grew homesick and lonely; they worried about the children or the spouse or the parent they had left behind. They and their families were sure that they could carry out the regimen at home just as well and probably better than in a sanatorium. Even after a patient died, the family saw no reasons for regret. "[My brother] seemed to gradually become weaker until on August 9th he left us," wrote Mrs. Lilla Davis. "He was so happy at being home once more that I cannot but feel we did right to bring him here to his old home [and] his old friends."[25]

Other patients, who lacked family and friends or perhaps had been rejected by them, turned to sanatoriums for care, board, and shelter, just as their earlier counterparts had turned to resorts and hospitals. For some, life at home was so unbearable that they begged for escape. E. R. Bush, for example, lived with her "very dissipated" brother and her sixty-four-year-old mother, whose meager earnings supported all three of them. "I can't fight everything in creation," she wrote to Flick at the end of a dreadful day; "I feel every day the importance of being in a San. and having regularity of living and freedom from worry."[26]

Lack of money also made life in a sanatorium seem desirable or even essential. Without a substantial nest-egg, a generous benefactor, or a supportive family and friends, a person had to work or seek institutionalization. Each course in its way provided a livelihood. While men and women sought care in institutions when they could not find work, they also looked for work when they could not get into institutions. The Pennsylvania Society, which had opened a Free Employment Bureau to help consumptives find suitable jobs, reported in 1911 that roughly a fourth of the people referred to it had requested work simply because they could not get institutional treatment. Ironically, the Society's own propaganda had probably worsened the problem of unemployment by raising fears of infection in the minds of both employers and co-workers. "I am so anxious to get well, and think I can recover with a few months treatment," wrote Mrs. D. P. Stackhouse. "With that dread disease tuberculosis it is almost impossible to get a situation. . . . Please consider this letter as confidential."[27]

In addition to money and family relationships—and interwoven with each of them—a third consideration affected decisions to enter an institution: the patient's chances of recovery. Although some families wanted to pay for the care of a dying consumptive in a sanatorium and many destitute patients died in the free institutions, most preferred a death at home. Insofar as hope, not circumstance, sent patients to sanatoriums, lack of it kept them at home or returned them there. When the outlook for life became bleak, paying for care seemed a bad investment, a waste of limited money and time. Men and women promised their spouses not to allow them to die among strangers, and tuberculous parents tried to remain with their children. "She says if she can regain her health she will leave her [two] children for others to care for, for a time," wrote a dispensary worker from Pittsburgh, inquiring about White Haven, "but if her case is hopeless she doesn't want to be separated from them and will do the best she can and then take them to the City Poor Farm as a last resort."[28]

Failure and Blame

Perhaps the leaders of the tuberculosis campaign had underestimated the strength of such social attachments; they had certainly overestimated the efficacy of the hygienic regimen. Their plan had seemed so clear, so logical. Men and women, diagnosed in the early stages of tuberculosis, would enter sanatoriums, comply with the treatment, improve, and then return home, where they would continue the regimen and help to inculcate their relatives and neighbors with healthful ideas. Their cures would symbolize the success of the movement and persuade others to seek early treatment. In reality, however, patients delayed getting treatment; they had conflicting needs and responsibilities. They were not always docile and compliant; they often left the institutions against medical advice; and, worst of all, they did not necessarily get well or stay well.

Leading physicians, who believed that recovery depended on proper discipline and who also needed that discipline for institutional harmony, tended to blame the patients themselves for the bad results. Flick interpreted lack of a patient's improvement as proof of something amiss—a weakness of character, an unfortunate failure in bodily immunity, bad environmental influences, or, most often, a lack of discipline. "I am sorry to hear that you have done so poorly since you have gone home and yet I am not greatly surprised," he observed to Mrs. Mary A. South. "It is a great pity that you did not follow my advice and content yourself at the Sanatorium until such time as in my judgment it would have been well for you to return home. It is the old story of people trying to form judgments in matters which they do not understand." "I am sorry to hear of the death of your sister," he wrote to the Rev. James M. Grant. "In looking over her chart, I find that I had made a doubtful prognosis . . . but did think that there was a possibility of helping her. I presume she was not able to carry out the treatment." Death from consumption, no longer signifying "divine visitation," as Flick had once expressed it, was now the result of human error.[29]

The tendency of physicians to blame the patients was by no means restricted to Flick. In 1912, Joseph Neff, director of Philadelphia's health department, reported a study of 3,028 patients discharged as improved or cured from various sanatoriums in the state. The study "revealed the fact that the majority did not follow in their homes the hygienic rules insisted upon in the institution, for which reason many relapsed and died." Neff hoped that a social worker could prevent such breakdowns by better supervision and enforcement of the rules. A report from the state concurred with Neff's interpretation. In a 1914 followup of state dispensary patients, those discharged for nonattendance did less well than those who had been discharged due to cure or arrest of their disease. The outcome proved "what is generally inferred," concluded the observer, apparently unaware that the two groups of patients could not be fairly or logically compared, "that indifference is the greatest enemy to any great movement for the welfare of the people, as well as to the success of the individual."[30]

This predilection for blaming patients reflected the faith that physicians placed in their methods. It also served to protect their authority even in failure, and it helped to sustain the confident optimism that seemed so important to sick and dying patients. Despite Flick's sometimes blunt and accusing manner, patients were grateful for the hope he held out to them. "Give her rest in mind and body and plenty of 'Flick cheer,'" wrote George Hiestand in reference to his sister-in-law, "and from my own experience I know she will have a complete recovery." Few if any physicians perhaps could continue a practice devoted to tuberculous patients if they lacked conviction that what they were doing worked, if they could not excuse their failures by placing blame on the patients and their almost inevitable lapses from the prescribed rules.[31]

Some of the patients at Mont Alto—most obviously those who edited and wrote for the magazine *Spunk*—used similar thinking to raise morale and bring order to the often unruly inhabitants of the state sanatorium. *Spunk*'s articles and quotations often preached optimism, cheerfulness, acceptance of the regimen, and the ability of men and women to will themselves to health. Fictionalized characters who behaved and believed this way typically recovered, while those who lost courage, groused about the treatment, disobeyed the rules, or went home too soon often relapsed and died. "Of course some cases will advance in spite of all and some are not diagnosed early enough," wrote Elmer E. McKee in 1916,

> but still there are many . . . who knew in time and failed to take the proper treatment or else did not stick at it long enough.
>
> In other words most far advanced cases can look back and see the turning point in their lives, a time when they stood at the crossroads trying to decide which road to take, and took the wrong one.
>
> All must admit that out of every ten patients who leave Mont Alto at least eight are making a mistake, a fatal mistake, going home too soon, wasting the time they did spend and wasting the state's money. This is the reason Mont Alto cannot point to more cures; the patients won't stick. A stranger listening to the reasons the patients give for going home would never imagine that a life was at stake; that these men were voluntarily giving up their only chance of life.[32]

Just as physicians and others blamed the patients for their lack of recovery, specialists in tuberculosis blamed the general practitioners. By thus explaining their poor results, they were defending not only their new, aspiring specialty but also the very legitimacy of the tuberculosis campaign. Flick, his colleagues, and physicians in the state system repeatedly criticized general practitioners for their late diagnoses and referrals, their ineffective, time-wasting treatments, and their skeptical views of the new scientific cures. Although the general practitioners rarely published their views, the profile drawn by the specialists suggests that their approaches may well have appealed to many patients. According to these descriptions, the general practitioners were more likely to treat their patients at home (where, of course, they could charge fees); they prescribed palliative medicines such as cough mixtures, opium, and alcohol; and they tended to use reassuring diagnoses such as bronchitis or a severe cold. In the early stages of disease, the general practitioner tried to persuade himself and his patients that nothing was wrong, noted Flick disapprovingly, and in the late stages "he contents himself with making his patient comfortable and easy of mind until death relieves him of his task."[33]

The Growth of Institutions

In spite of resistance to institutional treatment, the opportunities for tuberculous Pennsylvanians to obtain it grew steadily. Between 1904 and 1919, numbers of beds for tuberculous patients increased from 660 to 3,972. While private, philanthropic, and governmental facilities all participated in this growth, it was government that took an increasingly large role—32 percent of the beds in 1904, 50 percent in 1908, and 73 percent in 1919. Entrepreneurs, volunteers, and philanthropists could not by themselves meet the enormous needs, and the state, along with its two major cities, Philadelphia and Pittsburgh, took the lead in caring for the sick and protecting the public's health.[34]

The growth of institutions carried with it a change in the patterns of fiscal responsibility and social authority. Expenditures for the care of consumptives, vastly increased, shifted from patients and families to others— to charity and even more to government. Relief was thus expanded under the guise of medical treatment, but the patients who accepted it paid a price. As consumptives left their homes to enter hospitals and sanatoriums, authority over their lives shifted from themselves and their families to physicians, nurses, and others who ran the institutions. Control was rarely complete in the institutions, to be sure, and physicians and nurses tried to assert their authority elsewhere, including patients' homes, but the change in residence affected lives in important ways.

Despite the costs in terms of dollars and personal freedoms, the expanding system of care seemed, on the whole, like a good bargain. It met the hopes and needs of the sick and assuaged the fears of the healthy. Throughout the nation there was a growing faith in the expert, a new confidence that science, professions, and government, linked together, could solve society's problems. Supporting the system was good politics, good philanthropy, and good Progressive reform.

The campaign against tuberculosis moved with the spirit and momentum of its time, its sources of confidence several and strong. In an attack against a disease previously held to be hopeless, even modest successes seemed thrilling at first. Discovery of the tubercle bacillus had lifted the disease out of the mysterious and created a tangible target for intervention and control. The newly acquired knowledge of the cause and pathology of disease, of immunity and nutrition, and of the action of drugs, as Flick asserted, seemed to give medicine the power to make tuberculosis curable. Bacteriological advances in other fields supported this belief. Some of the leaders of the campaign, moreover, carried in their own bodies proof of success: Flick himself, of course, and Edward L. Trudeau, who, although he died of tuberculosis in 1915, had survived for more than forty years after his case had been pronounced hopeless. Even more convincing than individual examples were the apparent effects of the campaign on the population as a whole; rates of mortality from tuberculosis were falling almost everywhere in the nation.

Technical changes in the practice of medicine almost certainly contributed to the new optimism. Wider use of the stethoscope and of other techniques for examining the chest, together with staining the sputum for tubercle bacilli, led to earlier diagnosis. While early diagnoses were never frequent enough to satisfy the experts, they must have helped to create an illusion of success in at least two ways. First, early identification of a case automatically increased the time between diagnosis and death, thus falsely suggesting a longer survival than that of patients identified at a later stage.[35] Second, placing early cases in a group previously composed of advanced ones increased the proportion of patients who would have recovered anyway, even without treatment.

Overdiagnosis must also have played a role. The criteria that Flick and his colleagues used for early detection, when judged in retrospect, were not sufficiently specific. Healed tuberculosis was sometimes mistaken for active disease, and other conditions mimicked the dread consumption. Some such patients, falsely labeled as having active tuberculosis, appeared to make gratifying recoveries.[36] According to a niece who served as his secretary, Flick examined his patients through their clothing—a method not either then or now considered conducive to accurate observation. He "had such an uncanny ear," his daughter observed proudly, "that many of his delicate looking pupils refused to let him demonstrate on them in public, fearing he might make discoveries." X-ray examinations were seldom used or trusted during this period, and lack of bacilli in a person's sputum did not rule out tuberculosis. Who, then, could debate the master?[37]

Sanatoriums drew strength from the past as well as the present: from the old but persisting beliefs in a change of air and a healthful climate and from the desire to escape the dirty, crowded cities. Sanatoriums continued to advertise these attributes, physicians continued to mention them in their letters of referral, and patients still expressed interest in finding such places where they could go to recover. Through January 1910, the *Journal of the Outdoor Life*, echoing these ideas, published its news from institutions under the heading "Notes from Health Resorts." The therapeutic regimen itself, which had little if any direct relationship to turn-of-the-century science, was rooted instead in ancient medicine, hydropathy, and nineteenth-century health reform.

Despite the almost inexorable movement toward insitutionalization, a debate over the medical worth of the sanatoriums had already begun. By 1908, even some of the leaders in the campaign were expressing their reservations. At the International Congress that year, Livingston Farrand, executive secretary of the National Association, described the preventive value of sanatoriums as "practically negligible." Others questioned the cures. As some of the oldest and best of the sanatoriums began to publish their late results—from six to nine or even twenty years after the patients were discharged—it became increasingly clear that many apparent recoveries had been temporary. While patients seemed to improve in Pennsylvania's state sanatoriums, noted Albert P. Francine, their disease, when judged by x-ray examination, was often getting worse. Further, the unanticipated burden of unproductive yet infectious invalids who seemed to survive longer in the shelter of institutions created ever-increasing and worrisome costs. By 1912, attacks on the sanatorium movement were heard both abroad and in the United States. Among the critics was Thomas J. Mays, an old opponent of Flick's on the medical staff of the Rush Hospital. With statistics from thirteen U.S. cities over the years from 1875 to 1911, Mays argued that the campaign for isolation and disinfection was "proceeding on a blind trail"; it had not "accelerated one whit" the falling mortality rates in Philadelphia or elsewhere. Instead, he contended, the rates of death from tuberculosis were falling because of "the improvement of our physical and mental environment, and . . . the moral betterment of the human race."[38]

Almost no one, however—certainly not Livingston Farrand, not the Pennsylvania Society, not the health departments, not the specialists, and not the chiefs of the sanatoriums and hospitals—argued that the institutions should be closed. They would have destroyed their careers and defaulted on their implicit promises to provide for society's infectious sick and thus protect the public health. Halting their efforts was almost unthinkable. If institutions failed to cure, then they prevented; if they failed to prevent, then they educated; if they were less than completely successful, then their methods had to be changed. Perhaps pneumothorax or some of the new surgical treatments would improve results. There was still important work to be done. In 1916, 11,088 people died of tuberculosis in Pennsylvania, while many more had the disease, yet the state as a whole had only 3,818 beds for them. The risk of infection still threatened. Local hospitals, which would be more accessible to severely ill and dying patients, seemed essential. Establishing them was one task for the future; taking care of endangered children was another. Unexpectedly difficult times lay ahead and momentum was to falter temporarily, but the crusade had to go on.

Part III

Adjustments and Compromise,
1914–1938

15. Waiting Lists and Empty Beds

During the World War, there were no new initiatives in the tuberculosis campaign. Many physicians and other workers enlisted in the war effort and then endured the influenza epidemic of 1918. By the early 1920s, the mood of the nation had grown conservative, and Progressive reformers were banking their fires. The state health department, discouraged by the results of its tuberculosis work, had new leadership, a tighter budget, and increasing demands on its services. To conserve resources yet continue its tuberculosis program, health officials decided to reduce the number of advanced cases in the sanatoriums and admit more children instead. Treating and training children was becoming a popular project for schools, voluntary organizations, and health departments alike. The work was thought to prevent disease later, and the quick improvement shown by the children was gratifying.

To decrease the number of chronically ill adults in the sanatoriums and to shorten the waiting lists, health officials tried to persuade the counties to build their own institutions. Most counties, however, refused. Despite all the progress since the nineteenth century, the problem of poor consumptives was far from solved. Government leaders, like the Protestant Episcopal clergymen and like Flick in the early years at White Haven, preferred curable patients to the chronically ill.

In the 1920s and 1930s, as the number of paying patients decreased, the part-pay and private sanatoriums were struggling to survive. To fill its empty beds, the White Haven Sanatorium solicited increasing numbers of indigent patients from counties willing to pay its charges. The private sanatoriums—lacking patients, lacking philanthropic support, and unable to get adequate payment for county indigents—closed. Waiting lists for free beds in state sanatoriums, however, rose to record highs.

New therapeutic techniques brought a resurgent hope into the tuberculosis campaign during the 1930s. By collapsing a patient's lung, physicians believed that they could arrest the disease more quickly and make patients both non-infectious and able to work again. They could thereby shorten stays in the institutions, reduce the waiting lists, and still protect the public. With renewed enthusiasm and some federal funds, the state health department embarked on another major building program.

Retrenchment at the State Health Department

Between 1907 and 1916, Pennsylvania had built the largest state system for the care of tuberculous patients in the United States. Mont Alto—the nation's biggest sanatorium in 1916—accommodated 1,150 patients. With the additional beds at Cresson and Hamburg, the state could care for 2,210 people (see Graph 15-1). The health department's 115 dispensaries referred patients for admission and managed the care of some of them after discharge. For all these services, Health Commissioner Samuel G. Dixon had persuaded the legislature to spend enormous amounts of money. In 1915, after years of steady expansion, annual expenditures reached $1,558,400—69 percent of the health department's budget.[1]

The state had still not met the people's needs, however, and there was cause for discontent. At Mont Alto, where 51 percent of the patients had far-advanced disease in 1916, facilities were inadequate: half of these people lived in cottages built for early cases, a necessity that the medical director judged a disadvantage for both the patients and the sanatorium. The reasons that patients departed from Cresson were far from satisfactory: only 39 percent of them left on medical advice, while 48 percent left against advice, failed to return from leaves of absence, deserted without notice, or were dimissed for infractions of the rules. The others died in the sanatorium.[2]

Health officials started to question their methods. As reported by B. Franklin Royer, a physician who served under Dixon, the sanatoriums had been created in the expectation of curing incipient cases, but after ten years or so "it began to dawn on the clinicians . . . and the sanatorium workers . . . that something was wrong; that it was a very pretty promise in theory to talk about incipient cases, but quite another thing practically to get them. . . . About 5 percent of the cases sent in by the average practitioner could by a little stretch of the imagination, be called incipient."[3] Instead of the early cases, whose cure would benefit the commonwealth, the sanatoriums had attracted people with advanced disease. Although most of these returned home, improved or not, others became a drain on the state's resources.

Number of Beds

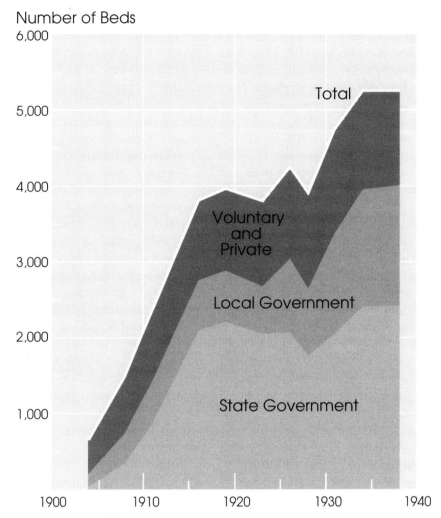

Graph 15-1. Beds for tuberculosis patients in Pennsylvania's hospitals and sanatoriums, 1904–1938, classified by auspices: (1) state government, (2) local governments, and (3) voluntary and private organizations. Numbers of beds are taken from directories of the National Association. The directories undoubtedly contain some errors, they omitted some small sanatoriums, and auspices are occasionally unclear.

In 1916, expenditures for the state's tuberculosis program dropped significantly for the first time; in the following year, admissions to the sanatoriums began to fall. Records are few, but the years from 1916 to 1919 were marked by epidemics, war, labor shortages, and changes in leadership. In February 1918, Commissioner Dixon died after a lingering illness. Royer became acting commissioner for the rest of 1918, and Edward Martin, a Philadelphia surgeon, was appointed to the job early in 1919. The state's expenditures were rising rapidly, an economic slump threatened its receipts, and the new governor, William C. Sproul, and his successor, Gifford Pinchot, were pressing for fiscal restraint. The Dixon years of optimistic expansion were over.[4]

In the summer of 1919, the health department began to promote new policies that reflected its smaller budget for tuberculosis. Commissioner Martin organized a military-style encampment at Mont Alto, to which the department's physicians and nurses from all over the state were summoned to hear and discuss the plan. Officials announced that the department would curtail the admission of far-advanced patients to its sanatoriums, shift the care of such patients to local institutions, and replace them in part with children. In 1920, it closed the two-hundred-bed hospital at Mont Alto, leaving this institution without facilities for care of the seriously ill. All these measures, officials explained, were medically sound and humane. They would shorten the sanatoriums' waiting lists, get hopeful cases into treatment more promptly, and allow incapacitated and terminal patients to spend their final months nearer their homes and families. By 1922, waiting lists for admission had shortened from six or nine months to two or three weeks. Albert P. Francine, now chief of the state's tuberculosis division, was pleased with the new efficiency of the sanatoriums: "many more children and curable types," he observed, "have been treated in 1921 and 1922 than heretofore."[5]

The health department, which had once set out to centralize the care of consumptives, was now trying to return some of it to local communities. Francine, like Flick before him, promoted the admission of advanced and dying patients to local hospitals. He and other officials, aided by "a quiet propaganda campaign" on the part of the state tuberculosis society, concentrated most of their efforts on county governments. Restricting admissions to the state sanatoriums was partly a tactic to make the counties accept responsibility for their own residents. In 1921, the legislature passed a law enabling each county to build and manage its own tuberculosis hospital, issue bonds to construct and equip it, levy a tax to maintain it, and charge fees if patients could pay.[6]

Efforts to shift expenditures from state to county governments also involved the dispensaries—a move that the state justified by the principle of local responsibility. For the state to initiate and maintain "a local institution, run for local welfare, under local administration," Francine asserted in 1921, "is foreign to our American ideals." Persuasion by state officials, reinforced by tuberculosis societies, helped to accomplish the change. In some reluctant communities, closing the dispensary forced the issue. It "aroused a strong and gratifying protest," Francine observed, and through the efforts of "the local tuberculosis society, the Red Cross, or civic body, or all three," the community offered "to supply quarters rent free, heat, light, and janitor service, if the [state health] Department would supply the doctor and the nurse, the necessary supplies, and reopen [it]." This arrangement was what the health department had hoped to achieve.[7]

In Philadelphia, the state proposed the transfer of state dispensaries to the city health department. Philadelphia agreed to take them as city clinics, and the transfer occurred smoothly in September 1923. Ward Brinton, one of the original Phipps physicians, took charge of the clinics. Unlike Flick, Brinton was enthusiastic about clinics and the role of nurses there. The success or failure of tuberculosis work, he declared in December 1923, depended more on the size and efficiency of the nursing service than on the medical work. The twelve city clinics were sufficient to their task, he noted, "but of nurses we need many. We should have eighty instead of thirty, and a hundred would be better." Brinton was echoing the words and goals of Mabel Jacques, the first tuberculosis nurse at the Visiting Nurse Society.[8]

The state health department also tried to economize in other ways. It postponed some repairs of its sanatoriums, stopped giving milk to dispensary patients, and tried to keep personnel costs under control. By the mid-1920s, all three sanatoriums were graduating nurses from their new two-year training schools. State officials described these schools as methods of rehabilitating their women patients, but the schools also helped to solve a labor shortage and may have saved the state some money.[9]

Saving the Wan and Sickly Children

As physicians became discouraged by their work with adults, some turned their attentions to children. Since around 1900, data had accumulated to show that tuberculosis developed in childhood. Autopsies revealed a rising prevalence of the disease during the first two decades of life, and a new and safer tuberculin skin test, introduced by Clemens von Pirquet in 1907, suggested the same phenomenon in living children. Except in their earliest years, however, children seldom died of tuberculosis; most showed no clinical evidence of the disease. How their bodies resisted infection and why some of them later developed disease in their lungs remained unclear. In 1913, H. R. M. Landis, now a leader at the Phipps Institute, listed some likely causes of the unfortunate outcomes: reinfection, unhygienic surroundings, poor food, low wages, physical fatigue, mental worry, an acute illness, and heredity. They made a disheartening set of obstacles to health. Physicians and their colleagues chose to concentrate on two narrow but feasible strategies: training children in healthful habits, and removing the most endangered, however briefly, to better surroundings. Their methods harmonized with those of the contemporary child-welfare movement, through which organized women and some physicians were trying to reduce infant mortality and improve the health of children.[10]

Training children in healthful habits was not a new idea, but around 1916 the National Association began to promulgate a more attention-catching method—the Modern Health Crusade. The Pennsylvania Society and boards of education joined the effort, urging children to keep their windows open, eat nourishing foods, wash properly, brush their teeth regularly, stand up straight, and get a good night's sleep. Titles such as "squire" and "knight" rewarded good performance, and costumed plays and pageants dramatized the lessons. In some of the schools, special nutrition classes taught selected children a healthful diet and a proper schedule for eating, rest, and play. Their weights were recorded weekly, and charts studded with stars rewarded their gains.[11]

Children at special risk of tuberculosis seemed to warrant more vigorous methods. Physicians classified these boys and girls into three sometimes overlapping groups: children thought to have mild but noncontagious infection, those known to have had contact with the disease, and those whose appearance or symptoms suggested either malnutrition or reduced resistance. These were usually the wan, thin sons and daughters of poor or working class families, whose frequent colds, open-mouthed breathing, nervous behaviors, or dull facial expressions, for example, suggested sickliness or even a "pre-tuberculous" condition.[12]

Teaching such children out in the open air seemed a logical way to protect them. The idea had originated in Germany, and in 1908 open-air schools were started both in Providence, Rhode Island, and in Boston. In 1911, the Henry Phipps Institute sponsored an open-air school in Philadelphia, and both the Pennsylvania Society and the city's board of educa-

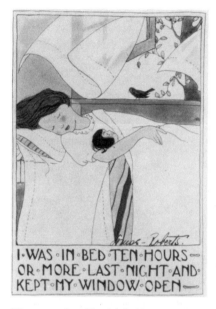 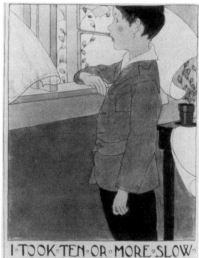

I·WAS·IN·BED·TEN·HOURS—
OR·MORE·LAST·NIGHT·AND·
KEPT·MY·WINDOW·OPEN—

I·TOOK·TEN·OR·MORE·SLOW·
DEEP·BREATHS·OF·FRESH—
AIR·TO·DAY·

Figure 35. Good health habits as portrayed in the *Yearbook of the Pennsylvania Society for the Prevention of Tuberculosis* (1919). From the Historical Collections, College of Physicians of Philadelphia.

tion adopted the method. The children, mittened and muffled up to their chins in blankets during the winter, took their lessons on roof-tops or in other open areas. They had regulated periods of rest and were given extra nourishment.[13]

Most radical among the programs to save the children were the preventoriums—institutions modeled in part on sanatoriums but designed to prevent tuberculosis, not to treat it. Alfred F. Hess, a New York City pediatrician, founded the first of these in Farmingdale, New Jersey, in 1909. Working through the tuberculosis clinics in New York City, Hess selected the malnourished children of the clinics' patients. His plan of treatment was simple: "Plenty of good food, a twenty-four-hour day in the open air, an intimate acquaintanceship with the fields and the woods, and a practical lesson in cleanliness and hygiene."[14]

In 1913, the Kensington Dispensary for the Treatment of Tuberculosis established the first preventorium in the Philadelphia area. Under the leadership of Sister Maria Roeck, a Lutheran deaconess, women of the Evangelical Lutheran Church had modeled this dispensary after that at the

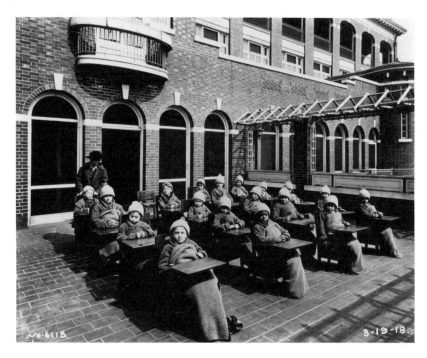

Figure 36. An open-air class in a Philadelphia school. Urban Archives Center, Temple University.

Phipps Institute. Opening in 1906, the dispensary served a working-class neighborhood in northeast Philadelphia, and in 1909 it started a special clinic for children. Needs of the boys and girls and their risks of future disease increasingly impressed the organization's physicians and leaders. "As one sees the children with their faces pale and wan," wrote Ida W. Hutzel, secretary of the board of managers, "one realizes that living, as most of them do among congested conditions, they cannot grow healthy and strong." The board resolved to find a farm where the little ones could be protected from the disease, the traces of which were beginning to show in their weakened bodies. Sr. Maria Roeck expressed the joy of watching as "the train pulled out to take the first of *our* children to *our* farm" in July 1913. Their destination was River Crest, a 140-acre farm on the Schuylkill River, west and a little north of the city.[15]

    In 1922, the state developed a similar program. The state had long accepted tuberculous children in sanatoriums, but now it wanted them earlier, before disease developed. The first children's camp opened at Ham-

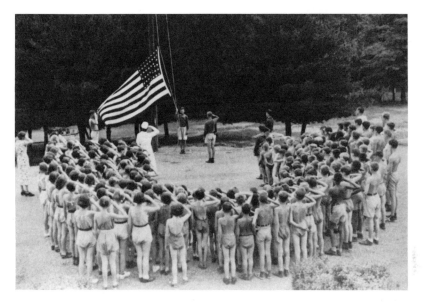

Figure 37. Flag ceremony at Mont Alto's preventorium. Courtesy of the South Mountain Restoration Center, South Mountain, Pennsylvania.

burg in 1922. "The State Health Department has gathered up a few of the broken bits of life from the small communities," wrote an observer for *Spunk*, the patients' magazine at Mont Alto, "and brought them up here [to Hamburg] into the hills to be mended and healed. Two hundred youngsters, frail and pale and under weight; not sick, but just at the place where a few more days or weeks may mean the difference between illness and h[e]alth. . . . They dwell in a city of tents, living in the open; eating of the best and most nourishing food; being examined and watched by skilled physicians and so guarded against the very beginnings of serious things." In 1924, the 200 children were moved from Hamburg to Mont Alto; Cresson could accommodate another 225. By 1929, one-third of the patients admitted to the state sanatoriums were children; physicians judged that only 5 to 6 percent of them had active tuberculosis of the lungs. The state had succeeded in changing its mix of patients.[16]

For the most part, the regimens at River Crest and the state sanatoriums resembled the one that Hess had developed at Farmingdale. Physicians and others also tried to correct the children's physical defects. Decayed teeth, infected tonsils, and even faulty vision, observed one physician from the Kensington Dispensary, were "capable of pushing the patient over the precipice, by reducing his resisting powers." The state, moreover, developed a program of heliotherapy—exposure to sunlight in gradually increasing doses. During the summer, the children dressed in the lightest possible garments and wore them "constantly at school and at play . . . during rainstorms as well as during the sunshine." Although William G. Turnbull, the medical director at Cresson, was cautious about attributing their gains to heliotherapy, he felt sure that they had "never been as happy or looked as well."[17]

Children rewarded their caretakers in a way that most adults could not: most of the children improved rapidly and convincingly. The results delighted the women at River Crest, gratified the physicians, and served to justify the policies and expenditures of the state health department. Annette S. Woll's observations of River Crest in 1919 illustrate the pleasures of watching the recoveries. "To see all these children (so pale and wan when they arrive) fairly blossom forth into round, brown, merry girls and boys here in this lovely spot does one's heart good." Physicians expressed confidence that even a few weeks at a preventorium had lasting results; it gave a boost to immunity that carried the child safely through to adulthood. In a report to the governor in 1928, Theodore B. Appel, secretary of health, referred with satisfaction to the preventoriums: "The hope for the future as far as prevention is concerned, lies in the treatment of the undernourished child."[18]

Waiting Lists for the State Sanatoriums

While the state succeeded in developing its preventoriums, it largely failed to stimulate the formation of local hospitals. By 1924, the voters of fourteen of Pennsylvania's sixty-seven counties had expressed themselves in favor of a local hospital, but only Beaver County had built one. In addition, Lackawanna County had taken over an existing sanatorium and the Allegheny County Home, founded in 1853, was also taking tuberculous patients. The next county hospital for such patients did not open until 1938.[19]

County officials strongly resisted spending their money on the care of the chronically ill. Unlike the state, which drew a large share of its revenues from corporations, the counties depended primarily on property taxes. County officials were very reluctant to raise the taxes of those who elected them, and other interests competed for dollars. In Lackawanna County, for example, the courthouse needed repairs and the motor club was demanding roads. In 1925, Schuylkill County successfully challenged the constitutionality of the state law on county hospitals. The law was amended, but the change made little difference. Physicians who had attended the state's encampment in 1919 could have anticipated such obstacles. In York, where the almshouse had just been condemned, J. S. Miller reported "no means of taking care of these advanced cases and the Poor Directors refuse to do anything." In Fayette County, O. R. Altman had also "found it impossible to deal with the Poor Board; they always do business from the standpoint of saving money and they look after themselves first, rather than after the people." For children, noted J. C. Reifsnyder, one could often raise money, but for "old tuberculous dying patients," it was much more difficult.[20]

Waiting lists for admission to the state sanatoriums again began to climb. In 1925, they included between six hundred and nine hundred applicants. Despite the state's attempts to select its patients, more than half of those in the sanatoriums had far advanced disease; some of them stayed for years. "For many of them, nothing can be done," complained William G. Turnbull, deputy secretary of health in 1926. "The admission of these hopeless cases is an injustice to the institution, to the early cases waiting admission, and often to the patients themselves. For others much can be done," he continued, making his values clear, "and these the institution welcomes."[21]

Slowly, however, if grudgingly, the state yielded to pressure. Although no one saved the letters from the patients or their advocates, many must have been written, just as Flick had received so many twenty years before. In a closely matched political struggle, popular demand for the care of advanced patients slowly overcame the medical preference for early, curable cases. "To the inexperienced it appears a simple thing to choose the hopeful cases and reject the hopeless," wrote Turnbull, but

> choosing is far from simple, either from the medical standpoint or the practical standpoint. The State sanatorium is established to serve the public and is dependent on public sentiment for its support. One far advanced, hopeless, helpless, homeless case in a community will stir up more public sympathy and excitement and a stronger demand for help than will a score of early and curable cases. This case cannot care for himself and there is no place locally where he can be cared for, therefore he must be admitted and admitted he is; to die far from everything dear to him.[22]

The Great Depression increased demands on state and local governments, not because of more tuberculosis but because of economic need. Although physicians preferred to view their institutions as places for treatment, the needy still used them for shelter and sustenance. As unemployment rose, more patients tried to enter the state institutions or to remain there longer, and growing numbers of children appeared on the waiting lists. The lists, which averaged 770 people in 1929, swelled to 911 in 1930, and to 1,331 in 1931. In August 1932—a month when large numbers of children typically applied for the preventoriums—1,610 applicants of all ages were waiting for admission. The state added new units that accommodated 400 patients, and during the summer months it provided 100 additional beds for children. By 1934, the capacity of the state system had risen to 2,414. Between 1926 and 1938, some local governments, most notably Philadelphia and Pittsburgh, also increased their beds for tuberculous patients (see Graph 15-1, p. 271).[23]

Although physicians worried that deaths would rise again because of the Depression, mortality continued to fall (see Graph 15-2). By 1934, the number of beds for tuberculosis in Pennsylvania exceeded the number of deaths reported—an accomplishment scarcely dreamt of three decades before. Leaders of the campaign, however, were still not satisfied. As deaths had declined and beds had multiplied, the National Association had raised its standards. In 1916 it had advocated one bed for every two annual deaths; in 1929 it recommended two beds for every death (a goal that Pennsylvania had not yet achieved), and by 1942 the recommended ratio was to rise further, to 2.5 beds per death.[24]

Empty Beds

While the state was trying to deal with its excess of patients during the 1920s and 1930s, the part-pay and private sanatoriums had empty beds. Middle-class and well-to-do people developed tuberculosis less frequently than did poor people, and the falling rates of the disease further reduced the numbers who both needed care and would pay for it. Other patients whose resources permitted, moreover, still preferred treatment at home.

Between 1915 and the late 1930s, Flick and his colleagues struggled to keep their sanatorium at White Haven solvent and busy. They continued the nursing school, hired their tuberculous patients as workers after discharge, and in every way possible tried to control expenditures. Costs increased, however, and charges rose accordingly: from twelve dollars a week in 1915 to twenty-one dollars in 1925. In 1919 the sanatorium bought its first x-ray machine, and in 1926 the board offered the service to its visiting physicians. By charging fifteen dollars to take a chest x-ray of patients in town, it hoped to make the unit self-supporting.[25]

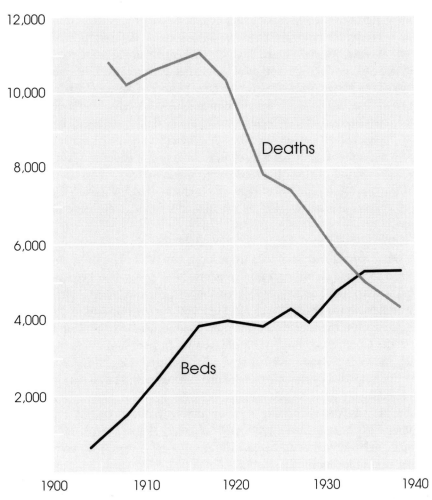

Graph 15-2. Reported annual deaths in Pennsylvania from tuberculosis in all forms, 1906–1938, compared to the number of beds for tuberculosis patients in hospitals and sanatoriums, 1904–1938. Figures are plotted for years in which the National Association published directories. Mortality figures before 1906 are not available.

Empty beds increased the costs per capita, and the management tried a series of changes to keep them occupied. In 1915, the board dropped the title of "Free Hospital for Poor Consumptives" from its letterhead, leaving only "The White Haven Sanatorium Association." Dr. Neale had suggested this change to increase the number of patients. "Poor people feel that they are being humbugged" because of the charges, he noted, and those "more able to pay object to the stigma of being objects of charity." In 1916, the board decided to pay its visiting physicians for their work. Although it may have merely wanted to stabilize its medical staff, maintaining a loyal cadre of physicians was one of the typical ways that contemporary hospitals attracted patients. In 1926, when the average number of patients had dropped to an eleven-year low, the sanatorium began to advertise. At about this time, the duration of stay began to creep upward. During the early 1920s, the average patient (who stayed for more than three months) remained for about eight months; by the late 1930s, this figure was roughly a year. Over the same period of time, the sanatorium's death rate remained fairly stable, fluctuating around an average of 16 percent. The institution that had once evicted its patients after six months now found it desirable to keep them.[26]

Keeping such patients helped the sanatorium only when someone paid for their maintenance and, for this purpose, the White Haven Sanatorium turned increasingly to local governments. New Jersey had been slow to build sanatoriums, and White Haven solicited patients there—with some success. Nevertheless, 1926 was a bad year; the patient population dropped to 150. In July, the sanatorium made an overture to the commissioners of Luzerne County, of which White Haven was a part, and offered to take their indigent consumptives in return for its usual charge. The commissioners, surprised by the offer, responded affirmatively. They were opposed to building a county sanatorium, they did not have the money for it, and other demands were pulling them in different directions. By the year ending early in 1928, Luzerne County was paying almost a third of the costs of patient maintenance at the sanatorium; all local governments combined were paying for more than half of it.[27]

Until then, the number of paying patients had been fairly stable, but the next year it began to tumble; then came the Depression. By the mid-1930s, patients were paying for only 15 percent of the costs of maintenance, local governments were paying for more than 80 percent, and sponsors such as employers, labor unions, charitable organizations, and personal benefactors contributed the rest. The Free Hospital had largely returned to its original intent—the care of poor consumptives. Philanthropic contributions and endowment income covered the capital expenses of the institution and made up any differences between the payments received for maintenance and the sometimes higher costs.

The agreements between the sanatorium and the county governments illustrate a curious but typically American blend of voluntary and public efforts. Each party in the arrangement subsidized the other and served its own interests at the same time. The White Haven Sanatorium received payment for its services and, through the steady supply of patients, fulfilled its philanthropic function—the care of the sick. The counties also saved money. By using the White Haven Sanatorium, they avoided large capital expenditures; the voluntary organization had already made that investment.[28]

County support proved so successful that by late in 1931 the sanatorium had a waiting list that included more than forty patients from Luzerne County alone. When the county commissioners began to press for prompter admissions, Flick proposed a new solution: "Perhaps we could 'farm out' patients to the private sanatoria which I understand are nearly empty." On December 12, 1931, he requested Anna L. Morris, White Haven's superintendent, to find out if such an arrangement was feasible.[29]

During the previous fifteen years, there had been many changes in the private sanatoriums. Elwell Stockdale had died of tuberculosis in 1917, Margaret G. O'Hara had died of heart disease in 1923, and management of their institutions had passed into different hands. The falling rates of tuberculosis and the declining economy had hurt the private sanatoriums, and to some observers they were also falling behind in equipment. They lacked x-ray machines, laboratories, and surgical facilities, on all of which physicians were growing dependent. In 1931, when Flick made his proposal, the scarcity of patients was threatening the very survival of these institutions. Dermady would close by 1934, and by 1938 the national directory would list no private sanatoriums in or near White Haven.[30]

Nonetheless, Flick's idea did not succeed. In the opinion of Superintendent Morris, mixing county and paying patients was administratively tangled, socially unworkable, and economically unsound. On December 15, 1931, the superintendent expressed her concerns to Joseph Walsh, White Haven's medical director. Dr. Flick's " 'farming out' " proposal, she suggested, had "many complications, knowing as we do the class and type" of Luzerne county's patients. "Many of them come to us destitute and in a dying condition. We have been obliged to supply them with . . . necessities, such as pajamas, bath robes, hot water bottles, etc., and a great deal of medical care and nursing. I am wondering whether the smaller Sanatoriums would be equipped to take care of this type of patient. The fewer better class County patients would in all probability pull strings to get into the smaller Sanatoriums not only to avoid contact with the other class, but because they prefer to give the impression of going to a private sanatorium." Morris detailed some of the administrative questions raised by the proposal, including responsibilities for preventive supplies, laundry, x-ray services, and the transportation of doctors. And "would we be expected to take the very sick and destitute while the other Sanatoria got the lighter cases? And should the cases sent to the other places become too sick . . . or difficult to manage . . . would we be required to take them here?"[31]

Two days later, Morris responded directly to Flick. She had just had a discreet and unofficial conversation with Mrs. Stockdale, who was now managing Sunnyrest. Mrs. Stockdale had reported herself "at the end of her resources. Her place is in need of repairs and she has absolutely nothing," yet "she is not sure that she could take patients at $20.00 per week"—the rate that Flick had proposed. Once before, Sunnyrest had tried taking patients at $25.00 a week, but could not make it pay. "Mrs. Stockdale is also afraid the class of patients she would like to attract to Sunnyrest might object to the County patients." One New Jersey county, Morris added, already paid for two of Fern Cliff's eight patients at a rate of $3.25 a day. This rate, she had heard, did not cover the cost of maintenance. Morris suggested some preferable ways in which the White Haven Sanatorium could accommodate extra county patients, and the farming out plan was apparently dropped.[32]

Although county support had rescued the White Haven Sanatorium from fiscal disaster, it did not guarantee stability. New Jersey began to build more of its own institutions, and some of its county governments moved their patients to local care. Greater use by Luzerne County made up the difference, but Flick remained concerned. Declining rates of mortality from tuberculosis predicted the future, he believed, and the sanatorium would eventually have to broaden its field of usefulness.[33]

It was in the 1920s, when occupancy at White Haven was low, that Flick first expressed the idea of accepting nontuberculous patients. "We would like to get heart cases and working people broken down in health from overwork for our vacant beds," he explained. Perhaps businessmen could be persuaded "to send their employees . . . to the White Haven Sanatorium for a few weeks to recuperate. Such persons could be put into a good condition of health by rest and proper diet in a very short time." Acceptance of county patients obviated the immediate need for such a move, but in the mid-1930s, when occupancy drifted downward again, Flick started the legal action to amend the organization's charter. The sanatorium wanted to admit any patient who might benefit from a stay there, regardless of diagnosis. The state's welfare department objected; it still saw a need for sanatoriums and preventoriums but not for another general hospital. A compromise was reached and the charter was amended in October 1935. The amendment legitimized what the sanatorium had been doing for several years. During the year ending early in 1932, nontuberculous patients had first exceeded 10 percent of the total caseload and had continued in roughly the same proportions thereafter.[34]

Meanwhile, Joseph Walsh, the medical director, suggested to the visiting physicians that they readmit their patients for their summer vacations. "Dr. Flick and I have found that when these patients . . . took the sanatorium rest during this vacation period," Walsh observed, "they were benefited to a much greater degree than when they went to the seaside or mountain resorts." Competition between the sanatoriums and the resorts had not entirely disappeared.[35]

New Techniques, New Hope

During the 1930s, physicians and other leaders continued to debate the strategies for fighting tuberculosis. While state physicians still supported the care of children, others argued for additional hospitals, particularly in Philadelphia. Flick disputed both positions. It was the advanced consumptive, he believed, not the child who should be removed from the home to prevent tuberculosis. While it was fine to send children to the country on "a summer vacation," preventoriums could not be considered a means of fighting tuberculosis. Building additional hospitals, moreover, was simply a waste of money. There were thousands of vacant beds in Pennsylvania's general hospitals, he asserted, reiterating his 1909 argument; if only each of them would accept advanced cases, the waiting lists would disappear. Patients could get care nearer their homes, and both nurses and medical interns could acquire needed training in the disease. The separation of sanatoriums from the mainstream of health care had left them uninformed and inexperienced. If local governments would only pay these hospitals a sum of three dollars a day per capita, they would stamp out the disease. This plan would also help to save some of the hospitals that the Depression was pushing toward closure. As before, neither the hospitals nor the governments favored this idea.[36]

By 1933, Philadelphia's hospitals had, in fact, begun to admit tuberculous patients—even some who could not pay. On the average, however, these patients did not remain long. They came in for diagnosis, for surgical procedures, and for short periods of medical care, but not for the prolonged rest provided by a sanatorium.[37]

Among the patients with pulmonary tuberculosis who entered these hospitals, about a fourth expected to have collapse therapy. The oldest and most common of such procedures was artificial pneumothorax—the injection of air into the pleural space that normally surrounds each lung. This air, physicians hoped, would allow a tuberculous lung to collapse partly, thus to be freed of its usual breathing movements and allowed to rest. The walls of a tuberculous cavity within the lung might also come together and eventually heal. During the early 1930s, J. W. Cutler, chief of the pneumothorax clinic at the Phipps Institute, was trying this procedure in ambulatory patients. Although hindsight suggests that the benefits of the method were probably modest, his results seemed promising. Some of his patients promptly felt better, lost their fever, and coughed less, and tubercle bacilli disappeared from their sputum. No longer a hazard to others, such patients could convalesce at home, and even if they returned to work the diseased lung would remain at rest. A physician kept the lung in a semi-collapsed position by weekly or biweekly refills. Ambulatory pneumothorax, Cutler believed, would shorten a patient's convalescence, reduce the waiting lists for the sanatoriums, and protect the public's health.[38]

Not all patients, to be sure, were suitable candidates for the procedure, and among those who were, some had scar tissue that prevented the desired collapse. Others developed complications: infection, coughing up blood, and even sudden death. Nevertheless, pneumothorax gave the physicians something to do for long-continuing illness. According to one doctor quoted by *Spunk*, unaided bed rest seemed like a poor competitor; it did "not seem to be a method of attack but rather a method of passive resistance."[39]

When pneumothorax was unsuccessful, physicians could now turn to various kinds of surgery. They could sever the scar tissue that was preventing collapse or they could damage the nerve that supplied the diaphragm (the most important breathing muscle), thus reducing respiratory movements. Most radically, when other procedures failed, they could do a thoracoplasty: a surgeon excised some ribs so that the chest wall sank in on the underlying lung, thus decreasing the lung's mobility and possibly closing a cavity. This procedure had a higher rate of complications, but when it succeeded and when a person with advanced disease went home again, uninfectious and able to work, the resulting deformity seemed to be worth it.[40]

The promise of surgery, which had spurred the development of general hospitals since the nineteenth century, was finally affecting the treatment of tuberculosis. The new procedures instilled a fresh enthusiasm in the caretakers and in those responsible for the institutions. In 1933, the Philadelphia General Hospital established a thoracic surgery unit. In 1938, the White Haven Sanatorium converted half of the ground floor of its administration building into a surgical division with an operating room, a sterilizing room, four recovery rooms, and all the necessary equipment. By this time, one-third of the patients at the sanatorium were already getting collapse treatment.[41]

Between 1935 and 1938, the state launched a major modernization program. A new Democratic administration had come to power in Harrisburg; the department of health had a new secretary, Dr. Edith MacBride Dexter; and some federal Social Security funds were becoming available for health-related purposes. The state purchased two mobile field units, each equipped to perform tuberculin skin tests and x-ray examinations and each designed to make earlier diagnoses among high-school and other students. More ambitious and more expensive were Dexter's plans for the sanatoriums. According to a blatantly political pamphlet published in 1938, the department had found conditions in its sanatoriums deplorable. Masonry walls were crumbling, wooden buildings were fire traps, and the Dixon cottages were long outmoded. The department set out to rebuild and expand the sanatoriums and reduce the waiting lists. In 1938, ground was broken for a fourth sanatorium in western Pennsylvania. At Mont Alto, a "huge infirmary with accommodations for 715 patients" and "a magnificent preventorium" were both nearing completion. At Hamburg, where the state had concentrated its most advanced cases, the "all-enduring monument" of the work was taking shape—a new Division of Chest Surgery. An architect's sketch illustrated the new $150,000 surgical building—a "miracle house wherein . . . many persons are wrenched from the jaws of death . . . and given the opportunity for new life." The cycle of hope, medical promise, and institution-building was starting anew.[42]

From the turn of the century, the tuberculosis movement had had a profound impact on the lives of many Pennsylvanians. The degree to which people experienced these changes, however, varied considerably. Among the least affected, paradoxically, were those who had the highest rate of mortality from tuberculosis: the Pennsylvanians who were also black. They were unusually cautious about entering institutions, and were often excluded from them. For the sake of black people and for the protection of white society, tuberculosis leaders decided that different approaches were needed.

16. "P.S. I Am . . . Colored"

"While reading The Washington Times I notice the description of your Sanitarium and the Wonderful Work you are doing for the Consumptive," wrote Robert D. Freeman to Flick in 1906. "I Write to ask you would you take me at your Sanitarium. I am a Poor boy Afflicted With the Muscular Rheumatism and Lung trouble." For about two years, Freeman had had a cough and weakness, which had not responded to medical treatment, and he was "just able to get about out of doors. My father have spent most all of his Money for Doctors Bill and Medecine and he is not able to do any thing more for me. Beside he have four more Children to take Care off. If you would take me at your Sanitarium and cured me I would worked and do all I could to pay my way. Please see If you can help me in anyway." At the end of his three-page letter, Freeman added a single but very important line: "P.S. I am a Colored boy. Do you take Colored People?"[1]

The postscript made a world of difference. By 1910, Protestants, Catholics, and Jews in Philadelphia could all find sanatoriums that would admit them and honor their religious preferences. Fairly well-to-do consumptives could choose a private sanatorium; the poor could go to the Philadelphia General Hospital or to Mont Alto; and others could go to White Haven or to other institutions that partially subsidized their care. But black men and women—despite an unusually high tuberculosis death rate—had the fewest options for treatment, and they used even those reluctantly. For various reasons, relatively few tuberculous blacks were getting care in the institutions that were treating whites.

Leading white physicians gradually realized that untreated and unsupervised tuberculous blacks were a threat to the health of whites, as well as to the health of other blacks, and that special programs were needed to treat them and control the spread of infection. In 1914, H. R. M. Landis started a dispensary system in Philadelphia through which black nurses and physicians took care of black patients. In 1933, Flick initiated a tuberculosis ward at the Frederick Douglass Memorial Hospital, the older of the city's two black hospitals. Both arrangements served the interests of the white physicians while they also provided treatment for black patients and helped to train their caretakers.

Black physicians responded to these initiatives for their own reasons. Henry M. Minton, the first and most prominent physician to participate in Landis's program, found opportunities in it for black doctors and nurses; the work was a source of racial pride. If acceptance of a segregated system troubled him, he published no record of it; accommodation was a path to advancement. For Nathan F. Mossell, the founder and medical director of the Douglass Hospital and a staunch antisegregationist, the tuberculosis ward offered the only hope of saving his institution. Accepting the ward prolonged the life of the hospital, but the aging Mossell had to resign.

Black and White in Philadelphia

During the nineteenth and early twentieth centuries, society restricted the options of black people in virtually all phases of life—education, housing, employment, medical care, and recreation. Most important was the exclusion of blacks from desirable jobs. In the 1890s, when the black scholar W. E. B. Du Bois studied Philadelphia's seventh ward, then the center of the city's black population, he found 61.5 percent of the working males and 88.5 percent of the working females in domestic or personal service. Only 8.2 percent of the black workers were engaged in manufacturing and mechanical industries, while 46.9 percent of the white workers were so employed.[2]

Nevertheless, blacks in Philadelphia had made notable progress during the nineteenth century. A relatively successful, educated, and proud elite had emerged, some of whom could trace their roots to colonial times. A cadre of well-trained black teachers taught black children (but not white children) in both public and private schools, and the rate of illiteracy was comparatively low. In the 1890s, Du Bois observed that 81 percent of the blacks in the seventh ward could read and write. This percentage had risen considerably since 1850, and was higher than rates reported for the Italians, Russians, Poles, Hungarians, and Irish.[3]

Regardless of education, status, or capabilities, blacks who wanted to practice medicine faced serious obstacles. White medical schools accepted only a few black applicants. Even after 1913, when Pennsylvania legally required a year of internship for medical licensure, white hospitals rarely accepted a black graduate for this experience. In addition, white hospitals rarely accepted blacks on their medical staffs. Because medical practice was becoming increasingly specialized and dependent on hospitals in the twentieth century, exclusion from postgraduate training and inability to admit patients to hospitals were major impediments to professional success. They limited the quality of black physicians' work, their professional reputations, and their incomes.[4]

In addition, black physicians endured the discourtesies and humiliations of a predominantly white, racist society. As late as in the 1930s, Virginia M. Alexander, a well-educated black physician, reported aloofness and frankly insulting comments from white physicians, nurses, and hospital employees. Although black physicians who were known to the staff of a friendly institution were often treated graciously and could share in information about their patients, such a reception was seldom assured. Their opinions were sometimes ignored or dismissed. At the Philadelphia General Hospital, Dr. Alexander observed, the "contempt with which some resident doctors treat a note from a colored doctor is strikingly noticed by patients and doctors alike. Such remarks as 'Who is Dr. X? Is he colored?' and with that the note is sometimes chucked or a notation is made on the patient's [chart:] 'patient referred by Dr. X (colored).' These exceptions stand out very clearly in the minds of most patients, and possibly of all colored doctors."[5]

Black women who hoped to become nurses faced similar barriers. A survey in the mid-1920s showed that only 54 out of 1,642 accredited training schools in the United States admitted black students. Of these 54 schools, 25 were connected with hospitals or departments of hospitals for black patients. If a black woman had the courage to apply to a predominantly white training school, she was usually refused regardless of her qualifications.[6]

Black institutions emerged in response to white discrimination. In the fervor of Reconstruction, men of both races had cooperated in founding two medical schools where blacks were welcomed—Howard Medical School in Washington, D.C., and Meharry Medical College in Nashville, Tennessee. Additional black schools followed, but none had the resources to meet the rising standards for U.S. medical schools. Black hospitals and training schools for nurses also developed, partly filling the needs for education, clinical experience, and the care of patients. Among these institutions were two in Philadelphia: the Frederick Douglass Memorial Hospital and Training School, founded in 1895, and the Mercy Hospital and School for Nurses, which opened in 1907. Both hospitals welcomed patients of all races, but they served mainly the black community.[7]

In Philadelphia, this community was changing rapidly. In 1890, it consisted of fewer than forty thousand people, 3.8 percent of the city's population. During the 1890s alone, however, it grew by 60.4 percent. Most of the new residents had come from the South, fleeing oppression and seeking opportunities in the North. The migrants, as Du Bois described them, tended to be young, their largest age group between twenty-one and thirty years old. Typically originating in rural areas, they moved in stages to southern towns, then to cities, and on to Washington and north to Baltimore or Philadelphia. Ever since the social upheavals during and after the Civil War, tuberculosis had become common among Southern blacks, and the age of the migrants made them especially susceptible.[8]

Although black Philadelphians had long patronized white physicians, many distrusted white institutions. Du Bois, among others, reported a fear of hospitals, bred partly out of the brusque manner and lack of sympathy with which blacks had been treated, common in the lives of all poor people. For blacks, this fear was probably part of a larger experience of white oppression, bad in the North and worse in the South: systematic discrimination, loss of political rights, economic exploitation, personal assaults, lynchings, and an increasingly strict Jim Crow segregation. If a person was sick, still unfamiliar with the ways of the city, and ever unsure of a welcome, it seemed safer, indeed often was safer, to rely on the familiar and trusted— the family and perhaps other advisers and healers who had long practiced among blacks. Du Bois, who shared the values of orthodox medicine, disparaged the "old class of root doctors and patent medicine quacks with a lucrative trade among Negroes," but sick or troubled men and women, including some with tuberculosis, used them for decades.[9]

In 1935, blacks in Philadelphia still had reason to be wary of white institutions. Although most of them expressed a preference for one of the white hospitals and many seemed satisfied, according to a survey reported by Dr. Alexander, others had cause to complain: "'Treatment . . . is not pleasant. The authorities are prejudiced.'" "'White patients get better attention.'" "'I wouldn't go back . . . because of the segregation there.'" The lamentable "lack of regard for human suffering" that Alexander had witnessed among the white student nurses on the General Hospital's tuberculosis wards had made her "positively heartsick."[10]

Blacks and Tuberculosis

Tuberculosis was a major problem among blacks. In 1900, Philadelphia's rate of death from all forms of the disease among "colored" people was 447 per 100,000; the rate for whites was 198 per 100,000. Observers tried to explain this difference but often disagreed. Some argued that the black race was predisposed to the disease by heredity, while others pointed to environmental or personal causes such as poverty, crowding, and unhygienic habits. Du Bois blamed environmental rather than hereditary factors. "It must be remembered that Negroes are not the first people who have been claimed as its [consumption's] peculiar victims," he observed; "the Irish [too] were once thought to be doomed by that disease—but that was when Irishmen were unpopular."[11]

Despite this high frequency of tuberculosis, hospitals and sanatoriums often excluded blacks, and neither money nor personal recommendations could assure them acceptable care. In 1905, Livingston Farrand, executive secretary of the National Association for the Study and Prevention of Tuberculosis, wrote to Flick about "the wife of a very prominent member of the negro race" who had the "unqualified endorsement of a number of the most prominent men" and whose husband was "extremely anxious to have her admitted to some sanatorium. . . . He is able to pay ten or fifteen dollars a week," but Farrand had not been able to find a place for her. Flick obtained a single offer—from Mrs. Wilson, the proprietor who had the greatest need for business. She could take the patient, Mrs. Wilson replied, but "subject to certain restrictions." The woman "of course could not dine with the other patients, but could have her Dinner served in her room—In that manner the other patients would not be offended—or she hurt."[12]

In 1923, when data were first available, only twelve of Pennsylvania's twenty-nine tuberculosis institutions admitted blacks. Among these twelve, the state sanatorium at Mont Alto segregated patients by race and Jefferson Hospital's chest department admitted blacks to its wards only. Private sanatoriums were the least likely to accept black patients. Two motivations seem likely: the proprietors were acting out of their racial prejudices or, eager to attract a clientele, they were catering to what they thought white patients would prefer. Most tuberculous men and women were white, and no private institution in Pennsylvania could succeed without them.[13]

In the early twentieth century, a number of tuberculosis institutions did accept black patients: the Rush Hospital, the White Haven Sanatorium, the Henry Phipps Institute, the state sanatoriums, and the Philadelphia General Hospital. Flick, who had felt the stings of prejudice himself because of his religion, had made sure that every institution that he helped to found was open to all, regardless of race, creed, or color. When Elwell Stockdale was asked about admitting a black patient to White Haven in

1901, he replied with "the usual thing. . . . we care nothing for color. is this correct?" Flick's reply, though not recorded, was surely affirmative.[14]

When institutions accepted black patients or even encouraged them to come, utilization remained low. In the early years of the Phipps Institute, the proportion of black patients was consistently smaller than seemed indicated by the prevalence of the disease among blacks. From 1904 to 1906, Flick repeatedly expressed his concerns about the reluctance of blacks to use the Institute. Its location made it easily accessible to them, and he and his staff had tried to attract them. Compared to whites, Flick observed, "the colored . . . people are more loath to become a public charge and are more disposed to help themselves. They will not go into a public institution if they can manage to crawl around."[15]

Traditional black fears of white-dominated institutions undoubtedly contributed to the low utilization, and so did individual experience. Institutional death rates among blacks with tuberculosis were typically higher than those for whites. As one black physician, Harold E. Farmer, later observed, the relatives and neighbors who had watched patients go off to a sanatorium, only to worsen or die, often concluded that institutionalization was dangerous. Also, the milk regimen, wherever it was used, must have made a large proportion of black patients sick. A deficiency in intestinal lactase, the bodily substance that digests milk sugar, is now known to be common among otherwise healthy black adults. Even one glass of milk can cause abdominal cramping, bloating, and the excessive passage of gas by rectum. This condition, unknown at the time, may help to explain why some of the black consumptives who came to the Phipps dispensary never returned.[16]

In addition to the high death rate and the sometimes unsuitable regimen, blacks who entered institutions faced racial insults and humiliations. At the very least, they had to adapt themselves to a place where most of the patients and all of the physicians and nurses were white. White patients had ways of making their attitudes known. *Spunk*, the patients' magazine at Mont Alto, although otherwise silent on racial issues, published occasional racist jokes. These included characters with names such as Sambo, Rastus, or First and Second Nigga, and this "Conversation . . . between the rural editor and the colored porter":

> Editor—Well, Charles, did you go to church yesterday?
> Porter—Yessah, Boss, yessah; I allus goes to church: I'se one ob de pillers ob de church.
> Editor—What did your minister preach about?

Porter—Well, Boss, I didn't 'zackly ketch der applercation ob de connection,
      but it wuz sumpin' erbout de 'Possle Paul pintin' de pistol to de 'Fezians.
Editor—That will do, Charles, you may sweep the press room floor.[17]

At the White Haven Sanatorium, white patients sometimes objected to washing the dishes or cleaning the bathrooms for their black counterparts (when this was part of their work program), and one father was disturbed by his son's having to sleep on a cot near a "dying Negro."[18]

Despite such racist complaints at White Haven, Flick had resisted segregation; he feared that it would lead to the exclusion of blacks. During the fall of 1914, however, Miss Anna L. Morris, superintendent of the sanatorium, had allowed the white patients to separate themselves from blacks in the cottages. Neither Flick nor any member of the board of directors had apparently learned of the segregated pattern until the blacks as a group objected and insisted upon their rights.[19]

When Morris, at Flick's request, tried to return some black patients to the now all-white cottages, forty-two white patients sent an "emphatic protest" to Flick. To "be forced to mingle with negroes" was unjust, they proclaimed, and if the superintendent persisted in her efforts, they would have to seek treatment elsewhere. Flick defended the sanatorium's policy of nonsegregation, but to no avail. A few days later, on December 4, the white patients increased their threat:

> If we were to go down to our respective homes, and make it known there that the cause of our leaving this institution was on account of being compelled to live in the same quarters with Negroes, we feel sure that it would cause many prospective patients giving preference to some other institution where such conditions would not exist. As there is nothing in your advertising literature sent to patients . . . that they would be expected to associate with Negroes; we think it is an injustice to live in daily contact with them. We have no personal enmity against Negroes, we merely desire there [*sic*] segregation, as we do not think it desirable for the Black and White Races to mix.[20]

The protest struck at the institution's most vulnerable point, its economy. Although the patients paid only part of the cost of their maintenance, their fees and their numbers gave them power. The sanatorium needed them and others like them to maintain a reasonable rate of occupancy and keep its costs per capita under control.

The conflict pitted Flick against his board of directors, his ethical principles against the survival of the institution. At first, he tried to manage the crisis through Anna Morris. He ordered her to enforce the rules, regardless of who might leave the sanatorium, but Morris failed to take the necessary action. On December 12, when Flick went to White Haven, he could not regain control. In an emergency meeting on December 18, the board decided to exclude black patients. Flick cast the only negative vote. The next day he asked that no more patients be assigned to his care, and on December 23 he tendered his resignation from the medical directorship. He continued, however, as president. The sanatorium returned to its normal state, with one exception. In a pragmatic retreat from principle, it listed a new rule on its application form: "No negroes will be admitted to the Sanatorium."[21]

White leaders knew that they were failing in their efforts to reach black consumptives, treat and instruct them, and thus control the danger they represented to white society. Some, like Flick at the Phipps Institute, were puzzled and frustrated. Mabel Jacques, the tuberculosis nurse for the Visiting Nurse Society, grew hostile and accusatory—unable to understand or to deal with her black patients. When her tuberculosis class for blacks failed in 1909, she lashed out against them. Black patients, she declared, were

> the most difficult people with whom we have to deal . . . absolutely refusing to alter their manner of living. Occasionally we run across a family or an individual willing to do as we wish, but they are the exception. The Philadelphia negro is, as a general rule, insolent and overbearing, with a smattering of education to mingle with the superstitions and prejudices of his race, and constantly on the defensive against any suggestion regarding his mode of living that may benefit him. That he has consumption he will rarely ever admit, but the same man who denies it may quite cheerfully tell you that he has tuberculosis. Mention milk, eggs and fresh air to him and he is ready to almost throw you bodily out of his home. It is for the negro more than for any other race that we need strict legislation for he can seldom be persuaded; he must be forced.[22]

Almost two decades later, William G. Turnbull, Pennsylvania's deputy secretary of health, could describe little, if any, progress toward attracting and keeping black patients. "We who are in the State work are perfectly willing to admit that we are not handling the negro problem in any adequate way," he acknowledged in 1928. Tuberculous blacks were still too few in the state sanatoriums, and they stayed there only half as long as their white counterparts. "I do not know what should be done. . . . I have little hope of accomplishing much in an institution that is predominantly white. . . . In spite of all the workers can do for the comfort of the colored patient, he does not feel at home. An uncomfortable colored patient is not a contented patient. . . . It appears to me, in spite of the disadvantages of race segregation, more could be accomplished by the establishment of separate divisions, where they could be under supervision of nurses and physicians of their own race."[23]

A Segregated Dispensary System

Turnbull undoubtedly knew of the separate dispensary system that H. R. M. Landis had started for blacks in 1914. Landis had graduated from Amherst College in 1894 and from Jefferson Medical College in 1897. During an internship at Philadelphia Hospital, he developed tuberculosis and went to Saranac Lake for treatment. After returning home, he joined the medical staffs of the White Haven Sanatorium and the Phipps Institute, and became a skilled clinician with wide-ranging interests in social issues. Cultured and aristocratic in taste yet comfortable with acquaintances in all walks of life, he was widely liked and respected as a colleague, teacher, and leader. In 1914, he was director of the Clinical and Sociological Department of the Phipps Institute. As Charles J. Hatfield later recalled, Landis "felt that white doctors and nurses perhaps did not understand the workings of the Negro mind, its fears, superstitions, [and] dislikes."[24]

In 1913, Landis had become president of the Whittier Centre, a new voluntary organization of whites that aimed to study and meet the needs of the colored people. The founders wanted "the colored man and the colored woman [to] play a part and come to the fore" in any effort to help them. As Landis expressed the idea in 1914, "If the race is to rise it must be through and by its own members. In no other way can it become self-reliant and independent." Black success through self-help, with good will and assistance from whites, was the contemporary strategy for progress promulgated by Booker T. Washington, founder and principal of the Tuskegee Institute. Although some black leaders opposed segregation and pressed for civil rights more aggressively, Washington's accommodative approach was dominant: it appealed to many members of both races.[25]

Leaders of the Whittier Centre decided to focus their efforts on public health, and to start by hiring a competent black visiting nurse. It seemed, as Landis remarked, that a black nurse could more easily gain access to the homes of other blacks, that she could "go with immunity, day or night, into districts in which it would not be safe for a white woman," and that she could establish "a greater degree of confidence" among black patients than white nurses had been able to achieve.[26]

Mrs. Elizabeth W. Tyler, a graduate of the Freedman's Hospital Train-

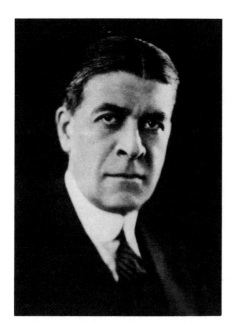

Figure 38. H. R. M. Landis. Historical Collections, College of Physicians of Philadelphia.

ing School in Washington, D.C., started the new work on February 1, 1914. She was superbly qualified for her position. She had done private-duty nursing, had taught physiology and hygiene at the college level, and had been the first black visiting nurse on the staff of the well-known Henry Street Nursing Settlement in New York City. She was now assigned to work with the Phipps Institute and was asked to find blacks who might be tuberculous and who therefore needed diagnosis and possibly treatment. "How to do this was a serious question," Tyler wrote in her first report to the Whittier Centre on October 1, 1914.

> On visiting the colored churches one could hear the telltale cough, note the symptoms in physique and carriage, but this was not the time nor place to win the confidence of those who needed advice.
>
> One could meet those on the street who looked ill and evidently were ill. When questioned one was almost invariably assured that the person suspected was in perfect health. This was manifestly not the way to reach them. It was finally agreed that a house-to-house investigation alone would reveal the true health conditions of the colored people in this city. These investigations began in those blocks nearest Phipps Institute. . . . The worker had not gone far when she discovered that in very many families visited there was one or more persons who were not well. This was not discovered as the result of the perfunctory question, "Is there any illness in this family?"

> One must first become acquainted with some member of the family, and these confidences were subsequently revealed.[27]

Tyler's approach exemplified the visiting nurse at her skillful best. When she first called upon one family of five, she reported, the mother, Mrs. W., would not give details of her family life. The worker understood and the visit ended, but with an invitation to return. Only on the third visit was Mrs. W. "willing to talk freely about her family problems," which included economic difficulties, a sick child, and a husband with symptoms of tuberculosis. After her first eight months of work, Tyler reported having "intimate knowledge" of 327 families, or 1,084 people; she had found 263 people ill, of whom 138 had either tuberculosis or manifestations suggesting it. Tyler tried to persuade those who might have the disease to go to the Phipps dispensary; others she referred to appropriate agencies.[28]

Her methods succeeded, and the Pennsylvania Society for the Prevention of Tuberculosis agreed to pay for a second nurse, Miss Cora H. Johnson, to work at the Phipps Institute. By the end of 1914, Landis could report that the number of black patients at the Institute had more than doubled—from 57 new patients the year before to 121. They were also returning for care rather than disappearing after the first visit.[29]

The increased work load justified the next step in Landis's plan, and in 1915 the Institute gave a part-time appointment to Dr. Henry M. Minton. Minton, a member of a prominent Philadelphia family, was born in 1870. He graduated from the Phillips Exeter Academy in 1891 and from the Philadelphia College of Pharmacy in 1895. He conducted the first black-operated pharmacy in the city, was the first pharmacist at the Douglass Hospital, and then studied medicine. After graduating from Jefferson Medical College in 1906, he joined the medical staff of the Mercy Hospital. With Minton's good work at the Institute, together with that of the nurses, use of the Phipps dispensary by black patients continued to rise. Despite a leveling-off period during the World War, the dispensary counted 245 new black patients in 1920, and in 1921 it added two more part-time black physicians to its staff.[30]

Other organizations followed the Landis model. According to the Pennsylvania Society, the efforts of the two nurses brought more black patients to hospitals. Jefferson Hospital employed a black physician for its chest department, and later it added a black nurse to care for the extra patients there. Meanwhile, the Pennsylvania Society, pleased with the results, decided to pay for a black nurse, Miss Jane C. Turner, to work with the Visiting Nurse Society of Philadelphia.[31]

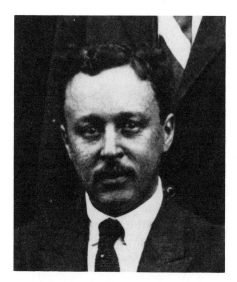

Figure 39. Henry M. Minton.
Mercy-Douglass Hospital and
School of Nursing Collection,
Center for the Study of the History
of Nursing, University of
Pennsylvania.

The Philadelphia Health Council and Tuberculosis Committee, which emerged out of the Pennsylvania Society in 1919, helped to extend the system further. The Council's missions included fighting tuberculosis, for which it received its own income from the Christmas Seal campaign. In 1922, the Health Council, along with the Phipps Institute, the Whittier Centre, and the Chest Department of Jefferson Hospital, established a Negro Bureau to coordinate the work among blacks. The Bureau offered educational programs for the black community, and it staffed up to four numbered clinics, each modeled on Landis's plan. The clinics for blacks at Phipps and at Jefferson became the Negro Bureau Clinics No. 1 and No. 2 respectively.[32]

Landis, who held key positions in most of these organizations, promoted the work with a two-part argument: blacks had an excessively high rate of tuberculosis, and those who had the disease were a menace to the white community. In their work as servants, cooks, and laundresses, for example, blacks came into frequent and intimate contact with whites and exposed them to infection. The disease among whites, therefore, could not be controlled without attending to "the Negro problem."[33] The rhetoric echoed the language used in the tuberculosis campaign a generation or so before. Then, it was chiefly the poor who had threatened the dominant community; now, it was "the Negro." In both instances, physicians were reflecting popular anxieties. They were also using them, even increasing them, to further their campaign. Appeals to fear and self-interest, not just to sentiment or humanitarianism, seemed better able to effect change.

As fear of poor consumptives, many of whom were immigrants, had helped to fuel the earlier work, so reaction to the black migration stimulated the efforts to care for blacks in the 1920s. Although this migration was evident by 1900, an even greater number of blacks arrived in the city during the war years of 1916–18 and again in 1922–23. The census reported a 58.9 percent increase in the city's black population between 1910 and 1920, and another 63.5 percent rise during the subsequent decade. By 1930, 219,599 blacks constituted 11.3 percent of the city's residents. As southern, rural, and poorly educated migrants pressed into the city, they unsettled both the whites and the old-Philadelphian blacks. They increased the need for housing, strained the resources of charitable organizations, and created concern about the spread of contagious disease. According to Sadie T. Mossell, whose study earned her a doctorate in 1919, the migration increased the move to segregate the school system and helped to close the restaurants, theaters, and white churches to black residents who had long used them.[34]

The growing black population, however, also created opportunity; it increased the economic base for black businesspeople and professionals. In health care, as in commerce, churches, and schools, segregation itself could be advantageous to middle class blacks by protecting them from white competition. Through the Landis plan, black professionals gained positions where none had been before. In 1924, Minton reviewed the qualities that, in his opinion, made black physicians and nurses successful in their tuberculosis work. "The members of these two professions know the innermost thoughts, ambitions and peculiarities of their own people," he asserted, "and receive from them that response and confidence which would be impossible in a program from which they were omitted." The professionals had gained prestige, influence, and usefulness; the race, a sense of pride. The work, Minton continued, "has given to the colored community a group of their own men and women who, representing a great movement, are regarded as authorities and as such are welcomed into their churches, lodges, [and] public gatherings, and by their newspapers, that they may bring a message. There is in the Negro race today a growing sense of racial consciousness which makes these people feel proud of any creditable work that is propagated by members of that race—and to the same degree of pride there will exist an interest in this work." Minton urged that black physicians and nurses be involved in considering all health problems that affected black people. "Recognition begets pride," he concluded, "the hope of recognition begets ambition, and proper ambition will make better men and women of all of us."[35]

By this time, Minton had advanced in his own career. He continued his work at Phipps, and in 1921 he also became the superintendent of the Mercy Hospital and Training School. His own success and connections eased the way for others. Some of the interns at Mercy and some of the graduate nurses from its training school went on to jobs at the Phipps Institute or at other clinics of the Negro Bureau. At least two additional Mercy graduates joined the Visiting Nurse Society of Philadelphia.[36]

Again, as in the early 1900s, the Phipps Institute had devised an arrangement that provided care for poor tuberculous patients and that also helped physicians and nurses to acquire the training and the experience they needed to advance their careers. Late in 1921, the Institute also began to participate in undergraduate nursing education. Landis proposed that the senior students at Mercy Hospital each rotate for two months through the Phipps, where they would be trained in tuberculosis work and in other aspects of public health nursing such as home visiting, prenatal care, and the care of babies—all services that the Institute now offered. Their instructors included Minton, Miss Lulu Warlick, superintendent of nurses at Mercy, and later Miss Fannie Eshleman, a white nurse who in 1923 became director of social service at the Institute and warmly supported the project. The Visiting Nurse Society provided the students with two additional months of experience.[37]

A clinical conference that Landis began at the Institute in 1934 helped to create an esprit de corps among staff members of both races. For each case discussed at the weekly or semiweekly meeting, the nurse presented a full socioeconomic history, the physician then described the medical details, and the x-ray films were shown. " 'The Clinical Conference was well known throughout the city,' " Eshleman observed, " 'and the nurses were proud of their contribution.' " The conference was serving the needs of the nurses much as the Monday evening conferences had served the early Phipps physicians.[38]

Research, like education, was linked to patient care. As the numbers of black patients climbed in the 1920s and 1930s, exceeding the numbers of whites by 1934, white physicians began to study racial variations in tuberculous disease. When compared to whites, for example, black patients were found to have greater numbers of bacilli in their sputum, and post-mortem studies suggested that cavities developed more quickly in their lungs. The record system in the dispensary was reorganized to clarify how the disease spread through several generations of both black and white families. The dispensary, the laboratory, and the pathology department were all serving each other, as Flick had envisioned in 1903.[39]

Despite the increasing sophistication of their training and their growing responsibilities, black physicians and nurses still faced two important obstacles. First, they were working in a segregated system in which they could only take care of black patients. Second, they were blocked from taking full and independent charge of their own work. Although Minton became the supervisor of the Negro Bureau, he and other black physicians and nurses functioned under white authority.[40]

Inadequate training of blacks, according to Landis, necessitated white direction. He considered physicians especially deficient—the "weak link" in the system. "For a time the feeling was entertained that it would be possible, eventually, to turn the entire responsibility of the Negro Bureau over to the Negroes themselves," he observed in 1926. "This idea has been abandoned, for the present, at least. The race is too inexperienced to walk entirely alone. They still need guidance. How long this will be necessary, it is now impossible to say. The better trained their doctors become, the nearer will they come to handling their own health problems. But this, I feel, is something that lies in the distant future."[41]

Landis's explanation was oversimplified. Although many blacks were poorly trained, and although life in a segregated and prejudiced society may have ill-equipped them to compete with their white counterparts for supervisory or independent positions, whites also had a racist predilection for automatically judging blacks as less capable, not quite up to standard. Such racist beliefs permeated white society. Physicians, biologists, anthropologists, and others had published a number of theories and observations that seemed to prove that blacks as a race were physically, intellectually, culturally, and morally inferior to whites. Popular views among whites supported the premise of white superiority and the propriety of white domination. Work relationships in a competitive society naturally reflected these beliefs, and to whites the very idea that a black might take authority over them seemed abhorrent, if not unthinkable. For blacks, the resulting block to promotion may well have persuaded potential candidates that the effort to compete for that promotion was not worthwhile.[42]

A Tuberculosis Ward at the Douglass Hospital

Flick took no part in developing the dispensary system for blacks. He considered it "a tantalizing service, dangling the cup of knowledge before them but with-holding the help which it makes them crave, telling them they have a curable preventable disease but keeping beyond their reach the means of [both] getting well and protecting those who are near and dear to them against the disease." What the "colored people" needed instead, he believed, was hospital care for tuberculous patients.[43]

The exclusion of blacks from White Haven in 1914 had troubled Flick, and late in 1932 he finally saw a chance to make a partial restitution. He was also hoping to realize one of his cherished dreams—a tuberculosis ward for advanced consumptives in one of the city's voluntary hospitals. At Flick's suggestion, Frederick M. Kirby, a well-to-do Wilkes-Barre businessman who had contributed large sums of money to White Haven, agreed to pay for such a ward in a black hospital at a rate of three dollars a day per capita. After considering both Mercy and Douglass Hospitals for his plan, Flick selected Douglass: it was weaker and more in need.[44]

Nathan F. Mossell, with the help of others, had founded the Frederick Douglass Memorial Hospital and Training School in 1895. Mossell was born in 1856 in Hamilton, Ontario, where his free-born parents had sought safety from the threat of slavery. In 1865, the family moved to Lockport, New York, where Nathan's father, a brick manufacturer, successfully protested segregation in the local school, thus enabling his children to get an integrated education. The young Mossell came to Pennsylvania in the early 1870s, graduated from Lincoln University in 1879, and became the first black medical graduate of the University of Pennsylvania in 1882. His life in medical school was marred by student hostility and partial ostracism, but Mossell, never one to cringe before racial prejudice, did well scholastically and was applauded at length at the graduation ceremony. Like other black physicians, Mossell could not get an internship in Philadelphia, but the well-known surgeon D. Hayes Agnew arranged for him to become an assistant in the University Hospital's surgical outpatient department. Mossell later took postgraduate work in London and returned to Philadelphia prepared to practice surgery.[45]

The Frederick Douglass Memorial Hospital and Training School opened in October 1895 in a narrow, three-story brick house at 1512 Lombard Street, near the center of the seventh ward. It was the second hospital started and managed by blacks in the United States. Mossell and his colleagues attracted financial support from both the white and black communities as well as from the state, and in 1897 the training school graduated its first two nurses. Few hospitals ever succeeded quickly, however, and for Douglass the course was especially long and arduous. The very existence of a black hospital provoked negative reactions. It was "condemned by the whites as an unnecessary addition to a bewildering number of charitable institutions," Du Bois observed in 1899, and "by many of the best Negroes as a concession to prejudice and a drawing of the color line." Patients were slow to come. Although the hospital could accommodate twenty-one patients, it averaged only three in 1896, eleven in 1900, and thirteen in 1908. Even after the facilities were enlarged in 1909, fewer than half of the beds on the average were occupied over the next five years.[46]

Dissension among the physicians also threatened the institution's survival. The hospital had reserved the right to control who could do surgery, and during the first year Mossell, the chief of staff who undoubtedly made these decisions, performed two-thirds of the operations. Although the policy could be justified as a method of assuring the quality and safety of surgical practice, some of the physicians considered it dictatorial and exclusive—contrary to the very purpose of the institution. In 1905 the dissidents started to organize on their own, and in 1907 the Mercy Hospital opened on the corner of 17th and Fitzwater Streets, only three-fourths of a mile from Douglass.[47]

After the Mercy men split from Douglass, the latter suffered politically and economically. Faction fought faction within Douglass, and both the medical staffs and the boards of the two hospitals competed for patients and money. Powerful whites took sides, and increasingly favored Mercy. From about 1917 through the 1920s, two important agencies in Philadelphia—the Charities Bureau of the Chamber of Commerce and the Welfare Federation—withheld their endorsement of Douglass, thereby decreasing the hospital's chances of raising money. In 1917 and again in 1919, the State Board of Public Charities tried to remove Mossell as head of the hospital. The black community rallied to raise funds for Douglass and the board supported its leader, but the hospital's reputation was a mixed one, even among blacks. Although there were loyal and dedicated supporters, there were also tales of fiscal mismanagement, immoral conduct, and other improprieties. To what extent the stories were true or were spread maliciously is unclear.[48]

Mossell himself was a controversial figure—to some a hero and martyr, to others an autocrat who was blocking the progress of the hospital or blocking their own careers. When Miss Ethel Johns, a white nurse employed by the Rockefeller Foundation to study the status of black women in nursing, met him in 1925, she found him to be a "remarkable" man of "great physical force and vigour," one who discussed the efforts to oust him "with a good deal of humour. He really considers himself as standing for a principle," Johns continued, "that of racial equality."[49]

It was this principle, Mossell contended repeatedly, that had guided his life and made him so many enemies. He had founded the hospital as a protest against segregation, had named it for Frederick Douglass, and, like Douglass, had rejected white domination. Some powerful institutions, however, including the University of Pennsylvania and the State Board of Public Charities, had tried to make him subordinate, to tell him what to do. Around 1917, according to Mossell, the University had tried to send its few black medical students to Douglass for their obstetrical experience, thereby avoiding their own educational responsibilities by creating a segregated program. Mossell had refused, thus, he believed, turning the Chamber of Commerce and the Board of Public Charities against him. According to Bishop J. S. Caldwell, vice president of the board at Douglass in 1919, the state board thought Mossell was "too aggressive. They wanted a man selected who would be easier to handle."[50]

Mossell was "frankly scornful of Dr. Minton and Mercy Hospital," Ethel Johns reported in 1925. "He thinks they have sold their birthright of freedom for a mess of pottage, i.e., white recognition and support. 'Mercy is being used as a means of convenience by the University of Pennsylvania Hospital to provide a practise [*sic*] ground for colored medical students and interns.' He also says that [colored] private patients applying at the white hospitals are referred to Mercy, 'thus relieving an embarrassing situation.'" Mossell, in contrast, had refused to compromise.[51]

Mossell and Flick had much in common. Neither was a native Philadelphian; neither belonged to the dominant social group in the city. Both were intelligent, well-educated, and innovative physicians who, guided by strong principles, had broken barriers to create new institutions. In the process, they both saw powerful enemies in the University of Pennsylvania and in the state government. In 1932, they were both seventy-six years old, and they were both ill. Each for his own reasons was trying to save the Douglass Hospital.

The situation at Douglass would have daunted many a younger man. Occupancy rates were still low, income was meager, and bills were overdue. The state had been granting it a regular although modest appropriation, but in October 1931 the State Welfare Department (which had succeeded the Board of Public Charities) notified the hospital that its quarterly distributions of two thousand dollars would cease. Conditions at Douglass did not meet state standards, and the hospital would have to make certain improvements before it could get its money.[52] When an observer for the *Philadelphia Bulletin* visited Douglass in September 1932, she described it as

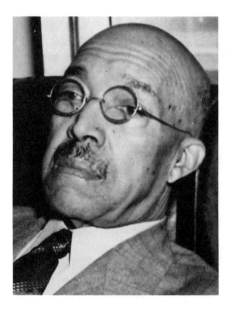

Figure 40. Nathan F. Mossell, ca. 1940. Mercy-Douglass Hospital and School of Nursing Collection, Center for the Study of the History of Nursing, University of Pennsylvania.

dirty—, linen soiled and mussy even in the rooms which are occupied. The walls have been painted recently in accordance with the requirements of the Welfare Department but in many places they are stained and broken. The floor coverings are worn through to the boards in many places and the carpets in a number of rooms are dingy and soiled looking. . . . The operating room was clean and well lighted but the sterilizing room adjoining had water on the floor where the pipes were leaking.

The patients all seemed cheerful and happy and the luncheon which was being served to them looked delicious and well cooked. The hospital is very dark and cheerless except in the rooms facing on Lombard st. It is not a hospital in which I would like to be ill.

Flick's proposal for a tuberculosis ward, with its annual income of fifty-five hundred dollars, was understandably welcomed: it might rescue the institution. With Kirby's money, Douglass made some necessary repairs and, late in January 1933, opened its new ward on the top floor.[53]

As Flick became more involved in the project, he began to sense an "organized influence" and a "subtle conspiracy" to oppose the tuberculosis ward and even to close the Douglass Hospital. Defamatory stories about Mossell and his hospital, which Flick was sure were false, were circulating both at City Hall and in Harrisburg. Flick himself had found Dr. Mossell and his medical staff "well educated and of rather a high type." As both friends and officials tried to divert his attentions to Mercy, Flick's suspicions

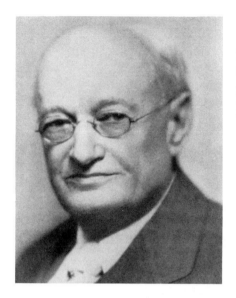

Figure 41. Lawrence F. Flick, ca.
1936. From Ella M. E. Flick, *Dr.
Lawrence F. Flick, 1856–1938* (White
Haven Sanatorium Association,
1940).

deepened. Because his health prevented his going to Douglass himself,
Flick had asked his longstanding colleague, Dr. Frank A. Craig, to serve as
his liaison. Craig assented at first, Flick noted, but then demurred, intimat-
ing that he would serve "if I would transfer the benefaction to the Mercy
Hospital with which the Phipps Institute already had some affiliation."
Craig at the time was assistant director of the Clinical and Sociological
Department of the University's Phipps Institute, where Landis was director and Minton still had an appointment. When Dr. Burgess Gordon, who
replaced Craig as Flick's liaison, tried to recruit some suitable patients from
the city's health department, Dr. Seth Brumm, chief of the Division of
Communicable Diseases and Tuberculosis, offered similar advice. Problems
at Douglass, Brumm counseled, made it wiser to give money, time, and
effort to Mercy; the latter was a willing and cooperative institution, and
both Minton and his staff were well trained. When Flick approached the
Rosenwald Fund for additional fiscal support, its director, Michael M.
Davis, responded in a similar vein. The "sinister influence" that led to such
advice, Flick concluded, was also withholding the state appropriation.[54]

Although Kirby's money and the new project temporarily raised the
hopes and spirits of the staff at Douglass, the status of the state appropriation soon became critical. In mid-March 1933 Flick learned that if the
remainder of the 1931–32 appropriation was not paid to Douglass before
April 1 it would lapse and never be paid. "This would be a catastrophe" for

the hospital's economy and for its chance of getting subsequent appropriations. Dr. Gordon and Dr. Charles A. Lewis, a staff physician at Douglass, went to Harrisburg to confer with Mrs. Liveright, secretary of the Department of Welfare. "Their report confirms what I have suspected and feared for a long time," wrote Flick to Mossell on March 23, namely, "that there is a determined attitude in the State Welfare Department to push the Douglass Hospital to the wall unless its management is reorganized and you withdraw from the superintendency of it. This creates a practical situation from which there is no escape." Mossell, Flick urged, should resign.[55]

It was a bitter choice for the proud and aging Mossell: to give up his title and leadership, or to witness the closure of the hospital that he had nurtured and ruled for thirty-eight years. Negotiations dragged out for months. As the welfare department had requested, the hospital reorganized itself, appointing Flick to its board in the process, and it tried hard to raise money. During the Great Depression, however, fundraising was exceptionally difficult, and unpaid bills accumulated. On May 26, the Philadelphia Electric Company turned off the hospital's current. "There were 11 consumptives on the fourth floor and between 20 and 30 sick people in the hospital," wrote Flick in a statement to the newspapers. "They were panic-stricken." Flick took the opportunity to increase his efforts to raise funds. On June 9, the White Haven Sanatorium Association agreed not only to contribute one thousand dollars to help repair Douglass but also to support ten beds for advanced consumptives. An agreement between the hospital and its leader was also reached. Mossell would resign from both the board and the executive committee, but his name would still be carried on hospital stationery as founder and emeritus medical director. Further, if the 1931–32 appropriations were received, he would be paid three thousand dollars for back salary and money that he had lent to the hospital. He would also get an annual pension of two thousand dollars. The government, with help from Flick, had finally achieved what some men of both races had wanted—the removal of Nathan Mossell. His hospital, however, survived the crisis. In 1934, the state released its 1931–32 appropriation, and added another for the next biennium.[56]

"The saving of this Hospital has been a noble work," wrote Flick to Kirby in September 1933, "and I am prouder of what I have done in it than of anything that I have been able to accomplish." In April 1937, the Douglass Hospital honored Flick with a plaque. Although Kirby had become too ill to contribute further, the White Haven Sanatorium Association was still supporting the tuberculosis ward, and Douglass was receiving its state appropriation. Mossell was rewarded less well. Despite his appeals and some letters by Flick to the board at Douglass, the hospital was slow in paying the money it owed him and probably never paid it in full. During the winter of 1934, Flick sent him a needed truckload of coal.[57]

Mossell's downfall, like his earlier difficulties, can be explained in several ways. His personal style of leadership—stubbornly principled, autocratic, loyal, and demanding of reciprocal loyalty—had won him "both loyal friends and bitter enemies." He had had the courage and strength to create and sustain a new black institution but had not been nimble enough to avoid being the target of factionalism and intrigue—from both outside and inside his institution. His style of interracial relations also worked against him. Radical activism and confrontation had helped to abolish slavery and a century later they were to play an important part in the civil rights movement, but during most of Mossell's adult life, the more common position among black leaders was considerably more conservative and accommodative.[58]

Politically and economically, accommodation was a more successful strategy for maintaining a hospital. Two black hospitals in Philadelphia exceeded the resources of the black community, and white support was needed. Mercy Hospital obtained it more successfully; it developed connections with the University of Pennsylvania, with politicians, and with funding organizations. In 1929, for example, it received $45,999 from state and local agencies, while Douglass received only $6,412.50. Lack of adequate fiscal support made Douglass and its leader, Nathan Mossell, vulnerable to other attacks.[59]

Whatever the explanations for the troubles at Douglass—personal, economic, political, or perhaps all combined—Mossell, like Minton at the Phipps Institute and in the Negro Bureau, was striving to advance himself and his colleagues in a racist, white-dominated society. Mossell confronted and fought segregation; Minton used a segregated system for racial advancement. Each man achieved more and advanced further than most of his contemporaries, but each was caught in a web of white restrictions, white interests, and white power. In 1913, H. R. M. Landis and Susan P. Wharton, writing for the Whittier Centre, described the relationship of whites and blacks in a way that was still pertinent years later: "Much of the work ostensibly done for both white and colored races together, ends—does it not?—in pushing the negro to the wall; 'with the best intentions.' The white races . . . somehow run off with the booty, with the interest, with the heart of the work whatever it is, with the fire that drives the engine. Watch the drift!—the way of least resistance, the easier way, wins—does it not?"[60] Even Landis, who had once hoped that blacks would "become self-reliant and independent," took an easier way by keeping control; integrating the clinics was out of the question. Flick won his long-sought "booty," a tuberculosis ward in a voluntary hospital. Given their racist environments and the mixture of goals that typically motivate human endeavors, however, perhaps each of the men achieved all that he could in his time.

While blacks were trying to better their place in a predominantly white society, tuberculosis was taking a smaller toll among people of both races. Flick, looking back over the decades between 1900 and 1930, attributed the falling death rates to institutionalization. His colleagues, however, rejected this argument as overly simpliflied.

Part IV

A Retrospective View

17. The Decline of Tuberculosis

Observers have long tried to explain the decline of tuberculosis but have yet to reach agreement. Since the 1930s, when Flick expressed his final opinions, scientists have clearly described how the infection usually spreads from person to person. The nature, size, and sources of the infectious particles are known, and the importance of ventilation has been proved. Much has been learned about the body's immune defenses, and some of the factors that impair them have been documented. Applying this knowledge backward through time, however, is fraught with interpretive dangers. It depends, for example, on reported death rates for years when diagnoses were often erroneous, and these rates were not usually adjusted for age, race, national origin, or economic status—all factors with which they varied. The death rates are probably more accurate, however, than measures of malnutrition, crowding, poor ventilation, and other contributors to the disease.

There are so many factors that affect the rates of tuberculosis that observers have often seen what they wanted to see. Their interpretations are affected by the knowledge and culture of their times, by their personal outlooks, and by their participation in related events. Explanations of the decreasing death rates have thus included a change in morality, altered personal habits, natural selection, socioeconomic improvements, and medical intervention. Flick attributed the falling rates to one particular kind of intervention, institutionalization. Using data from England and Wales, he publicly argued this view in 1890, and in 1932 he described the same phenomenon in Philadelphia.

Flick's explanation, which underscored the value of his life's work, was narrower than the ones endorsed by most of his colleagues. Few leaders of the tuberculosis campaign, however, excluded the impact of institutions. They had worked hard to establish the sanatoriums and hospitals that they thought would cure patients or, at the very least, prevent disease through isolation and education. They had also witnessed the falling death rates. In their minds and in their public pronouncements, the correlation of institutionalization with lessening mortality became at least partly a cause-and-effect relationship.

Flick's Argument

Late in 1931, the aging Flick began to gather data for a paper that would show again the value of segregating tuberculous patients. When repeated attacks of chest pain prevented his giving the paper himself, his son John read it to the Philadelphia County Medical Society on November 23, 1932. Between 1900 and 1930, Flick reported, Philadelphia's annual rate of death from tuberculosis had fallen from 354 per 100,000 living persons down to 81 (see Graph 17-1). Isolation of sick and dying patients in institutions, he argued, was the most important cause of this decline. Between 1900 and 1915 the number of tuberculous Philadelphians thus segregated had increased substantially, he explained, and the subsequent death rates had dropped sharply. Between 1916 and 1930, however, the number of segregated cases had diminished, and the decline in death rates had moderated accordingly. In addition, the patients isolated during these later years had had less-advanced tuberculosis. Their segregation, therefore, had had less impact. The preventoriums and the vast sums of money that the Pennsylvania Tuberculosis Society and the Philadelphia Health Council had spent on educational and other projects had had no apparent effect on falling mortality. With the "upwards of $500,000" that these organizations had earned by selling Christmas Seals in 1931, Flick concluded, they would have accomplished much more by supporting the institutional care of advanced consumptives instead.[1]

By criticizing the use of Christmas Seal funds, Flick created a stir among the doctors, and for the next two days the *Public Ledger* aired the argument on its front page. The timing of the controversy made it of special interest to the public. It was the eve of the Pennsylvania Society's annual fundraising campaign, and one hundred thousand letters promoting the Seals were just being mailed. The question, as the *Ledger* reported it, was basically one of strategy: should Christmas Seal money be spent on segregation or education? Society leaders defended their expenditures and their educational methods as entirely compatible with policies of the National Tuberculosis Association and with the opinions of prominent scientists. They agreed that isolation was valuable, but insisted that their Christmas Seal campaigns and their efforts to educate the public had been the leading forces in establishing sanatoriums and hospitals—that their work had persuaded state and local governments to make the necessary investments. Care of tuberculous patients was a public responsibiltiy, not a job for the tuberculosis societies. Several factors, not just isolation, caused the declining death rates. In addition to hospitals and sanatoriums, these included a

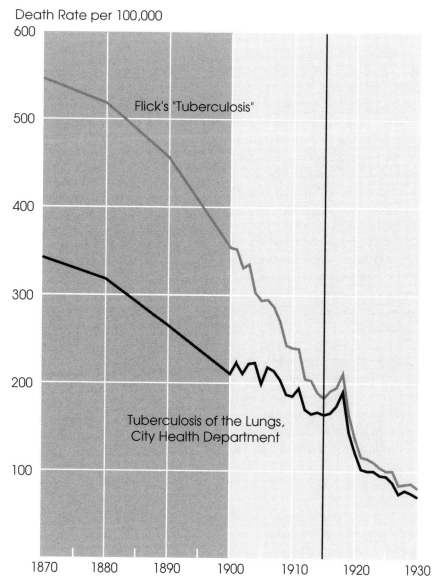

Death Rate per 100,000

Flick's "Tuberculosis"

Tuberculosis of the Lungs,
City Health Department

Graph 17-1. Flick's rates of death from "tuberculosis" in Philadelphia, compared with the city health department's figures for either consumption of the lungs or tuberculosis of the lungs, 1870–1930. From 1870 to 1900, figures are plotted every tenth year; from 1900 on, they are annual. The vertical line at 1915 separates the years 1900–1915, during which Flick thought that death rates were falling more rapidly, from the later period, when the decline of his "tuberculosis" slowed. Flick referred only indirectly to rates before 1900, shown in the shaded area.

higher standard of living, education of the public, and the work of health departments.[2]

Midst the flurry of controversy, no one publicly challenged the numbers that Flick had used for Philadelphia's mortality rates, but they were not the standard figures. Conventional statistical data must have created some awkward problems for the old crusader. As the Philadelphia health department reported it, the rate of death from tuberculosis of the lungs—the major infectious form of the disease—fell more slowly between 1900 and 1915 than during the decades before or after. This was the time, however, when Flick's influence had peaked and when he believed that the effects of his programs should have been evident.[3]

Flick, reasoning from his convictions, had substituted different statistics. In the early days of the Phipps Institute, J. Willoughby Irwin, one of the staff physicians, had examined the city's death rates between 1861 and 1903, and from them had tabulated figures for three mutually exclusive categories: tuberculosis, probably tuberculosis, and possibly tuberculosis. Death rates per 100,000 people for these three categories in 1900 were 214, 242, and 580 respectively. The first category—tuberculosis—included consumption of the lungs and some other organs, hemorrhage from the lungs, and scrofula. The second and larger category—probably tuberculosis— was quite diverse. Between 1870 and 1903, seven diagnoses contributed about 90 percent of it: marasmus (an emaciated condition usually but not necessarily described in young children), debility, inanition, inflammation of the brain, congestion of the brain, dropsy of the brain, and congestion of the lungs. The third, and very expansive, category—possibly tuberculosis—included many conditions, the most common of which were inflammation of the lungs (or pneumonia and bronchopneumonia, as it was later termed), inflammation of the stomach and bowels, convulsions, diarrhea, and typhoid fever.[4]

Flick had long believed that all the diagnoses in Irwin's second and third categories camouflaged many cases of tuberculosis, and in his 1932 paper he continued to use this classification. For the period before 1904— the year that Philadelphia instituted a new diagnostic nomenclature—Flick added together the deaths that Irwin had called tuberculosis and one-fourth of those in the other two categories. For 1904 through 1913, he added together the deaths from tuberculosis and half of those in the other categories. For 1914 on, he used the health department's figures for tuberculosis of all forms. The resulting numbers, as illustrated in Graph 17-1, trace a nicely declining curve, interrupted only by the rise in mortality rates that accompanied the World War and the influenza epidemic of 1918. When this rise is ignored, the slope of the curve is slightly steeper between 1900 and 1915 than it is during the later period. This difference is what he had apparently wished to document.[5]

In retrospect, Flick erred in both his data selection and his logic. His figures for tuberculosis death rates before 1914—grossly inflated—were never used by others. The most nearly valid numbers that he could have selected would have referred to disease of the lungs: consumption through 1903, and tuberculosis thereafter, shown in Graph 17-1. Diagnostic error should have been less in this category than in the other groups, and, because disease of the lungs was by far the most infectious form of tuberculosis, it was also the form most relevant to his argument. Most important of all, Flick failed to make clear that tuberculosis death rates, however derived, had been falling since 1870. Although he tabulated the annual rates from 1900 through 1930, he referred to the earlier decades in only a single, complicated sentence from which diligent listeners might later, if they cared to, compute the decennial rates for themselves. The data that he kept in shadow clearly refute the cause-and-effect relationship that he was trying to prove. Isolation could not have caused the decline in death rates that preceded it; there must have been other explanations. In 1913, H. R. M. Landis had called attention to a pertinent phenomenon that has long bedeviled attempts to explain the decline of tuberculosis: "'Figures like soldiers have a trick of obeying their own commander.'"[6]

We can only speculate on how Flick reached the conclusions that now seem so ill-founded. He knew that tuberculosis death rates had fallen late in the nineteenth century, and he knew that he was using statistical data that differed from those of his colleagues. It seem unlikely, however, that he was simply lying. More probably, he was so convinced that his views were right—intellectually, socially, and morally—that he adjusted the figures to match his beliefs. He had consecrated his life to the campaign against tuberculosis—an effort that he had once likened to "'the Crusade against the Saracens, for the recovery of the Holy Sepulchre.'" For Flick, perhaps, doubting the value of this work would have been like doubting the righteousness of that medieval mission.[7]

To dismiss Flick's thought and behavior as the self-justifying and deceptive machinations of a single individual, moreover, is to miss a more subtle, more important, and much more pervasive social process in which Flick was merely one participant. Physicians, nurses, politicians, social leaders, officials of the tuberculosis societies, and doubtless much of the public all believed that the tuberculosis movement was scientific, socially justified, and somehow effective. Even if some of the leaders differed over the best methods to use, their efforts to fight the disease had become an approved part of the social fabric. To have major doubts about the worth of the work was almost unthinkable. The gratifying fall in mortality rates helped to sustain this confidence, and the flaws in the logic that causally linked this decline to the measures implemented were typically overlooked or forgotten.[8]

Assessment of the Medical Interventions

Throughout much of the nation, as in Philadelphia, tuberculosis death rates were falling and had been falling since roughly the 1870s or 1880s. In England and Wales the rates were dropping as early as the late 1840s. Observers still argue over the reasons, and no single set of explanations applies to all nations or even to all regions in the United States. Institutionalization, however, was not the leading cause of Philadelphia's falling death rate. The decline of tuberculosis began before that form of segregation and continued fairly steadily thereafter until 1916. After 1920, as illustrated in Graph 17-2, the death rate fell somewhat more quickly. Institutionalization may have had an impact during this later period but it cannot be separated from other possible causes.[9]

While Flick was right in pointing to persons with advanced disease as the most dangerously infectious, and while segregating such people must have reduced the danger to others, it could not have done so by much in the first two decades of the twentieth century. Diagnoses were often made late in the course of illness, and institutional capacities, although rising, were very small in relation to the numbers of infectious people. Waiting times to enter the sanatoriums were long, and by the time applicants were admitted, they had probably already infected most of their close contacts. Durations of stay, moreover, were often short by mid-century standards, and most patients went home in a probably still infectious state. Many of them chose to leave the institutions of their own accord, and even Flick and his colleagues sent infectious men and women out of the White Haven Sanatorium after a six-months' stay. As late as 1939, 41 percent of the tuberculosis deaths in Pennsylvania occurred outside of institutions.[10]

If hospitals and sanatoriums failed to prevent the spread of infection during this period, did they prolong life or promote cure? In 1927, Flick did

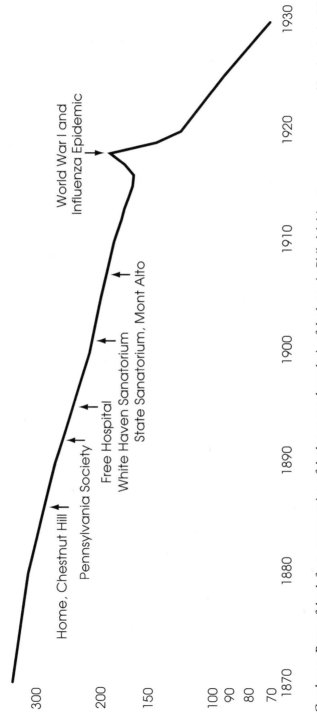

Graph 17-2. Rates of death from consumption of the lungs or tuberculosis of the lungs in Philadelphia, 1870–1930, as reported by the city health department and plotted on a semilogarithmic scale. With this scale, unlike a linear one, the slopes of the curve accurately represent the rates of change over time. Rates are plotted every tenth year between 1870 and 1900, every fifth year from 1900 on, except for the years 1915 to 1920. These are plotted annually to show the rapid changes that accompanied the World War and the influenza epidemic of 1918. Arrows indicate the beginnings of the Pennsylvania Society for the Prevention of Tuberculosis and of selected institutions.

not think so. "I treat very many cases of tuberculosis in their own homes and have done so for many years," he observed, "and my results in the homes of the patients are even better than my results in sanatoria. Incipient cases practically all get well under treatment at home, if properly treated, and even many advanced cases get well." A properly trained visiting nurse, he noted, could direct the care of a consumptive at home "with as good a prospect of recovery as can be had in a sanatorium."[11]

No one knows for sure whether Flick was right in his assessment of home care versus institutional care. Physicians during this period did not use controlled experiments in tuberculosis or in other comparable fields. Even if they had, diagnostic methods in the early decades were inadequate to ensure the comparability of experimental groups. A clinical history and physical examination, although valuable, did not clearly define the extent of a person's lung disease or even its nature. As a result, nontuberculous conditions such as bronchitis, emphysema, slowly improving pneumonia, and heart disease were sometimes mistaken for tuberculosis. Even when chest x-ray examinations became more available in the 1920s, clinicians still disputed their meaning. A rough generalization probably describes the situation as accurately as is possible: most persons with early disease recovered fairly quickly, while most patients with far-advanced disease died within about five years. For persons whose tuberculosis was moderately advanced, the chances of living for five years or so were about fifty-fifty. Results of care depended very much on the stage of the patient's disease.[12]

In hindsight, most ingredients of the therapeutic program must be judged ineffective; none had proven worth. The tonics, purgatives, creosote, and iodine that Flick recommended had no specific value, and they caused unpleasant, even harmful side effects. The outdoor life and open windows may have agreed with some patients (while they bothered others), and they diminished the risks of infection for caretakers and other close contacts. A beneficial effect on the course of disease, however, seems very unlikely. Common sense and clinical wisdom suggest that rest did help acutely ill, feverish, or exhausted patients. Rest, however, has never been scientifically tested in the absence of effective chemotherapy and, with it, has proved unnecessary. Implementation of rest, moreover, varied widely— from the rest and supervised work of the early years to very prolonged bed rest in the later decades. Severely malnourished patients probably did benefit from the food offered by sanatoriums and dispensaries. For some of these, it may have made a critical difference. Weight gain, however, did not necessarily indicate that a person's lung disease had improved. No evidence has ever supported the specific value of milk and eggs, although Flick still promoted their use in 1937. To the extent that patients took his advice, they may have contributed to the next great "epidemic" of the western world—insofar as current theories can be trusted—coronary artery disease.[13]

Institutionalization may have had other, less tangible advantages. The care and support of nurses, a trusting relationship with a physician, the confidence and hope that a sanatorium sometimes engendered, the comradeship of other patients, and escape from deleterious conditions at home or at work all may have contributed to recovery. Psychological factors have long been thought to alter the course of tuberculosis, but their actual impact on outcomes is not known. Assessing sanatorium care in psychological terms, moreover, is problematic. Although some patients clearly preferred institutional conditions to life outside, and may have benefited accordingly, others—homesick for families and friends, irritated by institutional regulations, and upset or discouraged by the company of other sick people—may well have reacted in opposite ways.[14]

Artificial pneumothorax, like the sanatorium, was never adequately evaluated. In the early years, physicians tried it on patients in all stages of the disease, including many who by later criteria would be considered very poor candidates. Of 1,000 patients admitted to institutions, estimated one authority in 1945, only about 500 were suitable for pneumothorax. Among these, it was technically possible in 375 and effectively accomplished (at least with further surgery) in 270. In 65 of these 270, however, it had to be stopped because of complications. Two years after the end of pneumothorax treatments, 180 would be judged as having arrested or apparently cured disease. Some of these would have recovered anyway. No more than 12 to 15 percent of the 1,000 patients, he concluded, probably benefited. Many years later, physicians recognized an infrequent complication of the repeated fluoroscopies required for the procedure: young women thus exposed to irradiation had an increased rate of cancer of the breast.[15]

Alternative Explanations

Many observers now attribute the decline of tuberculosis chiefly to socioeconomic changes—factors that some of Flick's colleagues had long acknowledged. Real income per capita in the United States rose from the 1820s to the Civil War, dipped during the 1860s, and rose even faster after that, through and beyond the end of the century. That people spent some of their increased income in ways that improved their health seems likely, but the means by which they did so remain unclear: they may have decreased their chances of becoming infected or improved their resistance, thus reducing their risk of developing disease. Changes beyond their ken or control, moreover, may have improved their health.[16]

The likelihood of becoming infected depends on the risk of inhaling infectious droplet nuclei. This, in turn, depends on the degree of sustained exposure to an infectious case, crowding of the environment, and ventilation, among other factors. Census figures and death rates do support a relationship between tuberculosis and crowded dwellings, and do so specifically in 1880 Philadelphia, but serial observations are lacking.[17]

Infection at home was clearly common, but there must have been other sources too. During the past quarter-century, researchers have repeatedly demonstrated that tuberculosis can spread wherever people are clustered together over time—in schools, in ships of the U.S. Navy, in prisons, in factories, in nursing homes, and in shelters for the homeless. One person with bacilli-laden sputum can alone start a small epidemic when conditions are ripe: congregate living, inadequate ventilation, and a susceptible population. Although twentieth-century observers have long blamed urbanization and industrialization for the high rate of tuberculosis in the nineteenth century, they have largely overlooked the growth of institutions as a likely contributor. Between the 1820s and the 1840s, Americans developed a new method of dealing with those whom they considered troublesome or simply dependent: they placed them together in large institutions. These were the penitentiaries, insane asylums, almshouses, orphan asylums, and reformatories. Institutional crowding was commonplace, living conditions were often dreadful, and, at least in the institutions for adults, consumptive inmates mingled freely with others. Because the disease, even if recognized, was not considered contagious, attendants in any of these institutions may also have been infectious. Men, women, and children who had migrated into the city from towns or rural areas, where tuberculosis was often less prevalent, could easily have contracted their first infection in these settings. Even inmates who had had a previous exposure could have been reinfected, although probably not as easily. In either case, they would have taken tubercle bacilli with them when they returned to the world outside.[18]

During the first half of the nineteenth century, the immigrant poor almost certainly had a comparable, or probably worse, exposure to tubercle bacilli. During most of this period, they traveled across the ocean in sailing ships that had been built for cargo. The passengers were packed into crowded quarters below deck, where the only air came down through the hatches. When seas were rough, the hatches were closed and there was no ventilation at all. Transatlantic-passage time averaged about five to six weeks, and much longer if the weather was stormy. Faster ships did make the trip during this period, but they were more expensive and did not carry the immigrant poor. Some of the hazards of the long voyage were well recognized at the time—starvation, epidemics of smallpox, cholera, and typhus fever, and the deaths of infants and children. No one, of course, noticed consumption; this disease, if contracted, would have become apparent only in subsequent months or years.[19]

Between the 1830s and the 1880s, the transatlantic voyage changed in ways that should have decreased the risk of tuberculous infection. New kinds of ships and new modes of propulsion reduced the duration of the trip. Sailing packets, which crossed the ocean in an average of thirty-four days, gradually replaced the cargo ships, and were in turn replaced by steamers. In 1856, steamships went from Glasgow to New York City in an average of fifteen and one-half days. Screw propulsion replaced paddles, and by the 1870s and 1880s some of the faster steamships were crossing the ocean in seven or eight days; others took longer, but less than two weeks. Sailing vessels, unable to meet the competition even for the steerage traffic, discontinued their services. Since the early 1800s, the duration of the transatlantic ordeal had been cut to about one-third.[20]

Because of improving ventilation during this period, fewer infections may have also occurred in U.S. homes, factories, and institutions. From the 1840s through to the twentieth century, health reformers, physicians, and others preached the evils of poor ventilation and the life-saving values of fresh air. Experiences in the Crimean War and the U.S. Civil War reinforced these ideas and undoubtedly led to better air supplies in at least some of the public institutions.[21] Technological changes improved the quality of stoves, furnaces, and ventilating devices, and manufacturers, often quoting the rhetoric of the reformers, marketed their new products aggressively. They promoted their use in homes, schools, prisons, hospitals, and various asylums where people were gathered together.[22] By the 1870s or 1880s, recommended minimal standards of ventilation had increased from four to thirty cubic feet per minute per person—and more in special circumstances. By this time, exhaust fans were used in factories to remove dust, moisture, and noxious gases. In the latter part of the century, states began to regulate industrial conditions. Massachusetts passed the nation's first dust-removal requirements in 1877, and Pennsylvania enacted its first law on the ventilation of factories in 1889.[23]

Average citizens, however, may have valued ventilation less than either warmth or economy. When fuel-efficient iron stoves began to replace fireplaces in the 1830s and 1840s, ventilation may have worsened in some settings. Open fireplaces had assured a natural draught, and reformers complained that people were sealing them up and huddling together around their stoves. How often they did so, whether or not they opened the windows, and to what extent devices such as airshafts, flues, and chimneytop ventilators counteracted the stagnant air have not been determined. By the mid-1860s, some affluent families were installing centralized hot-air furnaces equipped with ventilating ducts. These were expensive, however, and central heating did not become common among the middle classes until the twentieth century. In summary, ventilation probably did improve in the latter part of the nineteenth century, although not for everyone, and may have contributed to the decline of tuberculosis.[24]

While the risk of becoming infected with tubercle bacilli may thus have diminished during the latter half of the nineteenth century, the chance that a person, once infected, would then get the disease and die probably also decreased. The evidence supporting this idea too is necessarily circumstantial. Malnutrition severe enough to depress resistance, especially among the poor, seems likely in nineteenth-century America, although the data with which to assess it are scattered. Rickets, now known to result from a deficiency in vitamin D, was a widely recognized problem among children, and lack of food or even starvation brought the poor to the attention of various benefactors and reformers throughout the century. As income per capita rose, the people who could do so undoubtedly spent more on food.

Advances in preservation and transportation helped them to get it in greater abundance and variety. Philadelphians' use of ice in their homes became significant after 1830 and increased rapidly after 1855, when mechanization of ice-cutting lowered its price. By 1884, all but the poorest had iceboxes. Starting in the 1840s, railroads took foodstuffs from farms to increasingly distant markets, and better refrigeration improved their carrying capacities over long distances, especially in the 1880s. Refrigerator cars hauled increasing amounts of beef from the western ranges, and the prices of beef fell in the East. Improved techniques of canning further enhanced the distribution of meat, vegetables, and fruit. Although malnutrition persisted well into the twentieth century, the average diet certainly improved. The rising height of adult Americans in the late nineteenth and early twentieth centuries and the decreasing age at which girls started to menstruate tend to substantiate this conclusion.[25]

Additional stressful factors that may have affected resistance to tuberculous disease are almost hopelessly intertwined with each other and with factors that contribute to acquiring a first infection: warfare; economic, racial, and ethnic oppression; the psychosocial upheavals of immigration; and long, exhausting workdays. Many of these stresses have diminished since the nineteenth century, but whether, how, and to what extent any such changes have contributed to the decline of tuberculosis remain conundrums. The rising proportion of tuberculous people who were institutionalized in the 1920s and 1930s, along with the increasing length of their stays, may also have played a role in the falling mortality rates during this later period. There is no way to be sure.[26]

Some theorists attribute the decline—partly at least—to natural selection. Those who inherited the least amount of natural resistance to tuberculosis were more likely to die, they argue, while those with greater resistance, surviving in disproportionate numbers, passed their sturdier genes along to their greater numbers of children. This theory, well substantiated in animal populations, has further support from a study of human twins. Genetic transmission, however, is probably too weak a force by itself to explain the falling mortality rates. Even when tuberculosis was most prevalent in nineteenth-century Philadelphia, for example, it eliminated less than 1 percent of the population per year. Loss of such a small proportion of people could not significantly affect the genetic resistance of the surviving population, as one critic has observed, and cannot account for the rapid decline of the disease.[27]

The very high rates of tuberculosis among blacks in the past have often been attributed to low inherited resistance. Unlike Western white populations, according to this theory, African blacks had had little contact with the disease and were very susceptible to it when exposed to white societies in which it was prevalent. Although observers have clearly documented severe epidemics of tuberculosis among blacks (as well as among American Indians and Alaskan Eskimos), the causative factors can rarely be disentangled. These include heavy exposure to tubercle bacilli, recency of individual infection, crowding, poor ventilation, deprivation, and malnutrition. Whatever the explanations, the tuberculosis rate among blacks, although appallingly high in twentieth-century Philadelphia, fell much as did the rate among whites (see Graph 17-3). This fall occurred despite the fact that tuberculous blacks entered sanatoriums much less frequently than did whites.[28]

In 1938, the rate of death from tuberculosis of the lungs reached a new low in Philadelphia. Since 1876, when the Protestant Episcopal City Mis-

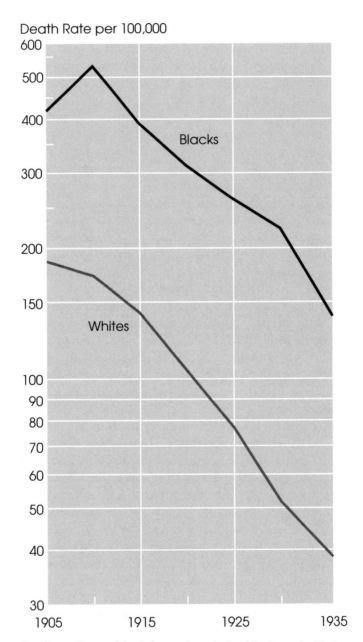

Death Rate per 100,000

Graph 17-3. Rates of death from tuberculosis of the lungs for blacks
and whites in Philadelphia, 1905–1935, as reported by the city health
department and plotted on a semilogarithmic scale so that changing
rates can be compared accurately. Rates are plotted every fifth year.

sion had started its work, this rate had dropped remarkably from 324 per 100,000 to 54. Just as impressive were the medical and social changes that had occurred over the sixty-two years—in the understanding of the disease, in diagnostic methods and treatment, in the caregiving system, in patients' choices, and in the identity of the caretakers.

18. Conclusions and Epilogue

The Changes

Between 1876 and 1938, the understanding of tuberculosis and the management of its victims changed in many ways. Physicians in the 1870s and 1880s thought of consumption as the result of hereditary predisposition, aggravated in some unfortunate way by a bad environment or improper living. About the predisposition they could do nothing. They could treat symptoms, they could try to strengthen a patient's body with better habits, nutrition, and tonics, and they could recommend a change in environment such as a trip to the country or a move to the West. Once the disease was clearly established, however, they considered the outlook bleak and probably hopeless. In the late 1930s, physicians understood tuberculosis as a bacterial disease that was communicable, preventable, and often curable. Although factors such as crowding and poor nutrition could predispose a person to it, the tubercle bacillus was the indispensable cause. Medical recommendations often included sanatorium treatment. This was usually considered the best method of curing the sick and the best way to protect others from infection. Surgical treatment, inconceivable in the earlier period, was offering hope to those who did not respond to the more conservative rest, nutrition, and fresh air.

Methods of identifying the disease improved. During the nineteenth century, diagnosis often depended on symptoms such as cough, weight loss, and fever, and only a small proportion of physicians could examine a patient's chest perceptively. The truly early case of tuberculosis was rarely recognized and, if suspected, could not be proved. By the late 1930s, tuberculin skin tests and x-ray examinations had become widely available. These helped in evaluating individual patients and in making surveys of apparently healthy populations. Bacteriological study of the sputum and other body fluids helped to clinch the diagnosis. As a result, physicians could identify the disease earlier and could recognize a larger proportion of all the cases. Most patients, however, still came to a doctor's attention later than was thought desirable.

The places where tuberculous men and women lived and were treated shifted significantly from homes to institutions. This change—never complete—varied with income and race. Poor consumptive Philadelphians of the 1870s usually lived and died at home. Some entered the Philadelphia Hospital, and a few went to the City Mission's House of Mercy. Gradually during the late nineteenth century and more rapidly during the twentieth, increasing numbers of patients entered the new tuberculosis hospitals and sanatoriums. More affluent patients sometimes stayed home during the nineteenth century, but often traveled in search of a better climate. By early in the twentieth century, some were going to private sanatoriums instead. By the mid-1930s, few well-to-do patients were left: the economic depression had reduced their incomes, and the disease itself had become much less common. The private sanatoriums disappeared. Throughout this time, tuberculous blacks entered institutions less frequently than did their white counterparts. Racial exclusion, segregated facilities, racist environments, and personal choices explain the different usage.

Concurrent with institutionalization came a change in the caretakers. Families and friends became less involved as others gradually took their places—the clergymen and their assistants, and then the physicians and nurses. Men and women from all walks of life were affected. Care of the sick—like a number of other traditional household functions—was shifting into the hands of those who specialized in the work. Before or during this time period, these functions included the growing and preservation of food, the baking of bread, the production of cloth and clothing, the education of children, and the care of the dead. In this case, however, the change was usually temporary. Most patients with tuberculosis—whether or not they recovered—left the institutions and went home again.

The sources of payment for care broadened remarkably over the six decades—from individuals and their families, to charities, and then to state and local governments. Care of the tuberculous, once largely a private matter, became mostly a public responsibility.

Goals, Flaws, and Outcomes

Three main goals justified the building of institutions for the care of consumptives. Religious and moral goals initiated the work; an institution would serve to correct the moral decay of an urban society and to save the souls of the hopelessly ill. By the 1890s, the goals were becoming more secular and medical. By segregating infectious men and women, institutions would prevent the spread of disease to others. Then cure emerged as an even more compelling goal. Cure had its own intrinsic value for the patient; it also promised to reduce the risk of infection and return the sick to productive lives. Both locally and nationally, prevention and cure were the dominant goals of the tuberculosis movement.

Linking the care of the sick to a fourth and even more ambitious goal—eradication of the disease through research—found expression in the Henry Phipps Institute, but this connection survived only in certain clinics and laboratories. The level of medical knowledge, the tools of research, and the traditions of funding were far too weak to support the care of inpatients for very long.

Prospective patients shared these goals to various degrees, but also had their own objectives in seeking institutional care. Some appreciated the relegous solace offered by the clergy, and others wanted to protect their relatives from further exposure to the disease. Probably most of the patients responded to the proffered hope of cure. The tuberculosis campaign had tapped into one of the strongest of human drives—the will to survive. In the case of many poor patients, however, it was need as well as hope that sent them to institutions. While they may have wanted medical treatment, they were also looking for basic subsistence and personal care.

When patients entered institutions, they and their caretakers made an implicit bargain. The sick would get medical advice, treatment, nursing care, food, and shelter. In turn, they would yield to institutional authority. At the Phipps Institute in its early years, poor patients also promised their bodies for research; in some other settings, they paid for their care with labor. More affluent patients paid with money. Their fees gave them a wider range of choices and greater power in negotiating with their caretakers, but the bargain was otherwise much the same.

Caretakers earned their own rewards by working in institutions. Many made a living from the work, but their incomes were usually modest. Nonmonetary rewards helped to pay for their efforts. The clergy, their assistants, the physicians, and the nurses often found gratification in helping their patients: they were fulfilling themselves through their service to others and perhaps through their service to God. Some physicians and nurses felt exhilarated because they were fighting the dread disease. They also earned knowledge, training, clinical experience, and a boost to their careers.

While the various bargains offered something to all participants, the tuberculosis campaign had some serious flaws in its strategy. Physicians overestimated their abilities to identify and institutionalize early cases likely to recover. They overestimated their abilities to cure the disease and to make infectious patients noninfectious. And they and the visiting nurses overestimated the ease with which they could influence patients' behaviors and habits. They also underestimated the conflicting needs, desires, and motivations of the sick. Physicians and their colleagues may have been confident in their recommendations, but tuberculous men and women pursued their own goals and pleasures. Although many desired treatment and cure, they also did what they wanted to do or what they thought they should do: they worked, they stayed at home with their children, they enjoyed themselves with their friends, and they often delayed entering an institution until they could work no longer and had used up their money. Had they still had money, they would have had to pay for their care; given the meager nature of home relief, they seemed to be making sensible choices.

The demands of the patients, reinforced by appeals from their advocates, helped to expand and shape the institutions. Waiting lists justified more beds, and patients' dissatisfactions with the hardships of early sanatoriums forced improvements in facilities. Pressures to accept advanced cases overwhelmed admitting policies and selection processes and helped to change the nature and goals of the sanatoriums. Although cure, or the hope of cure, continued to be a goal for patients and caretakers alike, the chronically ill and incurable became more acceptable. No institution could survive without them. The influence of patients and their advocates was not strong enough, however, to make institutions acceptable places in which most patients would live out their lives until they were cured or died. Many men and women left the institutions before they were healed and carried their infection away with them.

Because of these flaws in the strategy and because of the needs and desires of the sick, the tuberculosis campaign had a paradoxical result. Physicians and other leaders had tried to build an institutional system that would prevent and cure the disease, but neither goal, as can be seen in retrospect, was feasible on a broad scale. Although many of the sick did recover, there was no real medical cure. Both the long delays before institutionalization and the patients' return to their homes while still infectious seriously impaired prevention. No effects of the tuberculosis movement can be seen in the falling mortality rates at least until the 1920s and, even then, they are not clear. The campaigners created instead what many had tried to avoid—a system of care for the chronically ill.

Institutional care repaid society in several ways. It gave hope to thousands of tuberculous patients, at least for a time, and it partly relieved their families and friends of the financial and emotional burdens of caring for them. By segregating the infectious, institutionalization also alleviated some of the fears of contracting the disease—at home, at work, and in other public places. Through institutional activities, moreover, medical knowledge of tuberculosis slowly increased, and physicians and nurses were trained. The tuberculosis movement became a model for future campaigns against different diseases and other threats to the public's well-being. It linked voluntary, professional, and governmental interests in a joint effort to educate the public, prevent disease, train workers, and provide patient care.[1]

Persisting Characteristics

The tuberculosis campaign highlights some characteristics that still persist in the U.S. health care system. First, the curative goals of the new institutions competed and conflicted with caring for the chronically ill. To physicians and other leaders of the movement, cure seemed much more desirable: treatment of early, curable cases was briefer and cheaper than the care of those with advanced disease. As social policy, returning these men and women to productive lives helped to justify the expense. Cure also gratified the caretakers, enhanced the prestige of the doctors, and improved the image of the institutions. Patients themselves often preferred a place where others seemed to be getting better and where they could more easily sustain their hopes of recovery.

Care of advanced and incurable patients, however, did have support. Preventing the spread of infection served as by far the most compelling justification. Other support was obtained by linking the care of incurables to research and education. Most tuberculosis institutions, however, were far away from the organizations that might have sustained these goals— the major hospitals and medical schools. Sanatoriums developed instead mainly in rural areas, where land was less expensive, and where fears of city dwellers tended to keep them. One identifiable group of caretakers valued care of the chronically ill without trying to cure them or even prevent the spread of disease: the early Protestant Episcopal clergymen and their assistants. In addition, individual physicians and nurses cared for the sick and dying with compassion, and the visiting nurse Mabel Jacques tried to make her patients happy. Neither care nor happiness, however, were leading goals of the campaign.

In a second characteristic of the system, institutional care competed with home care and partly replaced it. Although the Reverend Durborow and Mabel Jacques tried to save the integrity of families by providing care at home, this goal never attracted wide support. The method was cumbersome: the clergy and the visiting nurses found the requisite travel tiring and probably inefficient. To most leaders of the tuberculosis movement, institutionalization seemed much more effective as a tool for prevention and cure: it segregated the patients from others, removed them from impoverished, unhealthful homes, and ensured greater discipline. Society was neither willing nor able to correct all the unfavorable home conditions or to provide adequate welfare assistance. Wary about the misuse of relief, it supplied the basic necessities mainly in institutions, where it could presumably control how the money was spent.

Care outside of institutions did persist in several forms and for different purposes. Physicians often treated private patients at home, thus preserving their practices and earning their usual fees. Clinics and dispensaries participated in the care of the poor at home, functioning primarily to make diagnoses, instruct the patients, select some for institutional care, and supervise them after discharge. For black people, care at home was often the only kind available. Institutions often excluded them, segregated them in a predominantly white setting, or otherwise made them feel unwelcome. Segregated clinics, staffed by black nurses and physicians, offered an acceptable way to be treated at home; they also avoided the racial mixing opposed by many whites.

Third, the system of care—segregated by race and stratified by income—reflected the larger social structure in which the system was imbedded. The state sanatoriums and the voluntary institutions did expand the options of the poor and working classes, but they did not challenge the social structure itself. Flick tried twice to do so, once when he resisted racial segregation at White Haven and once when he tried to send indigent county patients to the private sanatoriums. He failed both times. American society, with its inequalities and prejudices, had replicated itself in the health care system and was firmly entrenched there. Managers and patients both defended it.

Fourth, fear related to race and class and fear of becoming infected all played roles in the tuberculosis movement. Especially in the early years of the campaign, physicians and other propagandists used fear of infection to encourage hygienic habits, promote legislation, build institutions, and persuade patients to enter them and to accept the proper discipline. Campaigners argued that the public was thus protecting itself and that patients were saving themselves from death and protecting their families. Fear, however, was frequently hard to control, and victims of the disease also became the victims of fear. Men and women, stigmatized by the diagnosis, found their friends avoiding them and had more than the usual problems in finding jobs. Some, therefore, concealed the nature of their disease, even if it meant ignoring the proper precautions. Others refused to seek care in order to avoid the possible truth about their condition. Despite such problems, fear was a useful and probably indispensable tool. When campaigners portrayed the tuberculous poor and tuberculous blacks as dangerous to the rest of society, they were often trying to create a system of care for them. If people had not been made to feel anxious, they might have responded much less generously.

Fifth, as fear was important for a successful campaign, so was confidence in the methods. It came from knowledge of the tubercle bacillus, from the rising faith in science, from the documented recoveries of patients, and from falling mortality rates. These ideas permeated the campaign and its efforts at public education. All involved in the care of consumptives, moreover, needed such confidence in order to function. The tuberculosis societies and the health departments needed to communicate it if they were to gain support for their programs. Physicians needed it to treat their patients and give them a sense of hope. Nurses in private duty, in institutions, and in the homes of the poor needed to believe in the efficacy of their measures in order to teach their patients, take care of them, and feel safe themselves at the same time. Institutions needed to transmit this confidence if they were to attract and keep their clienteles. Patients, fearing death, wanted to believe that their caretakers could cure them, and their caretakers were thereby earning a living. With so much at stake, campaigners and caretakers—mutually supportive in their shared convictions—inevitably exaggerated their capabilities and those of medical science. When they had failures, they could always blame the lack of compliance by patients, continuing poverty and public ignorance, the inability of general practitioners to detect the disease early enough, and the still inadequate number of institutional beds. When long-term outcomes proved disappointing, prevention and education could justify the work, and there was always the hope of new and more successful treatments.

Decades have passed since tuberculosis was a major problem in the

United States, and there have been many changes in the general health care system. Diagnostic methods have improved, new medical treatments have been introduced and perfected, and partly (though not exclusively) because of these changes life span has lengthened. Expenditures have increased enormously, caretakers earn higher incomes, and both private insurance and public programs such as Medicare and Medicaid have helped to pay the costs.

Many chronic diseases still require our attention, however, and we use many of the same exchanges to cope with them. Research institutes offer free cancer treatments to people willing to participate in experiments, and hospices run by religiously motivated people take care of patients with incurable diseases. Medical centers still link their services to medical education and medical careers, and the poor are still more likely than the affluent to get their care from men and women in training, if care reaches them at all. Hospitals no longer train and use their convalescing women as nurses, but, as the nurses at least would argue, their salaries are still less than the work is worth.

The search for cure still competes successfully with the more custodial care of the chronically ill, and more resources are spent on institutional care than on care at home. Although visiting nurses still make their rounds through the cities, providing care, instruction, treatment, and personal support, they cannot entirely meet the need. In home care, as in institutions, the poor remain at a disadvantage; in the absence of insurance, some get little care or none at all.

Fear is still used in the health care system, and it still has destructive consequences. Although propagandists may use it more subtly than they did in the 1890s, they still create anxiety in the hope of persuading people to change their habits—in eating, sexual practices, and the use of tobacco, drugs, and alcohol. They are thereby trying to reduce the risks of cancer, heart disease, auto accidents, addiction, and AIDS, among other consequences—all desirable and sensible goals. Victims of disease, however, still become the victims of fear, shunned by their friends, barred from employment, and ineligible for insurance. Cancer and AIDS are examples. Yet fear of disease may be necessary in order to change human behavior. Even fear of the sick may help to create a system of care for those that the dominant society stigmatizes for some reason—poverty, drug addiction, or homosexuality.

Despite all our improvements in health care—indeed partly because of them—care of the chronically ill is becoming more important, not less so.

The most rapidly expanding segment of our population consists of men and women over the age of eighty-five—a group especially susceptible to chronic disease and disability. The mentally ill and the retarded need attention while AIDS, like tuberculosis, has added the threat of infectiousness to the burden of incapacity. Even tuberculosis is becoming more prevalent, especially among people with AIDS and among those who are poor and malnourished and live in crowded environments.

Many of our new treatments are halfway technologies, as Lewis Thomas has labeled them; they may lengthen lives, but they fail to cure.[2] Under these circumstances, different objectives such as comfort, physical function, and satisfying family and social relationships might be more appropriate. Whether they can attract a committed group of caretakers, a clientele, and the broad support of society, however, remains unclear. Cure or the hope of cure has powerful attractions, and distinguishing those who can recover from those who cannot is not always possible. Patients, relatives, and caretakers may disagree on the categorization. Costs are high, necessitating limits on eligibility and duration of care.

Any significant shift in the goals, methods, or possible leadership of the health care system would require major changes in funding and a persuasive campaign to alter public opinion and public values. The tuberculosis movement could well provide the prototype for such a campaign. Those who might undertake it would need inspiring leadership, committed professionals, a voluntary organization, promotion through cooperative media, training programs for the caretakers, and one or more methods of paying the costs of care. They would also need to believe in what they were doing, and transmit this conviction and confidence to others. At the same time, they would risk exaggerating their capabilities and promising the public more than is feasible. They might also try to control human behavior, impinge on personal freedoms, deflect resources from other desirable purposes within and outside of the health care field, and incur consequences that no one anticipated.

Whatever the changes we may wish to make, the system of care is inherently complicated; it serves many purposes and many users. Whether we merely tinker with it or try to alter it radically, we disturb some of the social exchanges bound up in it. We are now accustomed to thinking about health care in monetary terms such as costs per capita, reimbursement rates, and salaries. These reflect the economic aspects of some of the bargains negotiated over the past decades. As we debate costs and payment mechanisms, however, we should also recognize the less tangible exchanges—

what is at stake for both sets of players. For the caretakers, this includes money, of course, but also professional education, clinical experience, research, prestige, long and often discouraging hours of work, the risk of infection, pride in performance, the satisfaction of helping other, and a sense of personal worth. For patients, potential results of the bargain include cure, a sense of being cared for, receiving the basic necessities now known as welfare, separation from home and loved ones, anxiety, hope, and sometimes despair.

Epilogue

Flick spent his later years practicing medicine, writing, and enjoying his family, including his grandchildren. Although he suffered from diabetes, recurrent infections, and chest pain, and although his physicians placed him on bed rest for weeks at a time, he still managed to see a few patients, at least until the autumn of 1937.

Several organizations recognized the value of his life's work. Four colleges or universities awarded him honorary degrees, Notre Dame University gave him its Laetare Medal in 1920, and the Philadelphia County Medical Society gave him the Strittmatter Award in 1933. Two signs of recognition, however, never came: a Trudeau Medal from the National Tuberculosis Association, and the Philadelphia Award, a privately funded, annual honor that recognized outstanding contributions or achievements. Flick had repeatedly differed with officials of the National Association over the reporting of past events, and his stinging criticisms of the Pennsylvania Tuberculosis Society had undoubtedly caused some rancor. The probable obstacle to his receiving the Philadelphia Award, he confided to a friend in 1936, was his old nemesis, the University of Pennsylvania. If Flick was disappointed, he did not reveal it. "God has blessed my endeavors with results I am well satisfied with," he observed. "I have met with opposition but I am rather proud of the enmities I have made."[3]

He suffered deep losses during these final years, but there were quiet pleasures that connected him to his past. The death of his wife in 1934 was his greatest blow. His daughters remained a comfort, however, and so did his work. In 1937, he published his last book, *Tuberculosis*, designed as a guide for general practitioners. He also transliterated his old diaries from shorthand into readable form. Although many of his friends had died, he still maintained his correspondence and saw a few visitors. Joseph Walsh called on him regularly, and in 1935 the daughter of Agnes E. Moss (once the owner of the Hill Crest Sanatorium and now Mrs. Snowden) brought him some wild flowers from White Haven.[4]

Flick's last preserved letter was fittingly one to a woman who had asked for his medical opinion. "I am not in a physical condition to give you any advice," he replied on June 18, 1938, "as they have had to watch me for fear I would die the last three nights. However, I can see no objection to you taking insulin treatment. . . . I myself am taking four insulin injections a day." Though long resigned to his expected death, Flick was a therapeutic enthusiast to the end. He died at home on July 7, 1938, a month before his eighty-second birthday. According to his wishes, his body was autopsied at the nearby Pennsylvania Hospital. The examination showed evidence of diabetes mellitus, coronary artery disease, and healed tuberculosis in the upper portion of both lungs. It was the healing of his old disease that he had undoubtedly wanted to demonstrate. There was a sad but ironic sequel to this victory in death. In 1945, his eldest son, Lawrence, died of tuberculosis at the White Haven Sanatorium. The physician who had valued prevention even more than cure had failed to protect his own son from infection. The institution that he had founded in 1901, however, provided the needed care.[5]

Nathan F. Mossell, founder of the Frederick Douglass Memorial Hospital, survived Flick by eight years. In 1940 Lincoln University, Mossell's alma mater, awarded him an honorary doctorate of science, and in that same year he carried his class colors at the University of Pennsylvania's bicentennial celebration.[6] His portrait hangs in the medical school of the University of Pennsylvania, from which he had graduated as the school's first black physician in 1882. More than a century later, its place in the school's Office of Minority Affairs symbolizes both his pathbreaking leadership and the racial discrimination that still makes such an office necessary.

Like Mossell, Henry M. Minton died in 1946. Two years later, the Mercy Hospital and the Frederick Douglass Memorial Hospital merged. The institution, however, could not attract enough paying patients, and by the 1960s it could not find enough black applicants for its nursing school or its internships. Some of the white hospitals in the city were accepting blacks. In 1973, Mercy-Douglass Hospital closed. The name survives in nursing homes and in a variety of services to the elderly.[7]

Through the 1940s and beyond, Pennsylvania's annual rate of death from all forms of tuberculosis continued to fall; in 1956 it dropped for the first time below 10 per 100,000 people. During the 1950s it also disappeared from the state's list of the ten leading causes of death. In addition, chemotherapy started to have a decisive impact on mortality. In 1945, streptomycin was found to be effective in treating human tuberculosis. In 1952, isoniazid was shown to be even more useful, and it could also rather quickly make a patient noninfectious to others. Chemical cure and prevention both became possible for the first time.[8]

The number of beds available for tuberculous Pennsylvanians continued to rise until about 1942. Expansion of the state system, which lasted for several additional years, was the chief factor. Although the state's fourth sanatorium in western Pennsylvania never opened under state auspices, Pennsylvania did establish a new sanatorium in Philadelphia in 1952. Meanwhile, the numbers of beds under other kinds of auspices slowly decreased. The private sanatoriums had been the first to dwindle; next came the voluntary organizations. The interest in surgical treatment, however, counteracted the latter trend as some general hospitals opened small tuberculosis departments. Complicated facilities and a skilled staff were needed for major chest surgery, and for this purpose general hospitals welcomed tuberculous patients.[9]

Specialized tuberculosis institutions were nearing their end. In 1946, the White Haven Sanatorium was transferred to Jefferson Medical College as a gift. Members of the board believed that a medical school would improve the surgical services and the training of doctors and nurses. Demand decreased, however, and the sanatorium closed in 1956.[10] The state sanatorium at Hamburg followed in 1959, the one at Cresson in 1963, and Mont Alto in 1968.

Many of the institutions for the tuberculous adopted new missions to meet the needs of a changing society. Mont Alto now provides care for former mental patients still in need of intermediate or skilled nursing care. Hamburg serves the mentally retarded, and Cresson has become a prison. The Kensington Dispensary turned its attention to mentally retarded but trainable children, and its preventorium at River Crest became a residential facility for them. The Home for Consumptives at Chestnut Hill—now the All Saints Hospital—changed its focus to chronic diseases, then to rehabilitation. The sanatorium at Eagleville, initially called the Philadelphia Jewish Sanatorium for Consumptives, shifted its work to alcoholism and drug addiction. When the White Haven Sanatorium closed, the state bought the land and buildings to use for the care of the mentally retarded, but later it moved this program to different quarters in the town. The sanatorium itself fell idle. In the 1980s a private corporation bought the land that Flick and his colleagues had purchased in 1901. The sanatorium's powerhouse has been transformed into a restaurant, but except for some recent vandalism the property has not been otherwise altered.

During the mid-1980s one could still catch a glimpse of the sanatorium's past. Although auto traffic was blocked, one could walk up the driveway under the now-tall trees to the sloping plateau that looks over the Lehigh River. Weeds were high, but many of the old buildings were still standing. In the silence, it was easy to hear the ghostly voices: those of Elwell Stockdale, the tuberculous nurses and resident physicians, the medical staff who came from Philadelphia on their biweekly visits, and the chorus of patients—grumbling over their work assignments, singing in the kiosks, and asking for their mail from home.

Notes

A Note on the Flick Papers

The papers of Lawrence F. Flick include 169 bound volumes of letters, located in two places. The Historical Collections of the College of Physicians of Philadelphia holds 54 volumes of incoming correspondence labeled "Tuberculosis Letters" (LFCP in my notes). They date from the 1880s through 1908. A "Second Series" (SS) of 23 volumes are in the Department of Archives and Manuscripts, Catholic University of America, Washington, D.C. They too continue through 1908, but differ somewhat in source and content. The letters from private patients, for example, are almost exclusively in the "Second Series" while those dealing with the tuberculosis campaign are almost all in the "Tuberculosis Letters."

All letters to Flick from 1909 to 1938 are bound in another 57 volumes at Catholic University (LFCU). An additional four volumes, labeled "Miscellanies," contain mostly undated letters to Flick. Volume 1 is in Philadelphia, the other volumes in Washington. A card catalog at Catholic University provides an alphabetical index to all incoming letters.

Letters from Flick, 1903–1938, are bound in 31 letterpress copy books (LFLP). Each is indexed by addressee. These volumes are at Catholic University.

At the College of Physicians, two additional Flick collections supplement the correspondence. There are four scrapbooks of clippings (LFSB) and a large Pamphlet Collection that includes pamphlets, annual reports, announcements, advertisements, journals, and other such material. The Pamphlet Collection is soon to be cataloged.

In the notes that follow, all letters to Flick through 1908, unless otherwise specified, are in the "Tuberculosis Letters"; all from 1909 on, unless otherwise specified, are at Catholic University.

Abbreviations Used in the Notes

AMP	*Annual Message of the Mayor of Philadelphia*
AGPI—UPA	Archives General, Phipps Institute, University of Pennsylvania Archives
ARCH	*Annual Report of the Commissioner of Health of the Commonwealth of Pennsylvania*
ARFD	*Annual Report of the Frederick Douglass Memorial Hospital and Training School*

ARFH	*Annual Report of the Free Hospital for Poor Consumptives*
ARKD	*Annual Report of the Kensington Dispensary for the Treatment of Tuberculosis*
ARPB	*Annual Report of the Pennsylvania Board of Public Charities*
ARCM	*Annual Report of the Philadelphia Protestant Episcopal City Mission*
ART	*American Review of Tuberculosis*
ARVN	*Annual Report of the Visiting Nurse Society of Philadelphia*
BHM	*Bulletin of the History of Medicine*
CPP	College of Physicians of Philadelphia
CSHN	Center for the Study of the History of Nursing, University of Pennsylvania
ECS	Archives, Episcopal Community Services, Philadelphia
ES	Elwell Stockdale
FAM	*Fresh Air Magazine*
GG	George E. Gordon
GM	George E. Macklin
HP	Henry Phipps
HSP	Historical Society of Pennsylvania
JAMA	*Journal of the American Medical Association*
JNMA	*Journal of the National Medical Association*
JOL	*Journal of the Outdoor Life*
JW	Joseph Walsh papers, Historical Collections of the College of Physicians of Philadelphia
LF	Lawrence F. Flick
LFCP	Lawrence F. Flick papers (Tuberculosis Letters to Flick) Historical Collections of the College of Physicians of Philadelphia
LFCU	Lawrence F. Flick papers (to Flick), Department of Archives and Manuscripts, Catholic University of America
LFLP	Lawrence F. Flick papers (letterpress from Flick), Department of Archives and Manuscripts, Catholic University of America
LFPM	Lawrence F. Flick Pamphlet Collection, Historical Collections of the College of Physicians of Philadelphia
LFSB	Lawrence F. Flick Scrapbooks, Historical Collections of the College of Physicians of Philadelphia
LP	*Listening Post*
MJ	Mabel Jacques

MM	Mary Mahony
MBDH	*Monthly Bulletin of the Department of Public Health of Philadelphia*
NYPMJ	*New York Medical Journal and the Philadelphia Medical Journal*
PCA	Philadelphia City Archives
PHB	*Pennsylvania Health Bulletin*
PI	Phipps Institute
PMJ	*Pennsylvania Medical Journal*
RHPI	*Report (or Annual Report) of the Henry Phipps Institute*
RPS	*Report of the Pennsylvania Society for the Prevention of Tuberculosis* or its later names
SS	Lawrence F. Flick papers, Second Series, Department of Archives and Manuscripts, Catholic University of America
TACA	*Transactions of the American Climatological Association*
TRCP	*Transactions of the College of Physicians of Philadelphia*
TNA	*Transactions of the National Association for the Study and Prevention of Tuberculosis* or *Transactions of the National Tuberculosis Association*
TSCP	*Transactions and Studies of the College of Physicians of Philadelphia*
TSICT	*Transactions of the Sixth International Congress on Tuberculosis*
TUPA	Temple University, Photojournalism Archives
TUUA	Temple University, Urban Archives Center
UPA	Archives of the University of Pennsylvania
VN-CSHN	Visiting Nurse Society of Philadelphia Records, Center for the Study of the History of Nursing, University of Pennsylvania

Months have been shortened to their first three letters.

Introduction

1. Richard L. Riley, "Disease Transmission and Contagion Control," *American Review of Respiratory Disease* 125 (Mar 1982, pt. 2): 16–19. Bovine tuberculosis, transmitted from diseased cows by the ingestion of bacilli-containing milk, caused a small proportion of the deaths from tuberculosis in young children. Disease ac-

quired by this route usually involved nonpulmonary sites such as bones, joints, and the lymph nodes of the neck. Disease of the lungs in adults was rarely due to bovine tuberculosis. See William H. Park and Charles Krumwiede, Jr., "The Relative Importance of the Bovine and Human Types of Tubercle Bacilli in the Different Forms of Human Tuberculosis," *Journal of Medical Research* 23 (Oct 1910):205– 368, and Jules Freund and Gardner Middlebrook, "The Mycobacteria," in *Bacterial and Mycotic Infections of Man*, ed. René J. Dubos (Philadelphia: J. B. Lippincott, 1948), 302.

2. Arthur M. Dannenberg, Jr., "Pathogenesis of Pulmonary Tuberculosis," *American Review of Respiratory Disease* 125 (Mar 1982, pt. 2):25–27.

3. Dannenberg, "Pathogenesis," 26–29.

4. John S. Chapman and Margaret D. Dyerly, "Social and Other Factors in Intrafamilial Transmission of Tuberculosis," *American Review of Respiratory Diseases* 90 (Jul 1964):48–60; George W. Comstock, "Frost Revisited: The Modern Epidemiology of Tuberculosis," *American Journal of Epidemiology* 101 (May 1975): 369–73; and idem, "Epidemiology of Tuberculosis," *American Review of Respiratory Disease* 125 (Mar 1982, pt. 2):12–13.

5. Comstock, "Frost Revisited," 373–74; and idem, "Epidemiology," 13– 14.

Chapter 1. Doctor Flick and Tuberculosis

1. H. M. Neale to Lawrence F. Flick (LF hereafter), 4 Oct 1930 (for the quotation); LF to H. M. Neale, 8 Oct 1930; and Ella M. E. Flick, *Beloved Crusader: Lawrence F. Flick, Physician* (Philadelphia: Dorrance, 1944), 156. Flick owned buildings at 732, 736, and 738 Pine Street and probably lived in each of the latter two during the 1930s. His office was at 738 Pine.

2. LF to Frank Simpson, 9 Jan 1933, and LF to James J. Walsh, 9 May 1931.

3. LF to E. H. Flick, 16 Sep 1935, and LF to Sr. Mary Louis, 6 Apr 1934 (for the last quotation). See also LF to Ambrose Huebner, 15 Mar 1934; LF to Ralph M. Bashor, 24 Mar 1937; and Ella M. E. Flick, *Dr. Lawrence F. Flick, 1856– 1938* (n.p.: White Haven Sanatorium Association, 1940), 40–42.

4. LF to Sr. M. Cosmos, 8 Apr 1937; LF to Rev. Mother M. James, 11 Apr 1933; E. M. E. Flick, *Dr. LF*, 7, 23, 41; idem, *Beloved Crusader* 65, 365–82; LF to John Slevin, 25 Sep 1888, SS; John Slevin to LF, 26 Sep 1888, SS; and Joseph Walsh, "Memoir of Lawrence F. Flick, M.D.," *TSCP*, 4th ser., vol. 7 (Apr 1939): 118–19.

5. E. M. E. Flick, *Beloved Crusader*, 225, 9 for the quotations.

6. LF to Rev. F. Boniface, 8 Apr 1930; LF to Walter H. Abbott, 6 Nov 1930; LF to Norman J. Henry, 21 Sep 1933; LF to Arthur A. Bredenbek, 10 Aug 1936; Joseph Walsh to LF, 20 Mar 1930, 5 Jul 1936; LF to Joseph Walsh, 22 Mar 1930, 6 Jul 1936; LF to H. R. M. Landis, 10 Nov 1932; LF to Martha Tracy, 6 Apr 1935; LF to John B. Flick, 8 Apr 1937; LF to Franklin Printing Company, 16 Apr 1937; LF, *The Crusade against Tuberculosis in Philadelphia* (1932); LF, *The Pennsylvania Society for the Prevention of Tuberculosis* (1935); LF, *Tuberculosis: A Book of*

Practical Knowledge to Guide the General Practitioner of Medicine (Philadelphia, 1937); and "Short Life Story of Dr. Lawrence F. Flick and Brief Account of His Work in Tuberculosis," in *The Strittmatter Award, 1933, to Dr. Lawrence F. Flick* (Philadelphia Medical Society), 9–55.

7. LF, *Crusade*; LF, *Pennsylvania Society*, 16–24, 27–29; LF to Irvin P. Knipe, 22, 28 Mar 1927; LF to James J. Walsh, 4 Nov 1930, 9 Dec 1936; LF to Francis A. Faught, 18 Nov 1933; LF to J. Norman Henry, 10, 19 Apr 1934; LF to Henry M. Neale, 28 Feb 1935; LF to A. J. Cohen, 22 Mar 1935; and LF to Robert G. Paterson, 1 Apr 1935.

8. LF to Robert G. Paterson, 29 Mar 1934 (for the quotation), and E. M. E. Flick, *Beloved Crusader*, 288, 390.

9. Memorandum of John Flick Sr., 1888, LFLP, 1934, 95–96; LF to Thomas Sharbough [*sic*], 22 Feb 1934; E. M. E. Flick, *Beloved Crusader*, 20–41; and Cecilia R. Flick, *Dr. Lawrence F. Flick—As I Knew Him* (Philadelphia: Dorrance, 1956), 11–19, 44.

10. E. M. E. Flick, *Beloved Crusader*, 42–51 (44 for the quotations); idem, *Dr. LF*, 6; and C. R. Flick, *Dr. LF*, 45. There was less distinction between high school and college during this period than there is now. The college received the state's charter to grant academic degrees during Flick's years there (*Beloved Crusader*, 51).

11. E. M. E. Flick, *Beloved Crusader*, 51–55, and idem, *Dr. LF*, 6–7.

12. E. M. E. Flick, *Beloved Crusader*, 55–59; idem, *Dr. LF*, 7–9; and LF to H. M. Neal[e], 8 Oct 1930.

13. E. M. E. Flick, *Beloved Crusader*, 62–67, 114, and idem, *Dr. LF*, 9–10.

14. E. M. E. Flick, *Beloved Crusader*, 113–35, 149–50. Flick's first office was at 519 Pine Street. The Stones had moved from 415 Locust Street, where Flick had initially boarded with the family.

15. Ibid., 135–56; idem, *Dr. LF*, 14–19; and "Short Life Story," 9.

16. E. M. E. Flick, *Dr. LF*, 19, 21, and "Short Life Story," 10.

17. LF, *Development of Our Knowledge of Tuberculosis* (Philadelphia, 1925), 626–44 (for Villemin's work); Robert Koch, "The Aetiology of Tuberculosis," trans. Berna Pinner and Max Pinner, with an introduction by Allen K. Krause, *ART* 25 (Mar 1932):285–323; and James Tyson, *The Practice of Medicine* (Philadelphia: P. Blakiston, Son, 1896), 183. Tyson was not categorically denying infectiousness.

18. J. M. Da Costa, *Medical Diagnosis*, 5th ed., rev. (Philadelphia: J. B. Lippincott, 1881), 278.

19. Ibid., 282–84.

20. Ibid., 278.

21. Ibid., 284–85.

22. The first proponent in Philadelphia was William H. Webb, who in Feb 1878 read to the Sydenham Medical Coterie a paper, *Is Phthisis Pulmonalis Contagious, and Does It Belong to the Zymotic Group?* (Philadelphia, 1878). He argued affirmatively. Flick gave him full credit. A few other men publicly supported this view before Flick did. Flick inferred the contagiousness of tuberculosis from his own early contact with his stepmother's mother, who died of consumption ("Short Life Story," 10–11). Flick's chief articles on the topic were "The Hygiene of

Phthisis," *Proceedings of the Philadelphia County Medical Society* 9 (1888):24–35; "The Contagiousness of Phthisis (Tubercular Pulmonitis)," *Transactions of the Medical Society of the State of Pennsylvania* 20 (Jun 1888):164–82 (182 for the quotations); and "The Duty of the Government in the Prevention of Tuberculosis," *JAMA* 17 (22 Aug 1891):287–90. See also his comments in "Discussion on the Advisability of the Registration of Tuberculosis," *TRCP*, 3d ser., vol. 16 (1894):3–7, 24–27.

23. LF, "Hygiene," 30–31 (for the quotation), and LF, "Duty of the Government," 289.

24. LF, "Special Hospitals for the Treatment of Tuberculosis," *TRCP*, 3d ser., vol. 12 (1890):39–76 (64–65 for the quotations).

25. Esther G. Price, *Pennsylvania Pioneers against Tuberculosis* (New York: National Tuberculosis Association, 1952), 21, 24, 39–41, and, for the Philadelphia Board of Health, Edward T. Morman, "Scientific Medicine Comes to Philadelphia: Public Health Transformed, 1854–1899" (Ph.D. diss., University of Pennsylvania, 1986).

26. E. M. E. Flick, *Beloved Crusader*, 12–19; idem, *Dr. LF*, 37–43; C. R. Flick, *Dr. LF*, 45, 61, 63, 81–82; LF to Henry M. Neale, 12 Apr 1907, 18 Jan 1911; LF to H. R. M. Landis, 10 May 1911; LF to John J. Ferreck, 29 Apr 1914; LF to Mrs. Alfred Meyer, 20 Nov 1914; and LF to James J. Walsh, 21 Nov 1933. For the medical elite, see Leo J. O'Hara, *An Emerging Profession: Philadelphia Doctors 1860–1900* (New York: Garland Publishing, 1989), 295–322. For Flick's beliefs that prejudice against Roman Catholics had worked against him, see LF to Hugh T. Henry, 22 Nov 1933, and LF to James J. Walsh, 13 Oct 1930.

27. Charles E. Rosenberg, *The Care of Strangers: The Rise of America's Hospital System* (New York: Basic Books, 1987), 166–89; E. M. E. Flick, *Beloved Crusader*, 104–12; Price, *Pennsylvania Pioneers*, 22; *Strittmatter Award*, 6; Minutes, College of Physicians of Philadelphia, 6 Jun 1888; and Hall of the Pathological Society to LF, 26 Jun 1990, SS.

28. Discussions of LF's "Hygiene," 35–38 and "Contagiousness," 182–86; and "Discussion on the Advisability," 1–27.

29. Price, *Pennsylvania Pioneers*, 70–98, 147; S. Weir Mitchell, "Annual Address of the President," *TRCP*, 3d ser., vol. 15 (1893):lxxviii; and "Discussion on the Advisability," 1–27 (1, 2, 8, 11 for the quotations); and A. A. Cairns, "Division of Contagious Diseases," *AMP*, vol. 3 (1904):48. See also Daniel M. Fox, "Social Policy and City Politics: Tuberculosis Reporting in New York, 1889–1900," *BHM* 49 (Summer 1975):169–95.

30. Discussion of LF, "Special Hospitals," 76–86 (84 for the quotation).

31. "Short Life Story," 11–12 (11 for the first quotation); T. Mellor Tyson, "Rush Hospital for the Treatment of Consumption and Allied Diseases," in *Founders' Week Memorial Volume*, ed. Frederick P. Henry (Philadelphia: City of Philadelphia, 1909), 837–38 (837 for the other quotations); and E. M. E. Flick, *Beloved Crusader*, 277, 281.

32. Joseph Walsh, "History of the Pennsylvania Society," *RPS* (1906):3–4, and Price, *Pennsylvania Pioneers*, 57–60.

33. Flick wrote the first six of these tracts between 1892 and 1901. By 1896,

the society had distributed fifty thousand copies of the first tract and forty thousand copies of the second (*RPS* [1896]:5). The tracts were included in several of the reports and are compiled in Price, *Pennsylvania Pioneers*, 255–72. Their wording changed slightly over time.

34. Tract No. 1, "How to Avoid Contracting Tuberculosis (Consumption)," and Tract No. 2, "How Persons Suffering from Tuberculosis Can Avoid Giving the Disease to Others," both published in 1892 and reprinted in *RPS* (1902). The same themes appeared in later tracts, some of which were addressed to special audiences such as hotel-keepers and storekeepers.

35. Ibid. See also Morman, "Scientific Medicine," and H. W. Hetherington and Fannie Eshleman, *Nursing in Prevention and Control of Tuberculosis* (New York: G. P. Putnam's Sons, 1941), 198–225.

Chapter 2. The Quest and the Treatment

1. B. N. Farren to LF, 3, 11 Aug, 11 Sep 1893, all SS; Wm. Pepper to LF, 27 Nov 1893, SS; Bushrod W. James, *American Resorts; with Notes upon Their Climate* (Philadelphia: F. A. Davis, 1889), 19–23; Edward O. Otis, "The Psychological Factor in Selecting a Climate for Invalids," *TACA* 6 (1889):95–105; and "A Change of Air and Scene," *Philadelphia Medical Times* 16 (7 Aug 1886):823–24.

2. James A. Miller, "Climate in the Treatment of Pulmonary Tuberculosis," *ART* 18 (Nov 1928):523–50; Henry E. Sigerist, "American Spas in Historical Perspective," *BHM* 11 (Feb 1942):133–47; Perceval Reniers, *The Springs of Virginia: Life, Love, and Death at the Waters* (Chapel Hill: University of North Carolina Press, 1941); and William Burke, *The Mineral Springs of Western Virginia*, 2nd ed. (New York: Wiley & Putnam, 1846). For nineteenth-century concepts of the body in balance with the environment, and treatments that altered and corrected the imbalances, see Charles E. Rosenberg, "The Therapeutic Revolution: Medicine, Meaning, and Social Change in Nineteenth-Century America," *Perspectives in Biology and Medicine* 20 (Summer 1977):485–506.

3. Billy M. Jones, *Health Seekers in the Southwest, 1817–1900* (Norman: University of Oklahoma Press, 1967); Frank B. Rogers, "The Rise and Decline of the Altitude Therapy of Tuberculosis," *BHM* 43 (Jan–Feb 1969):1–16; John E. Baur, "The Health Seeker in the Westward Movement, 1830–1900," *Mississippi Valley Historical Review* 46 (Jun 1959):91–110; and Esmond R. Long, "Weak Lungs on the Santa Fé Trail," *BHM* 8 (Jul 1940):1040–54.

4. Letterhead of the Hygeia Hotel, Edward S. Dunn to LF, 12 Jan 1894, SS; *Block Island, Rhode Island. Ocean View Hotel* (Boston: Deland and Barta, 1883), 11, LFPM, vol. 80, no. 13[a]; and Charles E. Funnell, *By the Beautiful Sea: The Rise and High Times of That Great American Resort, Atlantic City* (New York: Alfred A. Knopf, 1975), 121.

5. Boardman Reed, "The Effects of Sea Air upon Diseases of the Respiratory Organs, Including a Study of the Influence upon Health of Changes in the Atmospheric Pressure," *TACA* 1 (1884):56; idem, "Winter Health Resorts—The Climate of Atlantic City and Its Effects on Pulmonary Diseases," *Philadelphia*

Medical Times 11 (18 Dec 1880):161–67; W. H. Geddings, "Notes on the Summer Climate of the White Mountain Village of Bethlehem," *Boston Medical and Surgical Journal* 101 (31 Jul 1879):155–61; idem, "Aiken and Thomasville as Types of the Inland Health Resorts of South Carolina and Georgia," *New York Medical Journal* 44 (25 Dec 1886): 707–13; and James, *American Resorts*, 158–65.

6. Frederick I. Knight, "The Opening Address," *TACA* 1 (1884):2–4 (2 for the quotations), and Alfred L. Loomis, "The Annual Address," *TACA* 2 (1885):2. See also Clarence C. Rice, "How the Therapeutic Value of Our Mineral Springs May Be Increased," *TACA* 3 (1886):163–73; and Paul H. Kretzschmar, "Public Health Resorts Versus Institutions for the Treatment of Bacillary Phthisis," *TACA* 5 (1885):71.

7. J. C. Wilson, "Remarks on the Climate-Treatment of Pulmonary Consumption," *Philadelphia Medical Times* 16 (26 Dec 1885):234, and Henry I. Bowditch, *Consumption in New England: or, Locality One of Its Chief Causes* (Boston: Ticknor and Fields, 1862; reprint, New York: Arno Press, 1977), 64–65.

8. *TACA*, 1884–1900, and Charles Denison, "The Preferable Climate for Phthisis; or the Comparative Importance of Different Climatic Attributes in the Arrest of Chronic Pulmonary Diseases," *Transactions of the Ninth International Medical Congress*, vol. 5 (1887):28–45.

9. LF, "The Hygiene of Phthisis," *Proceedings of the Philadelphia County Medical Society* 9 (1888):31–34 (33–34 for the quotation).

10. LF, "Hygiene of Phthisis," 33; LF, "The Treatment of Tuberculosis," *Medical News* 57 (15 Nov 1890):511–12; LF, "The Treatment of Tuberculosis," *Medical News* 75 (2 Sep 1899):299; LF, "Home Treatment of Tuberculosis," *Proceedings of the Philadelphia County Medical Society* 22 (1901):68–69, 83; LF, "Home Treatment of Tuberculosis," *Therapeutic Gazette*, 3d ser., vol. 18 (15 Jun 1902):366; and LF, *The Crusade against Tuberculosis: Consumption a Curable and Preventable Disease* (Philadelphia: David McKay, 1903), 216–22. The use of milk for consumption had a long tradition in folk medicine and was recommended by other physicians also.

11. LF, "Hygiene of Phthisis," 33–34; LF, "Treatment of Tb," 1890, 512; and LF, *Crusade*, 223–34. See also Anita Clair Fellman and Michael Fellman, *Making Sense of Self: Medical Advice Literature in Late Nineteenth-Century America* (Philadelphia: University of Pennsylvania Press, 1981).

12. Richard H. Shryock, *The Development of Modern Medicine: An Interpretation of the Social and Scientific Factors Involved* (New York: Alfred A. Knopf, 1947), 248–72; William G. Rothstein, *American Physicians in the Nineteenth Century: From Sects to Science* (Baltimore: Johns Hopkins University Press, 1972), 125–86; and Guenter B. Risse, Ronald L. Numbers, and Judith W. Leavitt, eds., *Medicine Without Doctors: Home Health Care in American History* (New York: Science History Publications/USA, 1977).

13. Harry B. Weiss and Howard R. Kemble, *The Great American Water-Cure Craze: A History of Hydropathy in the United States* (Trenton, N.J.: Past Times Press, 1967), and James C. Whorton, *Crusaders for Fitness: The History of American Health Reformers* (Princeton, N.J.: Princeton University Press, 1982). For Hermann Brehmer, see n. 34.

14. Weiss and Kemble, *Great American Water-Cure Craze*; Jane B. Donegan, *"Hydropathic Highway to Health": Women and Water-Cure in Antebellum America* (New York: Greenwood Press, 1986); and Susan E. Cayleff, *Wash and Be Healed: The Water-Cure Movement and Women's Health* (Philadelphia: Temple University Press, 1987). For hydrotherapy, see Simon Baruch, *The Uses of Water in Modern Medicine* (Detroit: George S. Davis, 1892), and idem, *The Principles and Practice of Hydrotherapy* (London: Bailliere, Tindall, and Cox, 1900), 347–58.

15. LF, "Treatment of Tuberculosis," 1899, 300 (for first quotation); LF, "Home Treatment," 1901, 71–72 (71 for second quotation); and LF, "Treatment of Tuberculosis," 1890, 510–14 (512 for other quotations). See also LF, "Some New Points in the Treatment of Tuberculosis," *Proceedings of the Philadelphia County Medical Society* 12 (1891):161–66; LF, "Treatment of Tuberculosis by Iodoform Inunctions," *American Therapist* 1 (Jul 1892):3–4; and LF, "A Further Report on the Treatment of Tuberculosis by Iodoform Inunctions," *Medical News* 60 (12 Mar 1892):288–91.

Creosote (also spelled creasote) and iodine, along with carbolic acid, spirits of turpentine, pine-needle oil, and other agents, were used as antiseptic agents in the treatment of phthisis. The use of creosote antedated Koch's discovery of the tubercle bacillus, just as Lister's antiseptic methods antedated Pasteur's germ theory in human disease. Speculations as to how the agents worked changed as the understanding of the disease changed.

16. LF, "Treatment of Tuberculosis," 1899, 300; LF, "Treatment of Tuberculosis," 1890, 513; and, for blisters and cupping, John V. Shoemaker, *A Practical Treatise on Materia Medica and Therapeutics*, 4th ed., rev. (Philadelphia: F. A. Davis, 1898), 283–86, 1044.

17. LF, "The Control of Tuberculosis," *Annual Report of the State Board of Health and Vital Statistics of Pennsylvania* 12 (1896):639–40. From the New York City Health Department, see also T. Mitchell Prudden, "Tuberculosis and its Prevention," *Harper's New Monthly Magazine* 88 (Mar 1894):631: "The things which cause them [infectious diseases] are no longer . . . mysterious emanations from the sick, or incorporate expressions of malign forces against which conjurations or prayers could alone promise protection, but they are particulate beings, never self-engendered, never evolved in the body, always entering from without—things which we can see and handle and kill."

18. Joseph A. Michel to LF, 6 Jul 1894, SS, and Elwell Stockdale to LF, 3 Jul 1897, 6 Jul 1897, SS.

19. Charles Rea to LF, 21 Oct 1898.

20. Eleanor N. Gilbert to LF, 21 Jul 1893, SS; and T. A. Gaffney to LF, 29 Jun, 2, 19, 23 Jul 1894, all SS.

21. A. A. Wertenbach to LF, 6 Jan 1898, SS, and Jno. J. Gilbride to LF, 14 Aug 1899.

22. Isaac H. Platt, "Suggestions Regarding the Management of Phthisical Patients at Health Resorts," *TACA* 5 (1888):122; Kretzchmar, "Public Health Resorts," 73–75; and LF, *Crusade*, 74–79, 232 (74–75, 232 for the quotations).

23. Elwell Stockdale to LF, "Friday" and "Sunday" [probably late summer, 1897], SS; Edward S. Dunn to LF, 12 Jan 1894, SS; A. A. Wertenbach to LF, 15

Apr 1899, SS; Mathias Hau to LF, 26 Mar 1900, SS; and T. A. Gaffney to LF, 19 Jul 1894, SS.

24. T. A. Gaffney to LF, 19 Jul 1894, SS, and Edward S. Dunn to LF, 12 Jan 1894, SS.

25. T. A. Gaffney to LF, 2, 23 Jul 1894, both SS, and Mathias Hau to LF, 26 Mar 1900, SS.

26. J. S. Campbell to LF, 24 Sep 1896; Wm. Beggs to LF, 9 Nov 1896; Joseph A. Michel to LF, 23 Jun 1896; and [Illegible] to LF 19 Jan 1897.

27. Geo. M. Chester to LF, 29 Aug, 23 Sep 1895.

28. *Philadelphia Inquirer*, 5 Mar 1899, sec. 1. Some of these advertisements, less specific than the samples quoted, promised improvement or cure of weak lungs, catarrh, hoarseness, cough, weight loss, and debility. Testimonials bolstered the claims. See ads for Hood's Sarsaparilla (*Philadelphia Inquirer*, 7 Mar 1895), and Dr. Pierce's Golden Medical Discovery (*Philadelphia Inquirer*, 4 Mar 1899). See also Samuel H. Adams, "Tuberculosis Nostrums," *TNA* 2 (1906):72–83.

29. Mrs. S. S. Erricson to LF, 30 Nov 1900, and J. Lewis Good to LF, 26 Nov 1900. For an ad by the American Koch Lung Cure, an organization that had branches in many cities (including one at 1334 Arch Street, Philadelphia), see *Philadelphia Inquirer*, 4 Aug 1901, sec. 1. See also "Exploiting the Consumptive" and "The Ways of the Koch Quacks," *Charities* 11 (8 Aug 1903):124–25; Gerald Keating, "Complete and Authentic Exposé," *Physical Culture* 9 (May 1903):443–48; and idem, "Coaching for the Koch Cure," *Physical Culture* 10 (Jul 1903):70–74.

30. Elmer E. Keiser to LF, 29 Nov, 8, 20, n.d. [ca. 21], 22 Dec 1897.

31. Robert Koch, "A Further Communication on a Cure for Tuberculosis," *Medical News* 57 (15 Nov 1890, Suppl.):521–26; Francis M. Pottenger, *The Diagnosis and Treatment of Pulmonary Tuberculosis* (New York: William Wood, 1908), 165–81; René and Jean Dubos, *The White Plague: Tuberculosis, Man and Society* (Boston: Little, Brown, 1952), 104–8; E[dward] L. Trudeau, "Results of the Employment of Tuberculin and Its Modifications at the Adirondack Cottage Sanitarium," *TACA* 9 (1892):18–23; Karl von Ruck, "A Contribution to the Treatment of Pulmonary Tuberculosis with Professor Koch's Tuberculin," *TACA* 10 (1893):169–79; and H. Longstreet Taylor, "Clinical Results from the Use of Tuberculin and Its Modification Antiphthisin (Klebs) in Pulmonary Consumption," *TACA* 11 (1895):74–85.

32. Annie A. Fitzer to LF, 3 Apr 1898.

33. Charles H. Pratt to LF, 4 Aug 1901, 19 Aug 1901, SS.

34. S. A[dolphus] Knopf, "Hermann Brehmer and the Semi-Centennial Celebration of Brehmer's Sanatorium for the Treatment of Consumptives; The First Institution of Its Kind (July 2, 1854–July 2, 1904)," *NYPMJ* 80 (2 Jul 1904):3–4; H. J. Corper, "The Centenary of the Birth of Hermann Brehmer," *Colorado Medicine* 24 (Jan 1927):16–19; Hugh M. Kinghorn, "Brehmer and Dettweiler: A Review of Their Methods of Treatment of Pulmonary Tuberculosis," *ART* 5 (Feb 1922):950–72; S. Adolphus Knopf, "Peter Dettweiler (1837–1937): Initiator and Promulgator of the Rest Cure in Pulmonary Tuberculosis, the One Hundredth Anniversary of His Birth," *Medical Record* 147 (18 May 1938):464–67; and Paul

Kretzschmar, "Dr. Dettweiler's Method of Treating Pulmonary Consumption," *New York Medical Journal* 47 (18 Feb 1888):175–80.

35. Edward L. Trudeau, *An Autobiography* (Philadelphia: Lea and Febiger, 1916), 73–131, 154, 169–70. In *Crusaders for Fitness*, 9, Whorton points out the "standard biography" common to most health reformers: illness, followed by discovery of a hygienic program that worked for themselves and then energized them to spread the message to others.

36. Paul H. Kretzschmar, "Institutions for the Treatment of Pulmonary Consumption in the United States," *TACA* 6 (1889):169–78; Vincent Y. Bowditch, "The Treatment of Phthisis in Sanitaria near Our Homes," *Boston Medical and Surgical Journal* 135 (30 Jul 1896):125–29; Edward O. Otis, "The Sanatorium or Closed Treatment of Phthisis," *TACA* 12 (1896):26–45; E[dward] L. Trudeau, "Sanitaria for the Treatment of Incipient Tuberculosis," *New York Medical Journal* 65 (27 Feb 1897):276–81; Irby Stephens, "Asheville: The Tuberculosis Era," *North Carolina Medical Journal* 46 (Sep 1985):456–59; Edward J. Nolan to LF, 15, 30 Aug 1893, both SS, and Mathias Hau to LF, 11 Jul 1899, SS.

37. Edward O. Otis to Elwell Stockdale, 31 Oct 1898, LFCP, and Elwell Stockdale to LF, 2 Dec 1898, SS.

38. Elwell Stockdale to LF, 2 Dec 1898, SS.

39. Elwell Stockdale to LF, 2, 28 Dec 1898, 13 Feb, 5 Mar, 1, 28 Apr 1899, all SS.

40. Elwell Stockdale to LF, 30 Jun 1899, SS: W. H. Vormann, ed., *Davos, Its Local, Physical, and Medical Aspects* (London: Provost and Co., 1882); Clinton Wagner, "Colorado Springs and Davos-Platz, as Winter Health Resorts, Compared," *Medical Record* 32 (29 October 1887):567–70; and D. B. St. John Roosa, "The Engadine and Davos," *TACA* 5 (1888):221–28.

41. Kretzschmar, "Public Health Resorts," 74.

Chapter 3. Helping Poor Consumptives

1. *ARCM* 7 (1877):17–18.

2. Nathaniel Burt and Wallace E. Davies, "The Iron Age 1876–1905," in *Philadelphia: A 300-Year History*, ed. Russell F. Weigley (New York: W. W. Norton, 1982), 471–96; Caroline Golab, "The Immigrant and the City: Poles, Italians, and Jews in Philadelphia, 1870–1920," in *The Peoples of Philadelphia: A History of Ethnic Groups and Lower-Class Life, 1790–1940*, ed. Allen F. Davis and Mark H. Haller (Philadelphia: Temple University Press, 1973); and Stephanie W. Greenberg, "Industrial Location and Ethnic Residential Patterns in an Industrializing City: Philadelphia, 1880," Alan N. Burstein, "Immigrants and Residential Mobility: The Irish and Germans in Philadelphia, 1850–1880," and Bruce Laurie and Mark Schmitz, "Manufacture and Productivity: The Making of an Industrial Base, Philadelphia, 1850–1880," all in *Philadelphia: Work, Space, Family, and Group Experience in the Nineteenth Century*, ed. Theodore Hershberg (Oxford: Oxford University Press, 1981).

3. *Annual Statement of the Guardians for the Relief and Employment of the Poor of Philadelphia* (December 31, 1870):16–17, 19–20, 47.

4. Isaac Ray, "What Shall Philadelphia Do for Its Paupers?" *Social Science Association of Philadelphia. Papers of 1873*, 1–14 (2 for the quotation). See also Charles E. Rosenberg, "From Almshouse to Hospital: The Shaping of Philadelphia General Hospital," *Milbank Memorial Fund Quarterly/Health and Society* 60 (Winter 1982):108–54.

5. For responses to the poor, see Paul Boyer, *Urban Masses and Moral Order in America, 1820–1920* (Cambridge, Mass.: Harvard University Press, 1978); Michael B. Katz, *In the Shadow of the Poorhouse: A Social History of Welfare in America* (New York: Basic Books, 1986); Priscilla F. Clement, "The Response to Need, Welfare and Poverty in Philadelphia, 1800 to 1850," Ph.D. diss., University of Pennsylvania, 1977; Eudice Glassberg, "Philadelphians in Need: Client Experiences with Two Philadelphia Benevolent Societies, 1830–1880," Doctor of Social Work diss., University of Pennsylvania, 1979; and Julia B. Rauch, "Unfriendly Visitors: The Emergence of Scientific Philanthropy in Philadelphia, 1878–1880," Ph.D. diss., Bryn Mawr College, 1974.

6. Deaths from phthisis reported at the Almshouse in 1870 totaled 166: 125 on the medical wards, 36 in the insane department, 3 in the children's asylum, and 1 each in the surgical and venereal wards (*Annual Statement*, 1870, 51, 57–90). The Board of Health reported 2,308 deaths from consumption of the lungs.

7. The Philadelphia Protestant Episcopal City Mission, *Plans and Appeal in Behalf of City Missions, by the Bishop of the Diocese, 1870*, 3, 4, 6 for the quotations, ECS. See also *ARCM* 1 (1871):5–7, 10 (1880):6–7; and Stanley R. West, "History of the Philadelphia Protestant Episcopal City Mission, 1870–1955," typescript, 3, 4, ECS.

8. *ARCM* 3 (1873):9, 11; 4 (1874):15; 6 (1876):3, 17–18 (17 for the quotation).

9. *ARCM* 6 (1876):18–19; 7 (1877):13–15; 8 (1878):35–38; 9 (1879): 51 (for the quotations); and Samuel Durborow, "The Home for Consumptives," copy, 1–3, ECS.

10. *ARCM* 7 (1877):15–18; 8 (1878):37–40; 9 (1879):50–56; 10 (1880): 14–16. Women who lived in the households where the patients boarded probably provided the nursing.

11. *ARCM* 11 (1881):14.

12. *ARCM* 9 (1879):27–28. See also *ARCM* 7 (1877):18.

13. *ARCM* 26 (1896):21.

14. *ARCM* 7 (1877):15, 8 (1878):40.

15. Durborow, "Home," 3, and *ARCM* 11 (1881):29–30. Angney recognized the contagiousness of consumption before most people did. He alluded to his own observations in households and to the experimental transfer of the disease to animals by inoculation with human sputum (presumably by French physician J. A. Villemin). At this time, the Mission was sending a few patients to the country for the summer—an action compatible with Angney's suggestions (*ARCM* 11 [1881]:8).

16. *ARCM* 12 (1882):40, also *ARCM* 11 (1881):31. In "Almshouse to Hospital," 127, Rosenberg notes that the example of the Almshouse helped to motivate the founding of private hospitals and dispensaries.

17. *ARCM* 13 (1883):30–32. I have assumed the writer here.

18. *ARCM* 16 (1886):12, and Durborow, "Home," 3, 5–12 (7–8 for the quotation).

19. *ARCM* 11 (1881):27–28; 16 (1886):84–85, 17 (1887):30, 70. A summary of all cases for a year through March 1882 shows that 11 out of 183 patients were discharged improved and one of them had returned to work (*ARCM* 12 [1882]:29–39).

20. *ARCM* 16 (1886):84–85 (85 for the quotations), and *ARCM* 17 (1887):30–31. The Report did not specifically mention Hell, but the phrase from Dante's *Inferno*, Canto III, line 9, would have been familiar to many of the Mission's readers: "ABANDON ALL HOPE YE WHO ENTER HERE." It was cut into stone above the gate to Hell.

21. Durborow, "Home," 11–12, and *ARCM* 17 (1887):28, 69, and *ARCM* 30 (1900):41. Locations of patients at the end of the fiscal year confirm a marked decrease in the numbers at home: from thirty-seven (93 percent) reported in 1886, to twenty-three (62 percent) in 1887, and to seven (32 percent) in 1888.

22. *ARCM* 17 (1887):68, 70, and 21 (1891):13. Use of gaseous enemas had been reported in France, and physicians at the Philadelphia Hospital were trying them with seemingly good results (Edward T. Bruen, "The Treatment of Pulmonary Diseases by Gaseous Enemata. A Preliminary Report," *Medical News* 50 [2 Apr 1887]:368–69). In "Notes and Comments," *Canada Medical and Surgical Journal* 15 (Mar 1887):509, Dr. William Osler, professor of clinical medicine at the University of Pennsylvania, reported: "In the medical wards of the Philadelphia Hospital an odd sight may now be daily witnessed. The resident physician, with large rubber bag full of gas, approaches the bed of a phthisical patient, who at once assumes the lateral decubitus [side-lying position], exposes the anus, when from two to three quarts of the gas are slowly injected into the bowel. This is the new treatment of phthisis . . . and already loudly vaunted." Flick traced the treatment to inhalation of "cow-house vapors" in the eighteenth century (*Medical News* 50 [7 May 1887]:530).

23. For contemporary changes in hospitals, see Charles E. Rosenberg, *The Care of Strangers: The Rise of America's Hospital System* (New York: Basic Books, 1987), 142–65.

24. Reports of Bolling (Chestnut Hill) and Angney (House of Mercy), *ARCM*, 1887–1890, and, for the quotation, *ARCM* 20 (1890):IV. Durborow died in the fall of 1888. Duhring took over in 1889.

25. *ARCM* 22 (1892):7, 29. Whitaker succeeded Stevens as bishop in 1887. For medical authority versus stewardship, see Rosenberg, *Care of Strangers*, 262–77.

26. *ARCM* 23 (1893):15–16; 24 (1894):17.

27. *ARCM* 24 (1894):20; 28 (1898):1.

28. One patient (1 percent of the total) was reported as discharged improved in 1877 (*ARCM* 7 [1877]:17). I have calculated the 1882 figures from the case reports. The 1890 figures are the Mission's. For these and the start of underlining, see *ARCM* 21 (1891):20.

29. The numbers cited come from statistics in ARCM, 1877–1990. They refer to all patients treated during the year in all segments of the Consumptive

Department. The term "discharge" includes "dismissals." For the Mission's fiscal problems, see *ARCM* 12 (1882):8–9, 13 (1883):13, 32.

30. "Report of Mrs. B. E. Nutt, Matron," *ARCM* 24 (1894):20, and A. F. Devereux to LF, 19 Mar 1895; also H. M. Fisher to LF, 17 Jun 1901.

31. *ARCM* 19 (1889):21; 21 (1891):16; 22 (1892):15, 22; 23(1893):15, 23; 24 (1894):24; 26 (1896):15, 29 (1899):50–51, 30 (1900):46.

32. *ARCM* 24 (1894):19; 25 (1895):23. See also *ARCM* 21 (1891):15, 23 (1893):21–22, 24 (1894):25; 30 (1900):43.

33. Ella M. E. Flick, *Beloved Crusader: Lawrence F. Flick, Physician* (Philadelphia: Dorrance, 1944), 175, 288–89. The City Mission tallied the patients' religions in its annual reports.

34. M. L. Coleman to LF, 2 Jan 1896.

35. Sr. Mary Borromeo to Rev. Dear Father [Joseph Scully], with a note from J. S. to LF, 14 Feb 1895, and E. M. E. Flick, *Beloved Crusader*, 289–94.

36. Sr. M. Borromeo to LF, 19 Aug 1897, 9 Jan 1899, 3 Feb 1899, 2 Feb 1900; Katharine Ball to LF, 21 Mar 1898; M. L. Coleman to LF, 16 Apr 1898; Sister Mary Borromeo, biographical materials, Archives, Sisters of St. Francis of Philadelphia, Aston, Pa.; and Sister Mary Borromeo, O.S.F., JW, vol. 13, CPP. Sr. Borromeo is credited with paying off a hospital debt of $150,000 and financing many improvements. According to the annual reports of St. Agnes' Hospital, payment from the Free Hospital (listed as the Sacred Heart League through 1898) rose steadily in both amount and percentage of income from 1895 to its peak year, 1899. For the five-dollar charge, see *ARPB* 28 (1897):82. In 1896, private rooms cost fifteen dollars a week and two-bed rooms eight dollars (Sr. M. Borromeo to LF, 31 Jan 1896). Between 1893 and 1900, occupancy at St. Agnes' varied from full to a quarter full (*ARsPB*).

37. Adele G. Tack to LF, 9 Jan 1899, and Sr. M. Borromeo to LF, 9, 22 Jan 1899.

38. Consumptive Patients, a list of those at St. Agnes' and St. Mary's, April 1899, LFCP, and Sr. M. Borromeo to LF, 19 Apr 1899. One man on Flick's list died before discharge. Four of the nine patients discharged had been at St. Agnes' for twelve to eighteen months; five, for two to six months. One patient, at St. Agnes' for two years, was not discharged.

39. *ARFH* 4 (1902):1 (for expenditures); *ARFH* n.d. [1899]:1; E. M. E. Flick, *Beloved Crusader*, 296; and Mary McManus to LF, 2 Mar 1898.

40. *ARFH* 2 (1900):outside back cover, and *ARFH*, n.d. [1899]:2.

41. *ARFH* 2 (1900):inside back cover (for the first quotation), also 2, and *ARFH* 3 (1901):inside back cover.

Chapter 4. Life As a Patient

1. *ARCM* 9 (1879):55, and J. D. Nevin to Miss Coleman, 14 Jun 1899, LFCP. In 1880, women's wages in Philadelphia were about 70 percent of men's wages within the same industries. Because women could not work in high-wage industries, their average income was proportionately even lower. See Claudia

Goldin, "Family Strategies and the Family Economy in the Late Nineteenth Century: The Role of Secondary Workers," in *Philadelphia: Work, Space, Family, and Group Experience in the Nineteenth Century*, ed. Theodore Hershberg (Oxford: Oxford University Press, 1981), 285, 308, n. 14.

2. Theodore Hershberg et al., "The 'Journey to Work': An Empirical Investigation of Work, Residence, and Transportation, Philadelphia, 1850 and 1880," in Hershberg, *Philadelphia*.

3. For examples, see *ARCM* 8 (1878):40, 13 (1883):37, 21 (1891):15; Alex. H. Davisson to LF, 31 Mar 1895; Mary L. Coleman to LF, n.d. [filed 10 Sep 1896], and 15 Aug 1897; B. C. Feran to LF, 18 Dec 1898; R. L. Smith to LF, 26 Aug 1889; Wm. Kieran to LF, 8 Jan 1900; John J. Duffy to LF, 19 Jan 1900; Mrs. Atherton to [Fr. Scully], 20 Apr 1900, LFCP; and H. A. Strecker to LF, 28 Mar 1901.

4. For examples, see Thomas Kearns to LF, 15 Feb 1895, and P. J. Mellon [?sp] to LF, 9 Jul 1900.

5. Mary Hurley to Mary Coleman, 29 Jan 1900, LFCP; Theodore A. Tack to LF, 1 May 1897; Henry M. Fisher to LF, 2 Dec 1895; Mary E. Ward to LF, 1 May 1898; and C. G. W. to Mary McManus, 2 Mar 1899, LFCP. The Little Sisters of the Poor, an order of Roman Catholic nuns, ran a home for the aged in Philadelphia; the "old mother" was probably an inmate.

6. Charles E. Rosenberg, "From Almshouse to Hospital: The Shaping of Philadelphia General Hospital," *Milbank Memorial Fund Quarterly/Health and Society* 60 (Winter 1982):108–54; John J. McKenna to LF, 24 Jan 1895; Henry M. Fisher to LF, 26 Feb 1899; Gerald P. Coghlan to LF, 4 Apr 1899; and Charles Wirgman to LF, 7 Apr 1898.

7. John J. Duffy to LF, 19 Jan 1900; Mary E. Ward to LF, 11 May 1898; and James C. McLoughlin [?sp] to LF, 7 Jan 1899. There are numerous other examples of need in LFCP, and in the *ARsCM*.

8. Chas. W. Naulty to LF, 27 Jul 1900, and Thos. Kearns to LF, 15 Feb 1895.

9. Thos. Kearns to Mrs. McManus, 19 Jan 1896, LFCP; Sr. Blanche to LF, 2 Aug 1903; M. A. Bradley to LF, 4 Sep 1900; Mary A. McManus to LF, 10 Sep 1897; Joseph O'Keefe to LF, 2 Nov 1901; Mary L. Coleman to LF, 28 Jan 1901; and B. C. Feran to LF, 8 Aug 1898.

10. Henry M. Fisher to LF, 4 Dec 1900.

11. Howard Greenwood to LF, 13 Jan 1901; Edwin S. Cooke to LF, 1 Feb 1899; M. A. McManus to LF, 22 Jul 1897; and Mary L. Coleman to LF, 12 Jan 1896. See also Owen McFarland to LF, 2 Sep 1897; Margaret A. Heraty to LF, 6 Feb 1900; A. G. Tack to LF, 6 Dec 1899; Mary L. Coleman to LF, 18 Sep, 18 Dec, 1896; Chas. W. Naulty to LF, 8 May 1900; W. H. Cline to LF, 20 May 1901; and William C. Currie to LF, 12 Sep 1900.

12. For the charges for care, see Mary L. Coleman to LF, 18 Sep 1896; Mary E. Ward to LF, 8 Feb 1898; and Edwin S. Cooke to LF, 1 Feb 1899. For burial costs, see Mary A. McManus to LF, 10 Sep 1897; Chas. W. Naulty to LF, 15 Mar 1900; M. A. McManus to LF, 4 Oct 1897; and Sr. M. Borromeo to LF, 30 Jan 1900. By 1896, the Home at Chestnut Hill charged those who could pay three

dollars a week (*ARCM* 26 (1896):13). It also expected the person responsible for the patient to pay the costs of burial (Form of Application, Philadelphia Protestant Episcopal City Mission, 189_, CPP).

13. This and the next paragraph are based on the *ARsCM* and the *ARsPB*. For the quotation, see *ARPB* 26 (1895):116; for the staffing, *ARPB* 27 (1896):127, 28 (1897):93.

14. *ARPB* 26 (1895):114 for the first two quotations, and *ARCM* 28 (1898):83 for the third.

15. In addition to the *ARsPB*, I have used here the annual reports of St. Agnes' Hospital; Sr. M. Borromeo to LF, 22 Oct 1901; B. Franklin Stahl, "St. Agnes' Hospital," in *Founders' Week Memorial Volume*, ed. Frederick P. Henry (Philadelphia: City of Philadelphia, 1909), 706–10; and Roberta M. West, *History of Nursing in Pennsylvania* (Pennsylvania State Nurses' Association, n.d.), 696–97.

16. Mary L. Morrison to LF, 6, 28 Jun 1901, and Josie C. Collom to LF, 25 Feb 1900; also Katie O'Byrne to LF, 26 Aug 1895, and Elizabeth O'Donnell to LF, 6 Feb 1899.

17. Mrs. Wm. F. Laird to LF, 9 Dec 1901, and Francis Fisher to LF, 30 Jun 1900. Although these kinds of complaints may seem straightforward, there were sometimes other sides of the story that did not support the complainant.

18. Chas. W. Naulty to LF, 23 Apr 1900; Michael J. McCaffrey to [Mary A. McManus], 3 Aug 1899, LFCP; and Cecilia Healy to Mrs. McManus, n.d., LFCP.

19. "Patient Records," vol. 1, 29 Apr 1899 through Dec 1901, ECS. In this volume, the resident physician at Chestnut Hill recorded admissions and departures, often with brief explanations. See also Sr. M. Xavier to LF, 12 Nov 1898, and Chas. W. Naulty to LF, 28 Mar 1900.

20. Chas. W. Naulty to LF, 30 Oct 1900. See also M. A. McManus to LF, 27 May 1899, and Chas. W. Naulty to LF, 26, 28, 30 Apr 1900.

21. *ARCM* 18 (1888):28.

22. Regina O'Leary to LF, 11 Sep 1900.

23. Regina O'Leary to LF, 2 Dec 1900.

24. Katie Leahy to LF, 25 Aug 1898. See also "Sanitarium Gabriels," *The National Hospital and Sanitarium Record* 1 (Sep 1897):6, and S. A. Knopf, *Pulmonary Tuberculosis: Its Modern Prophylaxis and the Treatment in Special Institutions and at Home* (Philadelphia: P. Blakiston's Son, 1899), 147–49.

25. Patrick O'Conner to LF, 8 Oct 1900; Laura S. Chapin to LF, 13 Jul 1898; Katie A. Leahy to LF, 22 Jul 1898; and George Schaaf to LF, 17 Feb 1900, SS.

26. A[nnie] E. Hackett to LF, 24 Aug 1899.

27. Annie E. Hackett to LF, 23 Dec 1899.

28. Annie E. Hackett to LF, 8 May 1900.

29. Sallie Morgan to LF, n.d.; Sisters of Mercy to LF, 4 Jul 1900; and [Annie E. Hackett] to LF, 9 Jul 1900.

30. Annie E. Hackett to LF, 30 Jun 1900.

31. [Annie E. Hackett] to LF, 9 Jul 1900.

32. Sr. M. P. H. Kieran to LF, 14 Jul 1900.

33. Annie Hackett to LF, 11 Jul 1900.

34. Annie Hackett to LF, 17 Apr 1901.

35. Sisters of Mercy to LF, 20 Jul 1901.
36. Sr. Mary P. H. Kieran to LF, 24 Jul 1901, and James McNamee to LF, 25 Jul 1901.
37. Sisters of Mercy to LF, 29 Jul 1901.
38. Regina O'Leary to LF, 10 Jul 1901, and James McNamee to LF, 17 Jul 1901.
39. Mary A. Becker to LF, 23 Dec 1901.

Chapter 5. A Camp in the Mountains:
The Beginnings of the White Haven Sanatorium

1. Vincent Y. Bowditch, "The Comparative Importance of Different Climatic Attributes in the Treatment of Pulmonary Consumption," *TACA* (1888):44–49; idem, "The Origin and Growth of the Sanatorium Treatment of Pulmonary Tuberculosis in Massachusetts," in *Tuberculosis in Massachusetts*, ed. Edwin A. Locke (Boston: Massachusetts State Committee for the International Congress on Tuberculosis, 1908), 65–73; and Lilian Brandt, comp., *A Directory of Institutions and Societies Dealing with Tuberculosis in the United States and Canada* (New York: Committee on the Prevention of Tuberculosis of the Charity Organization Society of the City of New York and the National Association for the Study and Prevention of Tuberculosis, 1904).
2. Guy Hinsdale to LF, 24 Jan 1895; *RPS* (1896):6, (1898):4, (1902):5; *ARFH* 10 (1908):5–7; and F. C. Johnson, "The Proposed Sanitarium for Tuberculosis at White Haven, Together with Some of the Reasons Why the State Should Lend Its Aid," *Transactions of the Luzerne County Medical Society* 5 (1897): 129–49.
3. Rosemary Stevens, "Sweet Charity: State Aid to Hospitals in Pennsylvania, 1870–1910," *BHM* 58 (Fall, Winter 1984):287–314, 474–95; Henry M. Fisher to LF, 31 Jan 1901; and Talcott Williams to LF, 24 Feb 1901.
4. *RPS* (1902):5; *ARFH* 9 (1907):1, 10 (1908):16, 11 (1909):1; *Proceedings of the Philadelphia County Medical Society* 21 (Jan 1900):1–32; and Benjamin Lee, "State Provision for the Treatment of the Consumptive Poor," *JAMA* 35 (20 Oct 1900):989–90.
5. "Hospital is Needed for Poor Consumptives," *Philadelphia Inquirer*, 14 Jan 1901; "Free Hospital for Consumptives," *Philadelphia Evening Telegraph*, 19 Feb 1901; G. L. Halsey to LF, 25 Jan 1901; S. W. Trimmer to LF, 24 Feb, 23 Jun 1901; Charles E. Voorhees to LF, 6 Mar 1901; Benjamin Lee to LF, 4 Jun 1901; Cyrus Woods to LF, 28 Jun 1901; "The Free Hospital for Poor Consumptives," handbills, [1901], LFPM, vol. 40, nos. 11, 12; and *ARFH* 9 (1907):2.
6. Elwell Stockdale (ES hereafter) to LF, 22 Jun 1901, 1 Apr 1899, SS. For length of his treatment, see ES, "The Diet at Sunnyrest Sanatorium, White Haven, Penn.," *JOL* 3 (February 1906):6.
7. ES to LF, 31 Jul 1901. The terms proposed by Stockdale (ES to LF, 9 Jul 1901) were seventy-five dollars a month and board.
8. LF, "A Year's Work at the White Haven Sanatorium of the Free Hospital

for Poor Consumptives," *Philadelphia Medical Journal* 10 (8 Nov 1902):678 (for quoted phrases); Johnson, "Proposed Sanitarium," 133–34; "Mike" [Fr. Michael Bergrath] to LF, 3 Jan 1901; G. L. Halsey to LF, 25 Jan 1901; topographical map of White Haven, Pa., U.S. Geological Survey, Washington, D.C., 1950; and maps of White Haven, Sanborn Map Co., 1903, 1908, 1927.

9. LF, "Year's Work," 678 (for the first quotations), and ES to LF, 31 Sep, 2 Aug 1901, and n.d. [filed 2 Aug 1901].

10. LF, "Year's Work," 680; LF to William B. Miller, 2 Oct 1901, LFCP; and LF to Henry M. Neale, 9 Apr 1936.

11. ES to LF, 15, 18, [26] Aug 1901.

12. ES to LF, 1, 6 Sep 1901, and LF, "Year's Work," 678. By "your rate for administration" Stockdale meant the institution's cost of administration. Flick took no money for his work there.

13. LF, "Year's Work," 680. Of the 156 patients admitted to the sanatorium during its first year, Flick judged only 9.6 percent as having incipient disease.

14. ES to LF, 10, 12, 18, 21, 27 Sep, 5, 9, 11, 14, 18, 30 Oct, 6 Nov 1901.

15. ES to LF, 8, 16 Nov 1901. Flick used nitroglycerine to treat or prevent bleeding from the lungs. Stockdale misspelled Dr. Snyder's name. Weight gains during the fall were partly deceptive. Stockdale learned in the spring, when the men were losing weight, that a seasonal change of clothing, including arctics, accounted for an estimated 2 1/2 pounds (ES to LF, 7 Apr, 25 May 1902).

16. ES to LF, 12 Sep 1901; Walter Reynolds to LF, 18 Sep 1901; [James] McNamee to LF, 18 Sep 1901; and Jay M. Brown to LF, 17 Sep 1901.

17. Benj. Montanye to LF, 20 Nov 1901; ES to LF, 26 Jan 1902; and *ARFH* 10 (1908):8. The *ARFH* (1902) cited different figures that were based on patients admitted. In 1909, the Free Hospital reported revised data based on patients discharged. I have used the latter.

18. ES to LF, 18, 21 Sep 1901, 24 Oct 1901.

19. M. S. Freas to Mrs. Eckley B. Cox[e], 28 Oct 1901, LFCP, and Mrs. Eckley B. Coxe, Benefactress, typescript, Sophia G. Coxe Home, Drifton, Pa.

20. ES to LF, 7 Nov 1901.

21. Henry M. Fisher to LF, 21 Nov 1901.

22. ES to LF, 29 Nov 1901.

23. ES to LF, 1 Jan 1902.

24. *ARFH* 4 (1902):2; LF, "Year's Work," 678; and H. McDevitt to LF, n.d. [filed 17 Jan 1902]. The Free Hospital was short of funds partly because state money was delayed. Receipts from the state for the year ending 1 Mar 1902 were only $3,750.

25. ES to LF, 18 Sep 1901.

26. ES to LF, 1 Oct, 29 Dec, 1901, 5 Feb 1902.

27. ES to LF, 25, 29 Dec 1901.

28. *ARFH* 4 (1902):6; ES to LF, 6 Dec 1901; and H. McDevitt to LF, n.d. [filed mid-Jan 1902].

29. ES to LF, 20, 25, 29 Dec 1901.

30. ES to LF, 7, 15, 25, 26 May, n.d. [filed 2 Jun], 4 Jun, n.d. [filed 10 Jul] 1902, and Regina O'Leary to LF, 15 May 1902.

31. ES to LF, 20 Aug 1902. For O'Hara's background, see p. 78.

32. ES to LF, 2, 27 Jan, 20 Aug 1902, and Anna G. Murphy to LF, n.d. [filed 23 Feb 1903].

33. LF, "Year's Work," 678, and John J. Campbell to Miss Rebecca Coxe, 12 May 1902, LFCP.

34. The boxes collected three to four thousand dollars a year.

35. Appeal letter, with letterhead of the Free Hospital for Poor Consumptives, to Mr. Willcox, 14 Oct 1901, LFCP, and *ARFH* 4 (1902):6.

36. "Curing Consumptives, and Seeing Them Grow Fat in a Month, at the First Open-Air Sanitarium in Pennsylvania," *North American*, 13 Oct 1901, sec. 6; "Cured of Consumption," *Philadelphia Record*, 17 Mar 1902; and "Cured Consumption in Seven Weeks," *North American*, 21 Mar 1902. For magazine stories, see, for example, Day A. Willey, "New Hope for Consumptives," *American Monthly Review of Reviews* 27 (Jun 1903):689–95. Letters from patients and their families, inquiring about the sanatorium, often referred to these articles.

37. ES to LF, n.d. [filed 2 Nov 1901], and 24 Mar 1902.

38. ES to LF, 2 Nov 1901.

39. *ARFH* 11 (1909):8–9.

40. John C. Nagle to ES, 1 Apr 1902, LFCP, and Solomon Solis Cohen to LF, 15 Jan 1903.

41. LF, "Year's Work," 679–81 (681 for the quotation).

42. Ibid., 678–79; *ARFH* 4 (1902):2; and ES to LF, 21 Sep, 9 Oct 1901, 15 May 1902. For the average annual costs of maintenance, see *ARFH* 4 (1902):3 and 5 (1903):3. Starting in Feb 1905, the expenses of the Philadelphia office were added to the reported costs of maintenance; a year later costs for earlier years were recalculated to make them consistent. By the new method, weekly costs of maintenance for the two years cited were $7.00 and $5.70 respectively (*ARFH* 8 [Feb 1906]:2).

43. During the years closing on 1 Mar 1902, and 28 Feb 1903, receipts of the sanatorium's maintenance fund from donations and contribution boxes rose from $6,677.20 to $21,844.69. For Coxe contributions, see ES to LF, 27 Sep, 20 Nov, 25 Dec 1901; S. G. [Mrs. Eckley B.] Coxe to ES, 8 Dec 1901, LFCP; [Mrs. Charles B. Coxe to LF], 14 Nov 1901; and E. M. E. Flick, *Beloved Crusader: Lawrence F. Flick, Physician* (Philadelphia: Dorrance, 1944), 308–309. See also Henry Phipps to LF, 26 Apr, 22 Oct 1902.

44. ES to LF, 11 Sep 1902, and Henry Phipps to LF, 14, 22 Oct 1902.

45. Edgar C. Gerwig to LF, 22, 26 Jul 1901; John E. Fox to LF, 12, 18, 20 Aug 1902; and Ward R. Bliss to LF, 2 Jan 1903.

46. ES to LF, 29 Jan, 13, 24 Mar, 3 Apr, 15, 28 May, 30 Dec 1902, 1 Jan [1903].

47. ES to LF, 30 Dec 1902, 1, 2 Jan [1903], 3 Jan 1903, and Guy Hinsdale to LF, 14, 29 Jan 1903.

48. From the year ending in Feb 1902 to that ending in Feb 1904, the number of patients admitted to the sanatorium annually increased from 69 to 516; the number admitted to other institutions by the Free Hospital decreased from 238 to 46. For members of the board and the medical administration committee, see

ARFH, 1902, 1903. See also Henry Fisher to LF, 19 Mar 1903, and J. Alison Scott to LF, 2 Mar 1906.

    49. Regina O'Leary to LF, 27 Jan 1903.

Chapter 6. Research, Training, and Patient Care: The Henry Phipps Insititute

    1. Ella M. E. Flick, *Beloved Crusader: Lawrence F. Flick, Physician, 1856–1938* (Philadelphia: Dorrance, 1944), 188–89; "Henry Phipps Institute," *New York Times*, 10 Jan 1903; John B. Roberts to LF, 10 Jan 1903; John J. Sullivan to LF, 11 Jan 1903; and Anastasia Davisson to LF, 10 Jan 1903.

    2. Kenneth M. Ludmerer, *Learning to Heal: The Development of American Medical Education* (New York: Basic Books, 1985), 29–38; Charles E. Rosenberg, *The Care of Strangers: The Rise of America's Hospital System* (New York: Basic Books, 1987), 157–65; and James Bordley III and A. McGehee Harvey, *Two Centuries of American Medicine, 1776–1976* (Philadelphia: W. B. Saunders, 1976), 187–200.

    3. Erwin H. Ackerknecht, *A Short History of Medicine* (1955; rev. printing, New York: Ronald Press, 1968), 175–85.

    4. Richard H. Shryock, *American Medical Research, Past and Present* (New York: Commonwealth Fund, 1947), 78–105, and Andrew Carnegie, *The Gospel of Wealth and Other Timely Essays* (Garden City, N.Y.: Doubleday, Doran & Co., 1933), 28–29. The two articles were first published in the *North American Review* in 1889.

    5. George W. Corner, *A History of the Rockefeller Institute, 1901–1953: Origins and Growth* (New York: Rockefeller Institute Press, 1964), 1–55, 94.

    6. James H. Bridge, "Captains of Industry, Part VIII, Henry Phipps," *Cosmopolitan* 34 (Dec 1902):163–67; *Dictionary of American Biography*, s.v. "Phipps, Henry"; *National Cyclopaedia of American Biography*, s.v. "Phipps, Henry"; *Autobiography of Andrew Carnegie* (Boston: Houghton Mifflin, 1920), 30–31, 131; Burton J. Hendrick, *The Life of Andrew Carnegie* (Garden City, N. Y.: Doubleday, Doran, 1932), vol. 1, 51, 54; and "Henry Phipps, Steel Man Is Dead," *New York Sun*, 22 Sep 1930, LFSB, vol. 4.

    7. Hendrick, *Life of Carnegie*, vol. 1, 132, 189–90, vol. 2, 44; H. R. M. Landis, "Henry Phipps," *RHPI* 22 (1930):2; Joseph Walsh, "Henry Phipps," JW, vol. 13; and Adolph Meyer to LF, 12 Jan 1931. For Phipps's frugality, see also Henry Phipps (HP hereafter) to LF, 1 May 1902, and 15 Sep 1903.

    8. E. M. E. Flick, *Beloved Crusader*, 176–77; HP to LF, 30 May 1904, SS; and James A. Gibson, *The Nordrach Treatment* (London: Sampson Low, Marston, 1901).

    9. E. M. E. Flick, *Beloved Crusader*, 178–80 (179 for the quotation); HP to LF, 26 Apr 1902; and Frank A. Craig, *Early Days at Phipps* (Henry Phipps Institute for the Study and Prevention of Tuberculosis, University of Pennsylvania, 1952), 5–8.

    10. E. M. E. Flick, *Beloved Crusader*, 180–88.

    11. "Henry Phipps Institute," *New York Times*, 10 Jan 1903; LF, "The Henry Phipps Institute for the Study, Treatment, and Prevention of Tuberculosis," *Phila-*

delphia Medical Journal 11 (31 Jan 1903):208–9; and LF, "The Work of the First Year," *RHPI* 1 (1904):3. Models for the Institute included the Pasteur Institute in Paris and the Emile Roux Dispensary in Lille, France, both visited by Flick during his European trip.

12. Joseph Walsh, "Speech at the Testimonial Dinner Given by the Staff of the Henry Phipps Institute to Dr. Lawrence F. Flick," 1 Feb 1910, JW, vol. 13.

13. Ibid., and LF, "Work of the First Year," 3–4.

14. LF, "Work of the First Year," 4–6, and LF, "The Hospital and Dispensary in the Warfare against Tuberculosis," *American Medicine* 9 (20 May 1905):826.

15. LF, "Work of the First Year," 6. For contemporary medical education, see Abraham Flexner, *Medical Education in the United States and Canada* (n.p.: The Carnegie Foundation for the Advancement of Teaching, 1910; reprint, Bethesda, Md.: Science and Health Publications, n.d.); Ludmerer, *Learning to Heal*, 47–101; and William G. Rothstein, *American Medical Schools and the Practice of Medicine: A History* (New York: Oxford University Press, 1987), 89–116.

16. George W. Corner, *Two Centuries of Medicine: A History of the School of Medicine, University of Pennsylvania* (Philadelphia: J. B. Lippincott, 1965), 192, 197, and Joseph C. Aub and Ruth K. Hapgood, *Pioneer in Modern Medicine: David Linn Edsall of Harvard* (n.p.: Harvard Medical Alumni Association, 1970), 16–17.

17. Craig, *Early Days*, 50–62; W. Taylor Cummins to LF, 22 Jan 1904; and Albert Francine to LF, 22 Jul 1904. See also LF, "Communities without Health Departments in the Crusade against Tuberculosis," *NYPMJ* 79 (11 Jun 1904): 1130–31, and Rosenberg, *Care of Strangers*, 166–79.

18. Quoted in Craig, *Early Days*, 51. In "Work of the First Year," 6, Flick noted that fear made organizing the medical staff more difficult.

19. Quoted in Craig, *Early Days*, 41.

20. Ibid., 9, 10, 38–39, 50–61; a review of all letters from staff members in the LF Papers, 1903–1909; and lists of staff, *ARsHPI*.

21. Biographical data for this and the next paragraphs come from W. J. Maxwell, comp., *General Alumni Catalogue of the University of Pennsylvania* (n.p., 1922); idem, *General Alumni Catalogue of Jefferson Medical College* (n.p., 1917); the *American Medical Directory*; Craig, *Early Days*; letters to Flick from the physicians; memoirs of thirteen of the men in *TSCP*; and Cecilia Flick, *Dr. Lawrence F. Flick As I Knew Him* (Philadelphia: Dorrance, 1956), 94–111.

22. Quoted in Craig, *Early Days*, 57–58.

23. *Dictionary of American Biography*, Suppl. 4, s.v., "Ravenel, Mazÿck Porcher," and LF to HP, 9 Oct 1903. See also HP to LF, 15 Sep 1903.

24. Albert P. Francine, "A Brief Account of Methods of Study and Treatment at the Henry Phipps Institute, Philadelphia," *PMJ* 10 (Sep 1907):943–44; Joseph Walsh, "The Methods of the Henry Phipps Institute for the Study, Treatment, and Prevention of Tuberculosis in Philadelphia," *Bulletin of the Johns Hopkins Hospital* 19 (Jun 1908):174; and Craig, *Early Days*, 14–15. For the honoraria, see LF to HP, 24 Dec 1903, 30 Mar, 16 Dec 1904, 30 Dec 1905; Geo. E. Gordon (GG hereafter) to LF, 19 Dec 1904; and LF to GG, 5 Jan 1906. During the first year, the same physicians staffed both hospital and dispensary, but the two positions were separated early in 1904 (LF to D. L. Edsall, 21 Jan 1904).

25. LF to HP, 30 Dec 1905, 12 Feb 1906, and LF to H. R. M. Landis, et al., 17 Feb 1906. Flick, following the model of the Rockefeller Institute, shifted responsibility for making proposals to the men themselves in 1909. A committee reviewed the proposals and approved promising ones. See Joseph McFarland to LF, 12 Jan 1909; LF to Joseph McFarland 14 Jan 1909; and "First Meeting of the Phipps Laboratory 'Staff,'" 25 Jan 1909, and "Second Meeting of the Committee on Problems," 1 Feb 1909, both JW, vol. 2. For physicians' difficulties in undertaking or completing their work, see Charles M. Montgomery to LF, 19 Feb 1906; E. John G. Beardsley to LF, 18 Apr 1907; Edward H. Goodman to LF, Feb 1908; and LF to Joseph McFarland, 16 Feb 1909.

26. LF, "The Treatment and Control of the Tuberculous Patient in His Home," *American Medicine* 8 (30 Jul 1904):187. Flick's mention of veterinary surgery referred to Leonard Pearson's work in bovine tuberculosis. Pearson was a member of the Institute's staff.

27. Francine, "Brief Account," 942–43; *RHPI* 2 (1905):411–38; LF, "Clinical and Sociological Report of the Year," *RHPI* 4 (1907):5–6; Walsh, "Methods," 174; and idem, "Speech at Testimonial Dinner."

28. Craig, *Early Days*, 12 and 57 (for the quotations), 51, 53–54, 59–60; Francine, "Brief Account," 945–46; and Walsh, "Methods," 174.

29. *RHPI* 2 (1905):411; LF to Amy McGuiness, 2 Mar 1906; Walsh, "Methods," 174; Charles J. Hatfield, "The Henry Phipps Institute for the Study, Treatment and Prevention of Tuberculosis," in *Founders' Week Memorial Volume*, ed. Frederick P. Henry (Philadelphia: City of Philadelphia, 1909), 842; and H. R. M. Landis, "Signed Consent to a Necropsy a Condition to Admission to Our Hospitals," *JAMA* 62 (3 Jan 1914):29–30.

30. Craig, *Early Days*, 57–58; John Gallagher to LF, 18 Dec 1903, 31 May 1904, May 1905; and F. N. Heaney to LF, 6 Nov 1904. See also Helen C. Jenks to LF, 9 Jan 1905; Milton Jackson to LF, 12 Aug 1905, SS; Talcott Williams to LF, 24 Nov 1905; and *RHPI* 2 (1905):411.

31. Walsh, "Methods," 175–76. See also Craig, *Early Days*, 17; and LF to Louis Gerstley, 15 Dec 1904. Only about a third of the hospital patients died in the Institute between 1903 and 1909; of these, 98 percent were autopsied (Landis, "Signed Consent," 30).

32. Edward L. Trudeau to LF, 6 Nov 1903; W. G. B. Harland to LF, 5 Jul 1906; and W. G. B. Harland, "Intratracheal and Intralaryngeal Injections," *International Clinics* 16th ser., vol. 2 (1906):288–98. In a letter to Joseph Walsh, 17 Mar 1908, JW, vol. 2, Charles M. Montgomery named three Institute patients "whose urine I am examining for albumin, all of whom I believe you are willing to treat with creasote so that we may get a few data about the relationship between creasote and albuminuria." Patients' responses are not known.

33. I have calculated all figures in this paragraph from tables in *RHPI* 2 through 6. Statistical data in *RHPI* 1 included nontuberculous and unsuitable patients. These were excluded from two-year summaries in *RHPI* 2. For first-year figures, I have subtracted second-year figures from those in the summaries. Unless otherwise specified, data refer to new tuberculous patients in the hospital and dispensary. The proportion of foreign-born patients increased from 39 percent in

1903 to 51 percent in 1909. Ireland led the list of foreign countries of parental origin, followed by Russia, Germany, Italy, and England. Jews came also from Austria-Hungary, Poland, and Romania (LF, "Work of the First Year," 11). Attempts to quantify earnings were stopped in 1908 because of inaccurate data (LF, "Clinical and Sociological Report," *RHPI* 5 [1908]:42). For filling the hospital, see E. M. E. Flick, *Beloved Crusader*, 191.

34. E. M. E. Flick, *Beloved Crusader*, 196; Walsh, "Methods," 176; "Report of Special Committee on Tuberculosis Nursing," Nurses' Associated Alumnae of the United States, *American Journal of Nursing* 11 (Aug 1911):973; and, for an overview of American nursing history, Philip A. Kalisch and Beatrice J. Kalisch, *The Advance of American Nursing*, 2nd. ed. (Boston: Little, Brown, 1986).

35. LF, "Hospital and Dispensary," 825 (for the first and third quotations), and LF, "Communities Without Health Departments," 1131.

36. Frank Heitler to LF, 29 Jul 1903 (for first quotations); P. Safran to LF, 17 Aug 1903; H. MacSorley to LF, 25 Sep 1903; Walsh, "Methods," 176; and E. M. E. Flick, *Beloved Crusader*, 196.

37. LF, "Cured Patients as Tuberculosis Nurses," *JOL* 8 (Jan 1911):4, and ES to LF, 14 Jul 1903. Phipps approved hiring "weak and necessitous" patients from White Haven (HP to LF, 3 Sep 1903).

38. ES to LF, 29 Jul 1903, and LF, "Cured Patients," 4–5.

39. LF, "Cured Patients," 5.

40. LF, "Cured Patients," 4, and the death record of Regina O'Leary, Record Series 76.22, PCA.

41. Charles [J]. Hatfield, "Nursing in Tuberculosis," *JOL* 4 (Oct 1907):322–24; LF, "Cured Patients," 5–7; LF to GG, 2 Sep 1904; Walsh, "Methods," 176–77; LF, "Work of the First Year," 6, 32; and LF to HP, 30 Oct 1905.

42. LF to ES, 18 Jun 1904; ES to LF, 21 Jun, 6 Jul 1904; Anne K. Sutton to Joseph Walsh, 25 Feb 1907, JW, vol. 2; A[nne] K. Sutton to LF, 21 Aug 1907, 5 May 1908; and Charles J. Hatfield to LF, 3 Jun, 23 Dec 1908.

43. For Flick's early, optimistic views of the dispensary, see LF, "Hospital and Dispensary," 825–26, and LF, "Communities Without Health Departments," 1131. Before the pupils, physicians taught patients both in the dispensary and in homes (Craig, *Early Days*, 15, 54–55).

44. LF, "Work of the First Year," 30.

45. *RHPI* 2 (1905):444 (for the quotation), and "Rules for Patients of the Henry Phipps Institute," n.d., CPP.

46. LF, "Municipalities in the Crusade Against Tuberculosis," *Medicine* 10 (May 1904):332, and LF, "Work of the Year," *RHPI* 2 (1905):43. See also LF, "The Essentials of the Crusade Against Tuberculosis," *New York Medical Journal* 85 (23 Mar 1907):530.

47. LF, "Hospital and Dispensary," 826. To provide milk, the Institute tried delivery by its own horse and wagon, by milk stations or depots, and by private milkmen. For the early years, see LF, "Work of the First Year," 30; LF to HP, 4 May 1904; LF to M. P. Ravenel, 20 Jun 1904; and LF, "Work of the Year," 3–4, 42.

48. *RHPI* 2 (1905):444.

49. Francine, "Brief Account," 944.

50. The first 'Inspectress' Report" form (*RHPI* 2 [1905]:430) did not list economic factors, but a later form included rent and income (Anne K. Sutton, "The Henry Phipps Institute Training School for Nurses," *TSICT*, vol. 3 [1908]:563). See also Walsh, "Methods," 174. Patients unsuitable because they were not poor enough were a problem from the beginning (LF, "Work of the First Year," 8). For this issue in other settings, see George Rosen, "The Impact of the Hospital on the Physician, the Patient and the Community," *Hospital Administration* 9 (Fall 1964):15–33, and Gert H. Brieger, "The Use and Abuse of Medical Charities in Late Nineteenth Century America," *American Journal of Public Health* 67 (Mar 1977):264–67.

Although Flick referred to case-finding in 1904 in "Communities Without Health Departments," 1131, the early dispensary seems to have been too busy to do much of it (LF, "Clinical Work of the Year," *RHPI* 3 [1906]:25). In 1909, Hatfield did mention it ("HPI," 841).

51. LF, "Hospital and Dispensary," 826.

52. Mrs. Mc Laughlin to "Dear Nurse," 27 Sep 1907, SS.

53. Mrs. John Schick to LF, 11 Jun 1909.

Chapter 7. Achievement and Disappointment at the Institute

1. GG to LF, 21 May 1903, and LF, "An Historical Sketch of the Henry Phipps Institute," in University of Pennsylvania, *An Account of the Exercises on the Occasion of the Opening of the New Building of the Henry Phipps Institue* (1913), 24–25 (24 for the quotation). See also Ella M. E. Flick, *Beloved Crusader: Lawrence F. Flick, Physician, 1856–1938* (Philadelphia: Dorrance, 1944), 192–96, 202.

2. GG to LF, 6 Jan 1904, and HP to LF, 6 Feb 1904. For communications among Welch, Osler, and Phipps (but not their content), see GG to LF, 10 Jun 1903, and HP to LF, 3 Sep 1903. Flick believed that Osler had come between him and Phipps and had diverted Phipps's support to Johns Hopkins.

3. LF to GG, 7 Jan 1904.

4. LF to HP, 2 Feb 1904, and HP to LF, 4 Feb 1904. For sickness, poverty, and crime, see also LF, "Work of the Year," *RHPI* 2 (1905):22.

5. LF to HP, 5 Feb 1904. Contributing to Flick's concerns at this time was Dr. Edsall's resignation (D. L. Edsall to LF, 3 Feb 1904).

6. LF to HP, 8, 22 Feb 1904; GG to LF, 17, 24 Feb 1904; LF to GG, 25 Feb 1904; and E. M. E. Flick, *Beloved Crusader*, 217 (for the quotation).

7. Edoardo Maragliano, "Specific Therapy of Tuberculosis and Vaccination Against the Disease," *RHPI* 1 (1904):197.

8. Ibid., 195–255, for the full report.

9. "Genoa Expert Says by Vaccination He Averts Consumption," *North American*, 29 Mar 1904; E. M. E. Flick, *Beloved Crusader*, 217–18; and Joseph McFarland, "The Beginning of Bacteriology in Philadelphia," *Bulletin of the Institute of the History of Medicine* 5 (Feb 1937):149. McFarland was recalling the atmosphere of the time, not the specific lecture.

10. LF to HP, 30 Mar 1904; HP to LF, 31 Mar 1904; and M. P. Ravenel to

LF, 12 Jun 1904. "Agglutination" refers to a clumping of antigen (derived from tubercle bacilli in this case) with specific antibody from serum.

11. LF to M. P. Ravenel, 13, 20, 23 Jun 1904; LF to HP, 23 Jun, 30 Aug, 7 Sep, 6 Oct 1904; GG to LF, 7 Jul, 10, 17 Sep 1904; M. P. Ravenel to LF, 17 Jun, 21, 31 Jul, 11 Aug 1904; LF to GG, 6 Jul, 6, 12 Sep 1904; Leonard Pearson to LF, 21 Jul 1904; HP to LF, 26 Oct 1904; and LF, "Work of the Year," 3–4. The building served also as a milk station and an extension of the pathological museum.

12. LF to GG, 6 Sep 1904; Andrew Innis to LF, 1 Sep 1904; and LF to HP, 22 Sep 1904.

13. LF to GG, 28 Sep 1904, and HP to LF, 6, 26 Oct 1904 (26 for the quotation).

14. Joseph Walsh, William B. Stanton, and H. R. M. Landis, "Clinical Reports on the Use of Maragliano Serum," *RHPI* 2 (1905):382–403; H. R. M. Landis, "Untoward Effects Following the Use of Maragliano's Serum," *TSICT*, vol. 1, part 2 (1908):816–19; and LF to Walter Reynolds, 23 Feb 1906.

15. LF, "Work of the First Year," *RHPI* 1 (1904):6–7; LF to HP, 7 Dec 1903; and HP to LF, 11 Dec 1903.

16. LF, "Work of the Year," 4, 48–49, and LF, "Clinical Work of the Year," *RHPI* 3 (1906):5.

17. LF, "Work of the Year," 47, and LF, "Clinical Work of the Year," 25. In early 1905, giving of milk was stopped when there was suspicion of its being sold but not when it was used by family members (LF, "Work of the Year," 42).

18. LF, "Clinical Work of the Year," 53–54 (54 for the quotation).

19. Ibid., 22.

20. LF, "Clinical and Sociological Report of the Year," *RHPI* 4 (1907):41, 44–45, and LF, "Clinical and Sociological Report," *RHPI* 5 (1908):38, 42 (42 for the quotation). The percentages refer to new patients. I cannot explain the drop in the percentage working; it stayed low through early 1910. Forms show no change in the work question. There was no coincident change in the proportions of hospital and dispensary patients or in the results of treatment. The drop preceded the financial panic of late 1907. That so many patients stopped work at about the same time because of milk seems unlikely. They might have failed to report work, or the physicians and pupil nurses might not have recorded work in order to help their patients.

21. LF, "Clinical and Sociological Report," 84, and Anonymous postcard to H. C. Wood, 22 Aug 1905, SS.

22. Milk List Phipps Institute Mar 1907, JW, vol 2; Joseph Walsh to J. Cohen, 23 Jan 1908, SS; E. H. Goodman to LF, 16 Apr 1908; and LF to E. H. Goodman, 18 Apr 1908. The numbers of patients receiving milk have been compiled from tables on "Aid Given," in the *RsHPI*.

23. LF, "Clinical and Sociological Report," 59, 83–85, and LF, "Present Status of the Tuberculosis Campaign and the Essentials for Thorough and Prompt Success," *New York Medical Journal* 91 (5 Feb 1910):262.

24. For views of the poor, see Josephine S. Lowell, *Public Relief and Private Charity* (New York: G. P Putnam's Sons, 1884; reprint, Arno Press, 1971); Michael B. Katz, *In the Shadow of the Poorhouse: A Social History of Welfare in America*

(New York: Basic Books, 1986), 66–80; and Andrew Carnegie, *The Gospel of Wealth and Other Timely Essays* (Garden City, N.Y.: Doubleday, Doran, 1933), 14–16, 19–21. According to Theodore H. Ingalls in "Three Men in Tandem," *Harvard Medical Alumni Bulletin* 37 (Fall 1962):19, Carnegie criticized Phipps's "'coddling' the consumptive poor." Phipps, said Carnegie, "'keeps spilling largesse, not bettering but spoiling humanity.'"

25. The number of new patients who received milk are tabulated in *RsHPI*, 1905–1910; the number of quarts distributed, 1907–1910. For the Institute's first year, Flick cited a cost for dispensary care of 85 cents per patient per week (about 12 cents a day) ("The Hospital and the Dispensary in the Warfare Against Tuberculosis," *American Medicine* 9 [20 May 1905]:826). Later costs (*RHPI* 3 [1906]:52 and 4 [1907]:103–4) were 8 and 9 cents per day respectively; more items were included in the latter figure. Inspections are tabulated in *RsHPI*. For Flick's 1904 recommendation, see LF, "Municipalities in the Crusade Against Tuberculosis," *Medicine* 10 (May 1904):332. The numbers of "old" patients in the dispensary, calculated from tables, *RsHPI*, show no significant change.

26. LF, "Clinical and Sociological Report of the Year," 107. For similar views on the importance of hospitalization, see Arthur Newsholme, "The Causes of the Past Decline in Tuberculosis and the Light Thrown by History on Preventive Measures for the Immediate Future," *TSICT*, special vol. (1908):80–109, and Livingston Farrand, "A Comprehensive Program for the Prevention of Tuberculosis," *TSICT*, vol. 3 (1908):236–44.

27. LF to GG, 12 Sep 1904; GG to LF, 10 Feb 1906; and LF to HP, 19 Jan 1914.

28. Flick reiterated this function of a dispensary in LF to Alfred Stengel, 31 May 1909. At about this time, the waiting list at the Institute had been exhausted and there were vacancies in all wards (Lillian G. Foley to Joseph Walsh, 3 Jun 1909, JW, vol. 2). Flick's earlier effort to reduce the patients' stay in the hospital to six months or less "so that their places can be filled with some one else" may have contributed (LF to Joseph Walsh, 21 Aug 1908, JW, vol. 2). It would not have contributed, however, to a similar situation that seemed to have been developing at the Rush Hospital at the same time (LF, *The Tuberculosis Situation in Pennsylvania in the Year 1909* (Philadelphia: Peter Reilly, [circa 1911], 13). The new state dispensaries and sanatorium, which opened in 1907, were more likely causes (see pp. 164, 167).

29. Joseph Walsh, "Memoir of Lawrence F. Flick, M.D.," *TSCP*, 4th ser., vol. 7 (Apr 1939):115.

30. LF to GG, 21 Nov 1904, and LF to HP, 27 Jan, 10 Feb 1905.

31. LF to HP, 21 Oct 1903, and Charles M. Lea to LF, 2 Nov 1903. See also Charles M. Lea to LF, 30 Oct 1903. The first annual report printed the lectures.

32. LF to HP, 6 Jul, 1 Aug 1904; LF to GG, 29 Jul (for first quotation), 13 Aug 1904; GG to LF, 11 Aug 1904; HP to LF, 13 Aug 1904; and Frank A. Craig, *Early Days at Phipps* (n.p.: Henry Phipps Institute for the Study and Prevention of Tuberculosis, University of Pennsylvania, 1952), 23.

33. E. M. E. Flick, *Beloved Crusader*, 205, 315–16 (316 for the quotation); "Henry Phipps Institute," *New York Times*, 10 Jan 1903; and D. J. McCarthy to LF, 13 Aug 1903.

34. Richard H. Shryock, *National Tuberculosis Association, 1904–1954: A Study of the Voluntary Health Movement in the United States* (New York: National Tuberculosis Association, 1957; reprint, Arno Press, 1977), 103–6. Flick's letters are rich with details of planning the Congress.

35. *TSICT* (1908). Architectural plans for the new building won a silver medal at the Congress. Exhibits based on the old dispensary and hospital won gold medals. The other prizes consisted of silver medals for "a unit package of preventive supplies," for a contribution to the pathological exhibition, and for the training school. Certificates of the prizes were reproduced in *RHPI* 5 (1908).

36. LF to GG, 30 Jan 1908. For the nurses' building, see LF to GG, 23, 26 Mar 1904; LF to HP, 27 Apr, 2 May 1904; and LF," Work of the Year," 3.

37. LF to GG, 5 Feb 1908, and LF to HP, 7 Feb 1908. Joseph Walsh, then assistant medical director, held four committee positions, Charles J. Hatfield four, Daniel J. McCarthy three, and H. R. M. Landis and Frank A. Craig one each (*TSICT*, vol. 5 (1908):2, 6, 7, 16, 17, and 19). Flick later acknowledged the distracting effects of this committee work, but only on the men's ability to present the Institute to its best advantage at the Congress (LF, "Historical Sketch," 27).

38. LF to Joseph McFarland, 1 Feb 1909, and Joseph Walsh to Charles J. Hatfield, 2 Jul 1909, JW, vol. 2. Letters to Flick document twelve of these resignations; changes in listings of the staff show others.

39. LF to GG, 17 Aug 1909, and LF to HP, 1 Nov 1909. See also LF to GG, 23 Jul, 13 Aug 1909; LF to John S. Phipps, 30 Jul 1909; and "Short Life Story of Dr. Lawrence F. Flick and Brief Account of His Work in Tuberculosis," *The Strittmatter Award, 1933, to Dr. Lawrence F. Flick* (n.p.: Philadelphia Medical Society), 38–50.

40. Ingalls, "Three Men in Tandem," 19; Craig, *Early Days*, 31–32; and Minutes of the Trustees, University of Pennsylvania, vol. 15, 4 Jan 1910, 34–35, UPA. Ingalls cited a third advisor, bacteriologist Theobald Smith, but Craig mentioned only Osler and Welch. Craig had access to "the early correspondence on file in the Institute, which was copied from the originals in the archives of the University."

41. Charles C. Harrison to HP, 16 Dec 1909, Provost Records, UPA 6.2H, UPA, and Charles J. Hatfield to LF, 27 Dec 1909, with a copy of the resolution. See also E. M. E. Flick, *Beloved Crusader*, 224, and "Short Life Story," 45–46.

42. Charles C. Harrison to GG, 7 Jan 1910, Provost Records, and E. M. E. Flick, *Beloved Crusader*, 10. Flick denied meeting with University personnel after mid-December (E. M. E. Flick, *Beloved Crusader*, 224–25). Clues to the change in leadership include "a conflict of strong personalities" (Esmond R. Long, "Memoir of Charles James Hatfield," *TSCP* 4th ser., vol. 20 [Jun 1952]:38), and "unfriendliness" to Flick of "the younger generation" at the University (E. M. E. Flick, *Beloved Crusader*, 226). Flick remained on good terms with Phipps. From 1914 to 1917 (and possibly longer), Phipps helped Flick financially with annual gifts of money (LF to Henry Phipps, 19 Jan 1914, 11 Jan 1917).

43. For University goals and responsibilities, see Report of the Committee Appointed by the Provost to Consider Plans for the Future Operation of the Phipps Institute, 2, 4, Archives General, Phipps Institute (hereafter AGPI), UPA; Minutes of the Trustees, vol. 15, 15 Mar 1910, 50–51, UPA; and Minutes of the Board of Directors of the Phipps Institute, 6 Jul 1911, AGPI.

44. Craig, *Early Days*, 25, 27–28, 31; *RHPI* 6 (1910):opposite 1; Paul A. Lewis to Cha[rle]s C. Harrison, 28 Apr 1910, AGPI; H. R. M. Landis to [Charles C.] Harrison, 28 Apr 1910, AGPI; and Alexander M. Wilson to Charles C. Harrison, 29 Apr 1910, AGPI.

45. "The New Phipps Institute," *FAM* 2 (Aug 1911):4–6.

46. Expenditures for the year ending Jan 1910, for Sep through Nov 1910, for Dec 1910 through Feb 1911, for the year ending 31 Aug 1911, and for Feb 1914, all in AGPI; Report of the Board of Directors of the Phipps Institute, 29 Sep 1910, AGPI; Minutes, Board of Directors, PI, 6 Jul 1911; "New Phipps Institute," 6; Minutes of Meeting of the University Committee on the Henry Phipps Institute, 11 Mar 1915, AGPI; University of Pennsylvania, the Henry Phipps Institute, an announcement, LFPM, vol. 137, no. 98; Charles J. Hatfield, "The Henry Phipps Institute," no. 98; Charles J. Hatfield, "The Henry Phipps Institute," *Pennsylvania's Health* [n.s.] 1 (May 1940):33–34; LF to D. J. McCarthy, 1 Jul 1916; and LF, *The Pennsylvania Society for the Prevention of Tuberculosis*, (1935), 21.

47. Report, Board of Directors, PI, 29 Sep 1910, 5 (for the first quotation); Minutes, Board of Directors, PI, 6 Jul 1911 (for the second quotation); and Minutes, Board of Directors, PI, 13 Dec 1911.

48. Report, Board of Directors, PI, 29 Sep 1910; Minutes, Board of Directors, PI, 6 Jul 1911; Minutes of the Board of Managers, Hospital of the University of Pennsylvania, 13, 20 Nov, 4 Dec 1913, 9, 16 Apr 1914, 27 May, 3 Jun 1915, UPA; and the following from the Archives of the Hospital of the University of Pennsylvania, School of Nursing: Rose M. Berchtold to M. S. Snyder, 25, 28 May 1915, the former with a petition from the Class of 1917; Marion E. Smith to J. William White, 3 Jun 1915; and newspaper clippings. See also Mary V. Stephenson, *The First Fifty Years of the Training School for Nurses of the Hospital of the University of Pennsylvania* (Philadelphia: J. B. Lippincott, 1940), 117–20. The Phipps training school probably closed in 1915 (Craig, *Early Days*, 22).

49. For examples of Lewis's work, see Paul A. Lewis, "Observations Bearing on the Possibility of Developing an Experimental Chemotherapy of Tuberculosis," *Bulletin of the Johns Hopkins Hospital* 28 (Mar 1917):120–25, and idem, "Chemotherapy in Tuberculosis," *American Journal of the Medical Sciences* 153 (May 1917): 625–40.

50. Charles C. Harrison to Henry Phipps, 16 Dec 1909; "$500,000 Is Phipps' Gift to U. of P. for Tuberculosis Fight," *North American*, 21 Dec 1909; "Dr. Flick Denies Friction Rumors," *Philadelphia Record*, 22 Dec 1909; LF to A. A. Watkins, 23 Dec 1909; LF to GG, 23 Dec 1909, 3, 6 Jan 1910; and LF, "Historical Sketch."

Chapter 8. Expansion at White Haven

1. Elsie Listebarger to LF, 4 Dec 1905. The second quotation is a composite of letters.

2. John J. Buckley to LF, 28 Jun 1902; Henry C. Lea to LF, 15 Feb 1904; F. J. Torrance to LF, 8 Jun 1903; James Elverson, Jr., to LF, 21 May 1902.

Torrance's Board of Public Charities would also have had to approve any state appropriation for the sanatorium.

3. The following income figures, rounded to the nearest dollar, are compiled and calculated from *ARFH* 10 (1908):3.

Annual Receipts, White Haven Sanatorium

Year through February	*Charitable contributions*		*Patients' board*		*State appropriation*		*Total net receipts*
	Amount	*%*	*Amount*	*%*	*Amount*	*%*	
1903	$29,722	42	$1,035	1	$39,335	56	$70,092
1904	19,766	29	0	0	49,065	71	68,831
1905	20,078	23	0	0	66,600	77	86,678

For the quotation and examples of political requests, see Theo. B. Stulb to LF, 2 Apr 1903; W. H. Berkelbach to LF, 5 Jun 1902; John E. Fox to LF, 12, 18 Aug 1902; Geo. H. Stevens to LF, 10 Jan 1903; Frederick Phillips to LF, 19 Mar 1903; P. J. Enright to LF, 27 May 1903; Robert S. Conklin to LF, 26 Apr 1904; George R. Patterson to LF, 16 Jul 1904; Geo. W. Dunn to LF, 16 Jul 1904; and Chas. E. Quail to LF, 23 Jul 1904.

4. *ARFH* 6 (1904):4–5; Henry F. Walton to LF, 16 Jul 1904; and LF to Henry F. Walton, 20 Jul 1904.

5. *ARFH* 5 (1903):4.

6. Annual reports listed the examining physicians: 37 in Feb 1902, 65 in Feb 1903, and 111 in Feb 1905. Physicians applied to Flick during the early years and to Joseph Walsh later.

7. *ARFH* 5 (1903):5, and 6 (1904):7. In June 1903, the state prohibited the sanatorium from taking any but bona fide Pennsylvania residents (LF to Henry C. Lea, 17 Feb 1904).

8. *ARFH* 5 (1903):4–5.

9. For patients' work in hospitals, see Charles E. Rosenberg, *The Care of Strangers: The Rise of America's Hospital System* (New York: Basic Books, 1987), 35–36. For advantages of work to patients, see M[arcus] S. Patterson, "Graduated Labor in Pulmonary Tuberculosis," *TSICT*, vol. 1, pt. 2 (1908):886–900; Linda Bryder, *Below the Magic Mountain: A Social History of Tuberculosis in Twentieth-Century Britain* (Oxford: Clarendon Press, 1988), 54–67; Hermann M. Biggs, "The Utilization of Work and Exercise in the Treatment of Pulmonary Tuberculosis at the Otisville Sanatorium," *JOL* 8 (Aug 1911):200–202; and "The Question of Employment," *JOL* 9 (Dec 1912):308–9. For the prevalence of work in U.S. sanatoriums, see "Employment of Tuberculous Patient," *JOL* 9 (Dec 1912):295–301.

10. ES to LF, 16 Feb 1903. Appropriation figures come from *ARFH* 10 (1908):18–19. Some earlier annual reports give somewhat different figures. The state and the Free Hospital had different fiscal years, making it difficult to cross-check sources. See n. 3 for contributions.

11. *ARFH* 6 (1904):3, 7 (1905):1–2, 8 (1906):3, and illustrations in all. See also H. R. M. Landis, "The White Haven Sanatorium," *JOL* 4 (May 1907):123–25. Other shacks were "double," i.e., two sleeping rooms connected by a dressing room. These accommodated eight men. The canvas-draped windows were later replaced by sliding glass.

12. For the staff, see *ARFH* 6 (1904):3, 44; *ARFH* 7 (1905):48; ES to LF, 11 Mar 1903; LF to Charles P. Noble, 23 Jun 1904; and Jas. H. Heller to LF, 6 Feb 1906. For work as desirable, see *ARFH* 8 (1906):6, and Landis, "WHS," 125.

13. ES to LF, 3 Jan [1903], 19 May 1903; J. B. Stockdale to LF, 26 Aug 1903; and *ARFH* 7 (1905):7, 48. A matron with experience earned a somewhat higher salary, e.g., twenty-five dollars.

14. Joseph Walsh listed the White Haven residents in his bound volumes of the *ARFH*, CPP, and noted the stage of their tuberculosis, their later careers, and the dates and causes of their deaths. Other sources include their letters to Flick and to Walsh (JW, vol. 1); *American Medical Directory*, 1909; W. J. Maxwell, comp., *General Alumni Catalogue of the University of Pennsylvania* (n.p., 1922); idem, comp., *General Alumni Catalogue of Jefferson Medical College* (n.p., 1917); and the Archives of the Medical College of Pennsylvania. After 1909 or 1910, most residents had less severe disease, and some were nontuberculous.

15. Joseph Walsh to A. C. Wentz, 12 Nov 1910, JW, vol. 1; G. Justice Ewing to LF, 23, 29 Mar 1903; and ES to LF, 23 Mar 1903.

16. ES to LF, 23 Mar 1903. Stockdale's observations were well-founded, but probably few U.S. sanatoriums had his desired staffing. By 1912, White Haven compared quite well with other sanatoriums, with 35 patients per physician ("Employment of Tuberculous Patient," 298–301).

17. For salaries, see LF to J. W. Walters, 18 Jan 1905; LF to Max H. Lubke, 16 Feb 1905; LF to Fergus J. O'Connor, 4 Nov 1908; Helen C. McDevitt to Joseph Walsh, 28 Mar 1908, JW, vol. 1; Medical Administration Committee to the Board of Managers of the Free Hospital for Poor Consumptives, 25 Nov 1908, 23 Apr 1909, JW, vol. 1; and Joseph Walsh to E. E. Holland, 1 Apr 1909, JW, vol. 1. Salaries differed a bit; some physicians, including a few without tuberculosis, earned more.

18. Mary E. Topham to LF, 30 Sep 1904; John J. Craig to Joseph Walsh, 18 Nov 1906, JW, vol. 1; and Walsh's annotated list of residents.

19. The seven physicians who served as visiting physicians at White Haven while also on the staff at Phipps were Joseph Walsh, Charles J. Hatfield, Daniel J. McCarthy, William B. Stanton, H. R. M. Landis, Frank A. Craig, and Mazÿck P. Ravenel. Others joined later.

20. Frank A. Craig, *The Story of the White Haven Sanatorium* (n.p., n.d.), 60. For the travel time, see the ad for Sunnyrest Sanatorium, *JOL* 2 (Jun 1905):113.

21. For the experience gained in treating early patients, see Frank A. Craig, *Early Days at Phipps* (Henry Phipps Institute for the Study and Prevention of Tuberculosis, University of Pennsylvania, 1952), 55.

22. ES to LF, 16 Sep 1903.

23. Henry M. Neale, "Sanatorium Treatment of Pulmonary Tuberculosis," *PMJ* 11 (Jan 1908):283.

24. D. J. McCarthy, "Sanatorium Discipline and Control of the Patient," in *Short Talks upon Work for Consumptives Delivered by the Medical Staff of the White Haven Sanatorium of the Free Hospital for Poor Consumptives* (1904), 10–11, in LF's collected reprints, CPP.

25. Norman Dain, *Concepts of Insanity in the United States, 1789–1865* (New Brunswick, N.J.: Rutgers University Press, 1964), 12–13; Gerald N. Grob, *Mental Institutions in America: Social Policy to 1875* (New York: The Free Press, 1973), 41–47, 88, 168–69; and Nancy Tomes, *A Generous Confidence: Thomas Story Kirkbride and the Art of Asylum-Keeping, 1840–1883* (Cambridge: Cambridge University Press, 1984).

26. White Haven Sanatorium of the Free Hospital for Poor Consumptives, Regulations, [1904], LFPM, vol. 40, no. 16 (for first and third quotations); George B. Kalb, "The Sanatorium Treatment of Tuberculosis," *PMJ* 9 (Jan 1906): 258–59; W. F. Wood to LF, 24 Jan 1908; and Henry M. Neale, "The Practical Treatment of Pulmonary Tuberculosis," *PMJ* 7 (Mar 1904):283.

27. "WHS, Regulations."

28. Ibid.; Kalb, "Sanatorium Treatment," 259; and *ARFH* 6 (1904):7.

29. ES to LF, 13 Jul, 3, 10, 15, 17, 22 Aug 1904, and, for his discouragement, 24 Mar, 12 Apr 1904. See also LF to ES, 23, 27 Aug 1904.

30. Edward Nocton, "Pennsylvania's Care for Consumptives," *The Era Magazine* 13 (Jan 1904):57–64 (57 for quotations), and Kalb, "Sanatorium Treatment," 259.

31. Lawrason Brown to LF, 30 May 1905, and Wm. H. Allen to LF, 16 Feb 1905. See also James Tyson to LF, 7 Nov 1903.

32. F. A. Craven to LF, 16 Mar 1903, and Mrs. Fred G. Day to LF, 1 May 1905.

33. The percentages are calculated from *ARFH* 11 (1909):8–11. For the duration of stay, see *ARFH* 22 (1920): back cover.

34. I have calculated these results from figures in *ARFH* 11 (1909):10–11. Of the 646 patients, 10 percent had not improved and less than 1 percent (3 patients) died. Costs per capita are calculated from figures in *ARFH* 11 (1909):6. For the bookkeeping change, see chap. 5, n. 42. For maintenance costs at other institutions, see *ARPB* 35 (1904):262–63, 277. Such comparisons must be made cautiously. Methods of calculating them were not standardized, and urban general hospitals naturally had higher costs than did a specialized rural sanatorium.

35. LF to LF (a form letter), 24 Sep 1904, LFCP; LF to Frank T. Gucker, 7 Nov 1904, LFCP; and *ARFH* 7 (1905):8, 10 (1908):3.

36. The proportions of patients with phthisis at St. Agnes' and St. Mary's are calculated from diagnostic reports of the medical wards in the respective annual reports. For Sr. Borromeo's encouragement of this move, see her letter to LF, 1 Mar 1903.

37. For the Jewish Hospital and the Lucien Moss Home, see Wm. B. Hackenburg to LF, 11 Dec 1895, 3 Feb 1900. I have calculated the proportions of patients with tuberculosis from the annual reports of the Jewish Hospital Association of Philadelphia.

38. Stage of disease was reported in *ARFH* 10 (1908):8–11. Patients in the

least-advanced group, "infiltration without softening," decreased from 40 percent to 29 percent between the years ending in Feb 1902 and Feb 1904. A changed classification in 1905 precludes further tracing.

39. W. J. Ashenfelter to LF, 8 Jul 1903; Robt. S. Maison to LF, 3 Jul 1902; ES to LF, 24 Mar 1904; and *ARFH* 5 (1903):4.

40. *ARFH* 7 (1905):10, and ES to LF, 25 May 1903.

41. ES to LF, 25 May 1903, 24 Mar, 13 Jul, 1904.

42. LF, "Communities without Health Departments in the Crusade against Tuberculosis," *NYPMJ* 79 (11 Jun 1904):1132 (for first and third quotations), and *ARFH* 7 (1905):10.

43. *ARFH* 5 (1903):4; ES to LF, 26 Jan, 16 Nov 1903, 11, 23 Aug 1904; H. R. M. Landis to LF, 22 Aug 1904; *ARFH* 6 (1904):6; and "A Friend" to LF, 15 Mar 1904. The gender of "Friend" is not known.

44. *ARFH* 7 (1905):11, also 6 (1904):8.

45. *ARFH* 7 (1905):10–11.

Chapter 9. Economy, Charity, and the State

1. National Association for the Study and Prevention of Tuberculosis, comp., *A Tuberculosis Directory* (New York: National Association for the Study and Prevention of Tuberculosis, 1916).

2. Elizabeth H. Thomas, *A History of the Pennsylvania State Forest School, 1903–1929* (Mont Alto, Pa.: Pennsylvania State Forest Academy/School Founders Society, 1985), 1–26 (7 for the uses of forests), and J. T. Rothrock, "Meeting an Emergency," *JOL* 3 (Dec 1906):464. Forestry became a division of the agriculture department in 1895, then a separate department in 1901. Rothrock was commissioner in both.

3. In her *History of the Forest School*, 18, Thomas's full phrase for Rothrock is "master of the use of the *fait accompli* and also at the art of the possible, a tool he used quite consciously." For the camp, see J. T. Rothrock, "Meeting an Emergency," 465–66 (465 for the quotations), and idem, "Outdoor Treatment of Tuberculosis at Mont Alto," *PMJ* 8 (Dec 1904):164–68; idem, *South Mountain Sanatorium Camp*, a pamphlet of the Pennsylvania Department of Forestry, [ca. 1904], LFPM, vol. 31, no. 13; and *Report of the Pennsylvania Department of Forestry* (1905–1906):80–96, 126–40. Financial support for Rothrock's camp came mainly from women, including Mrs. Eckley B. Coxe. Mont Alto is in Franklin County, roughly twelve miles southeast of Chambersburg.

4. *ARCH* 1 (1905–1906):4–6, 8–10; "Dr. Samuel G. Dixon to Be Health Commissioner," *Philadelphia Press*, 6 Jun, 1905; "Dr. S. G. Dixon, State Director of Health, Long Very Ill, Dies," *Philadelphia Press*, 27 Feb 1918; "Dr. Dixon Actually 'Died in Harness,'" *Public Ledger*, 27 Feb 1918; "'Thou Good and Faithful Servant,'" *North American*, 2 Mar 1918; Edward Martin, "Memoir of Charles B. Penrose, M.D.," *TRCP*, 3d ser., vol. 47 (1925):lxv–lxxiii; and Charles B. Penrose, Alumni Record File, UPA.

5. Newspaper sources, n. 4, and Samuel W. Pennypacker, *The Autobiography of a Pennsylvanian* (Philadelphia: John C. Winston, 1918), 380–81.

6. James M. Anders, "Memoir of Samuel Gibson Dixon, *TRCP*, 3d ser., vol. 40 (1918):xlix–lxvi; B. Franklin Royer, "Doctor Dixon's Work in Sanitary Science," *Proceedings of the Academy of Natural Sciences in Philadelphia* 70 (1918):127–38; *National Cyclopaedia of American Biography*, s.v. "Dixon, Samuel Gibson,"; "'86—Samuel G. Dixon, M.D.," *The Alumni Register, University of Pennsylvania* 20 (Apr 1918):609–12; Samuel G. Dixon, "A Discussion on Tuberculosis," *British Medical Journal* 2 (15 Sep 1906):609–11; Pennypacker, *Autobiography*, 284; and, for background, George Rosen, *Preventive Medicine in the United States, 1900–1975, Trends and Interpretations* (New York: Prodist, 1977).

7. *ARCH* 1 (1905–1906):17–18, 52 (52 for quotations).

8. *ARFH* 10 (1908):22 (for the quotation), and *ARCH* 2 (1907):6, 390. Flick wrote the initial version of the plank; it did not specify the agency that should develop the program.

9. *RPS* (1896):6, (1898):4, (1902):5, (1903):7–8, (1905):5, (1908):8; *ARFH* 10 (1908):5–7; and Howard S. Anders to LF, 10 Jan 1903.

10. J. T. Rothrock to LF, 12 Feb 1903, 18 Apr 1904; *ARCH* 2 (1907):17–19, 393, 404; and deeds of the purchase and sale filed in the Franklin County Court House. For Rothrock's private Mountain Side Sanatorium, see his "Outdoor Treatment," 165, and ads in *JOL* 2 (Jul 1905):147, 3 (Feb 1906):30. Rothrock's gain is unclear in amount, but cost of construction was low. Cabins at the forestry camp cost $40 each, and a forty-by-forty-foot assembly building with both a wide porch and windows on all sides cost $2,000 (J. T. Rothrock, "The History of the Big Chimney in the Assembly Building of Mount Hope," *Spunk* 12 [Feb 1921]:19).

11. Samuel G. Dixon to LF, 5 Mar 1908; Samuel G. Dixon, "The Government Control of Tuberculous Patients in Pennsylvania," *TSICT*, vol. 4, pt. 1 (1908):232–39; idem, "The Lesson of a State," *JOL* 5 (Feb 1908):1–5; *ARCH* 1 (1905–1906):33–34, 445; *ARCH* 2 (1907):17–21, 56–60, 99, 401–5; *ARCH* 4 (1909):230–32, 241, 268–96, 332–41, 407–11; B. Franklin Royer, "The Department of Health's Activity in Handling Tuberculosis in Pennsylvania," *PMJ* 16 (Feb 1913):383–89; and Thomas H. A. Stites, "The Tuberculosis Dispensary System of the Pennsylvania Department of Health: A Sketch of Its Organization and Methods," *PMJ* 12 (Jun 1909):698–702. For another politically masterful strategy, see Daniel M. Fox, "Social Policy and City Politics: Tuberculosis Reporting in New York, 1889–1900," *BHM* 49 (Summer 1975):169–95.

12. "An Act," 15 Dec 1904, LFCP; Joseph Walsh to a list of physicians, Spring 1905, JW, vol. 1; and *ARFH* 9 (1907):6.

13. *ARFH* 7 (1905):8. The charge was five dollars a week when a patient worked for one to four hours, and three dollars when a patient worked for four to eight hours.

14. *ARFH* 8 (1906):5–6, 9 (1907):7; LF to Cyrus E. Woods, 5 Mar 1907; and six monthly lists of patients discharged as unsuitable between Jul 1906 and 1 Mar 1907, JW, vol. 1. Monthly numbers ranged from 1 to 12 and averaged 7.5. About half of these patients were discharged within thirty days, a fourth in from thirty-one to sixty days, and a fourth after sixty days.

15. *ARFH* 7 (1905):8–9 (9 for all but the third quotation) and *ARFH* 8 (1906):5.

16. *ARFH* 8 (1906):6. Walsh wrote this annual report.

17. Rubin Krasnopolsky to LF, 4 Jun 1905; Mrs. Thos. J. Clark to LF, 30 Apr 1906; and Mrs. F. Dotts, Jr., to LF, 30 Sep 1906.

18. The sources of income, summarized below and rounded to the nearest dollar, are derived from *ARFH* 10 (1908):3 through 16 (1914). I have excluded end-of-year balances, loans, and repayments.

Annual Receipts, White Haven Sanatorium

Year through February	Charitable contributions		Patients' board		State appropriation		Total net receipts
	Amount	%	Amount	%	Amount	%	
1905	$20,078	23	0	0	$66,600	77	$86,678
1906	19,652	28	$16,224	23	34,461	49	70,338
1907	17,296	24	21,474	29	34,289	47	73,059
1908	14,537	19	32,677	42	30,787	39	78,001
1909	17,424	19	37,885	41	37,963	41	93,272
1910	50,103*	46	49,059	45	8,750	8	107,912
1911	25,673	30	61,057	70	0	0	86,730
1912	24,672	25	74,779	75	0	0	99,451
1913	48,660*	41	69,829	59	0	0	118,489
1914	29,378*	34	58,263	66	0	0	87,641

*Includes special funds for building and cottages.

Debt has been calculated from loans made and paid, summarized in *ARFH* 10 (1908):3. For the expansion, see *ARFH* 8 (1906):5–7, and 9 (1907):6–8.

19. *ARFH* 10 (1908):11–13.

20. *ARFH* 9 (1907):8–9, 10 (1908):22; A. Coleman Sheetz to LF, 24 Mar 1907; and LF to Edwin S. Stewart [*sic*], 1 May 1907.

21. C. D. Potter to LF, 14 May 1907; LF to Samuel G. Dixon, 21, 23 May 1907; Samuel G. Dixon to LF, 20, 22 May 1907 (20 for the quotation); and, for Potter, *Smull's Legislative Hand Book and Manual of Pennsylvania* (1907):843.

22. H. Z. O'Brien to LF, 29 May 1907; Minutes, Annual Meeting of the White Haven Staff, 23 May 1907, JW, vol. 1; and *ARFH* 10 (1908):23–24. In a conciliatory letter to the patients (Samuel G. Dixon to Joseph Highley, 31 May 1907, LFCP), Dixon explained that Mont Alto was full but that the state would try to increase its accommodations with tents to help them.

23. LF to H. Z. O'Brien, 1 Jun 1907; LF to Louis J. C. Bailey, 6 Jun 1907; "Open to Poor Consumptives," *Philadelphia Record*, 29 Aug 1907; *ARFH* 10 (1908):23–24; and Joseph Walsh to Edgar M. Green, 22 Jun 1908, JW, vol. 1.

24. H. Z. O'Brien to LF, 29 May, 23 Jul 1907, and Minutes, Annual Meeting of the White Haven Staff, 23 May 1907.

25. H. Z. O'Brien to LF, 19, 27 Jun 1907.

26. LF to Joseph Walsh, 25 Jul 1907, JW, vol. 1; W. F. Wood to Joseph Walsh, 24 Aug 1907, JW, vol. 1; Walter F. Wood to LF, 24 Aug 1907; LF to Walter F. Wood, 26 Aug 1907; and lists of matrons, orderlies, and pupil nurses, *ARFH*, 1904–1909.

27. LF to Walter F. Wood, 17 Oct 1907; Charles H. Miner to LF, 27 Nov 1907; LF to Chas. H. Miner, 29 Nov 1907; W. B. Stanton to "Dear Doctor," 17 Feb 1908, JW, vol. 1; *ARFH* 12 (1910):6 (for the quotations); Anna L. Morris, "White Haven Sanatorium Training School for Nurses," *ARFH* 15 (1913):9–11; and lists of graduate nurses, *ARsFH*. For problems in nursing care, including medication errors, tardy record-keeping, and overtime work, see Charles J. Hatfield to Joseph Walsh, 11 Nov 1907, JW, vol. 1.

28. Alex. Armstrong to LF, 27 Feb 1909, and fiscal reports in *ARFH*, 1904–1909. Expenditures on nursing exclude board and lodging.

29. LF to A. Guttmacher, 13 Jun 1908, and LF, "Work for Patients as an Economic Factor," *TNA* 5 (1909):182.

30. William B. Stanton, "Cooperation between the State and Private Corporations in the Crusade against Tuberculosis As Exemplified at the White Haven Sanatorium," *TSICT*, vol. 4, pt. 1 (1908):296; LF, "Work," 181–85; and Frederick L. Hills, "Work for Patients as an Immediate and Ultimate Therapeutic Factor," *TNA* 5 (1909):186–94. For complaints, see W. G. J. Baur and L. T. [?sp.] Gowell to LF, Jun 1908; Wm. Powick to LF, 24 Aug 1908; Alexander Armstrong to Joseph Walsh, 30 Dec 1908, JW, vol. 1; Miss Neal to LF, Jan 1909; and D. Saffer to LF, 30 Jul 1909. For the physicians' failure to place their patients on work after four weeks, see LF to J. Clinton Foltz (and others), 3 Mar 1909. For a survey of work in sanatoriums, see "Employment of Tuberculous Patient," *JOL* 9 (Dec 1912):295–301, with editorial comment, "The Question of Employment," 308–9. For stricter rest treatment, see Lawrason Brown, *Rules for Recovery from Pulmonary Tuberculosis: A Layman's Handbook of Treatment*, 2nd ed. (Philadelphia: Lea and Febiger, 1916), 20–32, 87–96; Joseph H. Pratt, "The Importance of Prolonged Bed Rest in the Treatment of Pulmonary Tuberculosis," *ART* 1 (Jan 1918):637–53; and Hugh M. Kinghorn, "Comparative Results Obtained in the Treatment of Pulmonary Tuberculosis," *TACA* 34 (1918):130–42. For abuse of work, see Samuel Wolman, "A Criticism of Tuberculosis Sanatoria," *Survey* 39 (17 Nov 1917):165–67.

31. "No Aid to Fight White Plague," *Philadelphia Record*, 23 Jan 1909; "White Haven Will Abolish Free Beds," a clipping attributed to the *Philadelphia Inquirer* 23 Jan 1909, LFSB, vol. 3; and *ARFH* 11 (1909):4.

32. *ARFH* 11 (1909):4–5 (5 for the quotation). See also LF to Jacqueline Harrison Smith, 19 Feb 1910; LF to Louis Gerstley, 1 Dec 1910; and *ARFH* 12 (1910):5–6.

33. *ARFH* 11 (1909):3.

34. LF to "My dear Doctor," n.d., JW, vol. 1; Minutes, Medical Administration Committee, 26 May 1909, JW, vol. 1 (for the last quotation); and Joseph Walsh to "Dear Doctor," 31 May 1909, JW, vol. 1. In LF to Wm. H. Wells, 23 Jun 1910, Flick noted two more reasons for the fee: to allow the examiner to make a full examination and a proper judgment, and "to discountenance free work for people who can afford to pay."

35. *ARFH* 12 (1910):1, 5 (1 for the first quotations); Alexander Armstrong to Joseph Walsh, 9 Apr 1910, JW, vol. 1 (for the Baker example); and LF to GG, 12 Jan 1910 (for the last quotation). Between Feb 1909 and Feb 1914, the number of patients treated per year dropped from 890 to 548, and expenditures for patient

maintenance rose from $7.88 per patient per week to $11.11 (calculated from *ARFH* 17 [1915]:back cover).

36. For sources of income, see note 18. Many letters seeking examiners in Jan and Feb 1910 are scattered through JW, vol. 1. They were targeted especially but not exclusively at New Jersey. Out-of-state physicians first appeared on the list of examiners in *ARFH* 12 (1910).

37. Sophia G. [Mrs. Eckley B.] Coxe to LF, 9 Aug 1909, and *ARFH* 13 (1911):1.

38. Death rates, calculated from figures in *ARsFH*, 1909–1916, are based on numbers of discharged patients who had remained more than one week. Department No. 3 had less than 13 percent of White Haven's patients during this period. Of all patients in the sanatorium, the proportion with cavities, the most-advanced category, peaked at 65 percent, as reported in Feb 1910. It then began to diminish, and was down to 34 percent by Feb 1916. Further analysis is complicated by changes in nomenclature. Between Feb 1910 and Feb 1916, however, the term "infiltration without softening" remained unchanged. The proportion of these patients (with the least-advanced disease) reached a low of 8 percent in Feb 1911, remained at 11 percent for the next two years, and then rose to 26 percent by Feb 1916. Ways to obtain incipient cases was a topic of a 1912 staff meeting (LF to Frank A. Craig, 29 Feb 1912).

39. *ARFH* 14 (1912):1, and Frank A. Craig, *The Story of the White Haven Sanatorium* (n.p., n.d.), 40. Craig was a visiting physician at White Haven from 1905 to 1946, and medical director from 1935 to 1946. Between Feb 1912 and Feb 1916, the *ARFH* classified patients within each department by stage of disease. The number of patients in Dept. No. 1 dropped from 268 to 5 (from 37 percent of all patients treated in the sanatorium to 1 percent).

40. *ARCH* 4 (1909):19, 30–31 (19 for the quotation) and 5 (1910):22–27, 50–51, 365, 402. On 1 Jan 1916, the sanatoriums counted 1,815 patients: 986 at Mont Alto, 355 at Cresson, and 474 at Hamburg (*ARCH* 11 [1916]:885, 914, 943).

41. LF to Samuel G. Dixon, 23 May 1910, and LF, *The Tuberculosis Situation in Pennsylvania in the Year 1909* (Philadelphia: Peter Reilly, n.d.), 11. This speech was delivered on 5 Oct 1910 in response to a paper by J. Byron Deacon, executive secretary of the Pennsylvania Society. The *PMJ* had deleted the more strident sections from Flick's comments, so he withdrew his response and published it privately.

42. LF, *Tb Situation*, 8–9 (for the quotations), 13.

43. Samuel G. Dixon to LF, 8 Mar 1907, and *ARCH* 2 (1905–1906):20, 403–5; 3 (1908):426; 4 (1909):29, 305–6; 5 (1910):365.

44. Minutes, York County Medical Society, 2 Sep 1909, LFPM, vol. 111, no. 138. Physicians suspected adenoids (enlarged tonsillar tissue in the back of the throat) of harboring tubercle bacilli and possibly being the portal of entry for the infection; they therefore recommended removal.

45. "Pennsylvania May Wipe Out Tuberculosis by 1918," *Public Ledger*, 23 Feb 1913, sec. 6 (for first quotations); Albert P. Francine, "The Development of the Tuberculosis Campaign in Pennsylvania, with a Discussion of Its Principles," *PMJ*

18 (Nov 1914):141–47 (142 for the quotation); Royer, "Department of Health's Activity," 382–85; and "Producers and Consumers," *PHB*, no. 18 (Dec 1910):5. For the Flick argument, see also LF, "Present Status of the Tuberculosis Campaign and the Essentials for Thorough and Prompt Success," *New York Medical Journal* 91 (5 Feb 1910):261–64; idem, "Advantages of Local Care and Treatment of Tuberculosis," *Interstate Medical Journal* 17 (Dec 1910):938–42; LF to G. A. Warfield, 9 Feb 1911; and Flick's testimony, "Proceedings of the Joint Committee of the Senate and House of Representatives," 12 Nov 1912, *Pennsylvania Legislative Journal*, Appendix (1913):5697. This debate was part of one that focused on responsibility for hospital care and the proper relationships among hospitals, government, charity, and private enterprise. See four papers, including one by Flick, presented before the Pennsylvania Medical Society and published in *PMJ* 13 (Jan 1910):250–78. For a later analysis, see Rosemary Stevens, "Sweet Charity: State Aid to Hospitals in Pennsylvania, 1870–1910," *BHM* 58 (Fall, Winter 1984):287–314, 474–95.

46. William G. Turnbull, "The State Sanatoria for Tuberculosis," *PMJ* 17 (Sep 1914):943–44 (944 for the quotation), and idem, "Pennsylvania State Sanatorium for Tuberculosis, No. 2, Cresson," *ARCH* 8 (1913):681. The state sanatoriums used milk as dietary supplements between meals. The dispensaries distributed milk and eggs, then gradually changed to cottonseed and olive oil. For Dixon's fluid, see, for example, *ARCH* 5 (1910):374–75, 6 (1911):943–56, 8 (1913):664–70. Work at the state sanatoriums included care of the lawns and walks, whitewashing, painting, grading, sodding, clearing land, landscape gardening, and making sputum cups (*ARCH* 5 [1910]:369).

47. For nativity, see *ARFH* 11 (1909):22, and *ARCH* 4 (1909):305. From *ARCH* 4 (1909):310, 312, 314, I calculate that 2.3 percent of the patients discharged from Mont Alto were black. According to the 1910 U.S. Census, White Haven Borough, 2.8 percent of the patients at White Haven Sanatorium were black. For occupations, see *ARFH* 11 (1909):21–22, and *ARCH* 4 (1909):316, 320–21, 326–27. For age, see *ARCH* 4 (1909):316, 321, 327, and the 1910 U.S. Census. For the stage of disease (Mont Alto and Cresson combined), see *ARCH* 8 (1913):93.

48. The land for the sanatorium at Cresson was a gift, and the land at Mont Alto was described as "worthless for anything but timber." The Mont Alto Iron Company had cut all usable timber three times for charcoal. A study in 1930 noted that the soil was "highly silicious, lacks fertility, and . . . offers about as poor an outlook for a forest as could be imagined" (John T. Auten, *A Soil Study of the Mont Alto State Forest*, Research Bulletin 4 [Harrisburg: Commonwealth of Pennsylvania, Department of Forests and Waters, 1930], 7–8). The state was acquiring this kind of land for from $1.68 to $3.75 per acre at the turn of the century (Thomas, *History of the Forest School*, 11, 19).

49. LF to Edwin S. Stuart, 14 Dec 1908; "Flick Asks State to Assist Fight on White Plague," *Philadelphia Inquirer*, 31 Mar 1909; LF to HP, 8 Apr 1909; LF to Benj. H. Shoemaker, 12 Apr 1909; Geo. E. Gordon to LF, 14 May 1909; and LF to Jos. S. Neff, 30 Jul 1909. After the hospitals declined, Flick wrote to Neff that there "seems to be a strong prejudice on the part of the medical professon against the general hospitals accepting consumptives." In addition, hospital leaders undoubt-

edly disliked the flat-rate reimbursement that was less than the cost of care. See Stevens, "Sweet Charity," 474–85.

Chapter 10. The Private Sanatoriums

1. ES to LF, 20 Nov 1901, 18 Feb, 13 Mar 1902. Other early private sanatoriums in eastern Pennsylvania included Bide-A-While, started by Dr. Wilfred B. Fetterman in Perkiomenville in December 1901. It took some of the Free Hospital's women patients but did not last long. The Rush Hospital for Consumptives and Allied Diseases opened a country branch in Malvern, Pennsylvania, in 1902. Rush accepted private and part-pay patients.

2. A. F. Stockdale to LF, 9 Jun 1902, SS; J. H. Dickenshied to LF, 4 Feb 1903, SS; Stockdale purchases and mortgages, recorded in the Carbon County Court House; *Souvenir of Sunnyrest Sanatorium*, [1904], LFPM, vol. 39, no. 49; *Sunnyrest Sanatorium, White Haven, Pa., for the Diseases of the Lungs and Throat* (n.p., n.d. [ca. 1909–1912]), pamphlet 722, CPP; *Sunnyrest Sanatorium, White Haven, Pa., for the Treatment of Tuberculosis* (n.p., n.d. [ca. 1909–1912]), pamphlet 7750, CPP; Lilian Brandt, comp., *A Directory of Institutions and Societies Dealing with Tuberculosis in the United States and Canada* (New York: Committee on the Prevention of Tuberculosis of the Charity Organization Society of the City of New York and the National Association for the Study and Prevention of Tuberculosis, 1904), 129; Philip P. Jacobs, comp., *The Campaign against Tuberculosis in the United States* (New York: National Association for the Study and Prevention of Tuberculosis, 1908), 123; and ads in *JOL* 2 (Jun 1905):113, 3 (Feb, Jun 1906):30, 200, 4 (Jul 1907):37.

3. Data on the McDonald family from the U.S. Census, Dennison Twp., 1900, 1910, and from a gravestone, St. Patrick's Cemetery, White Haven. August Maier, owner of the property in 1983, confirmed the location of the sanatorium. See also Mike [Bergrath] to LF, 3 Apr 1904; LF to M. J. Burgrath [*sic*], 4, 5 May 1904; M. J. Bergrath to LF, 6 May 1904; Mary Mahony to LF, 15 Jul 1904; and LF to Mary Mahony, 19 Jul 1904.

4. For Wightman (also spelled Whiteman) and Potts, see the U.S. Census, Philadelphia, 1900; *ARVN* 7 (1893) through 18 (1904), 24 (1910):15; Board Minutes, Visiting Nurse Society of Philadelphia, 30 Dec 1904, 6 Jan 1905, VN-CSHN; and Stephanie A. Stachniewicz and Jean K. Axelrod, *The Double Frill: The History of the Philadelphia General Hospital School of Nursing* (Philadelphia: George F. Stickley, 1978), 216.

5. LF to Helen W. Mauck, 8 Aug 1905. In the deeds, recorded in the Carbon County Court House, the main property is identified only by heaps of stones and the like. The smaller tract, purchased in 1906, was between Third and Fourth Streets. In 1912, Wightman bought Potts's share and, in 1918, sold it to Thomas M. and Sarah E. Bleuit for their Clair Mont Sanatorium. The house, still standing and pictured on an old postcard, was identified for me by Clayton Fox, White Haven.

6. Mary S. Bracken (daughter of Agnes E. Moss), interview with author,

Philadelphia, 5 Oct 1983; U.S. Census, White Haven Borough, 1910; and Genealogy of Mrs. Clarence Snowden [Agnes E. Moss], Hill Crest Sanatorium, JW, vol. 13.

7. Bracken interview; ES to LF, 19 May 1903; J. B. Stockdale to LF, 26 Aug 1903; Jas. H. Heller to LF, 8 Aug 1905, 11, 16, 24, 29 Jan 1906; LF to Agnes Moss, 2 Feb 1906; and Agnes E. Moss to LF, 31 Jan 1906.

8. Margaret McDonald to LF, 20 Jul 1906; LF to Margaret McDonald, 26 Jul 1906; Agnes E. Moss to LF, 15 Mar 1908; deeds in the Luzerne County Court House; and the Bracken interview. The 1910 Census indicates that Moss had mortgaged the house, but I could find no record of it in the Court House. The house still (1983) resembles its photo in *FAM* 1 (Jun 1910):back cover.

9. Kathryn Riordan, interview with author, Gwynedd, Pa., 6 Jan 1981; U.S. Census, Philadelphia, 1900, Springfield Twp., 1910; O'Hara's gravestone in Holy Cross Cemetery, Yeadon, Pa.; *Report of Philadelphia Polyclinic and College for Graduates in Medicine* 15 (1897):39; and Cecilia R. Flick, *Dr. Lawrence F. Flick As I Knew Him* (Philadelphia: Dorrance, 1956), 86. On 19 May 1902, O'Hara wrote to Flick from 30 W. 70th Street, New York City: "I have made arrangement with Dr. Baruch that I can go at any time with the privilege of finishing in the fall. At the same time he is kind enough to rush us through as much as possible. . . . I am much fascinated with the treatments here given, and I trust it will help me in my new work for the summer [at White Haven]." Dr. Simon Baruch, whose office was at 51 W. 70th Street, New York City, was a strong proponent of hydrotherapy in treating tuberculosis. In 1904, O'Hara specified the services of a "graduate in hydrotherapy," presumably herself (Brandt, *Directory*, 126).

10. Margaret G. O'Hara to LF, 25 May 1903, and Brandt, *Directory*, 126. The sanatorium was on the corner of Gowen Avenue and Sprague Street.

11. Lansdale and McGrath to LF, 19 Apr 1904; A. C. Abbott to LF, 20 Oct 1904; John I. Toomey to LF, 23, 25 Oct 1904; the Riordan interview; deed and mortgage in the Delaware County Court House; LF to George T. Osborne, 7 Apr 1906; photograph album of Kathryn Riordan; *Atlas of Delaware County East of Ridley Creek*, vol. 1 (Philadelphia: A. H. Mueller, 1909–1910), plate 24; and LF to Louis Gerstley, 13 Oct 1904.

12. Riordan interview and photo album. The E. T. Richardson Middle School now (1991) occupies the site. The trolley, south of the school, was built after the sanatorium opened and cut just south of the main house. Sinn Fein, an Irish nationalist movement with roots in the nineteenth century, was organized as a political party in 1905.

13. Mary M. Wilson to LF, 23 Sep 1904.

14. Mary M. Wilson to LF, 23 Sep, 18, 25 Oct 1904.

15. *Radnor-Wayne Sanatorium for Consumptives* (Philadelphia: Press of Ullrich Printing House, 1905) 7, LFPM, vol. 40, no. 48 (for the quotation); *Radnor-Wayne Sanatorium for the Cure of Tuberculosis* (n.p., n.d.), LFPM, vol. 55, no. 28; deeds and mortgage in the Chester County Court House; and Ellis Kiser, comp., *Atlas of Properties on Main Line Pennsylvania Railroad from Overbrook to Paoli*, 2nd ed. (Philadelphia: A. H. Mueller, 1908), plate 24. An intermediary, Robert S. Erwin, was involved in the sale. John Henry sold the land to Erwin, who resold it to

Stevenson on the same day. Erwin retained the mortgage in his own name. Stevenson was listed as the Radnor-Wayne's representative in the 1905 brochure. According to the U.S. Census, Philadelphia, 1900, he would have been twenty-five when he signed the deed. St. David's Golf Club now (1990) occupies most of this property.

16. *Sunnyrest Sanatorium*, pamphlet 7750, and Margaret G. O'Hara to LF, 7 Feb 1910 (for the quotations). In addition to promotions already cited, see Philip P. Jacobs, comp., *A Tuberculosis Directory* (New York: National Association for the Study and Prevention of Tuberculosis, 1911), viii; descriptions of the sanatoriums in directories of the National Association, 1904, 1908, 1911; ads in *JOL* 3 (Apr, Jul 1906):119, 241, 4 (Oct 1907):354; ad in *FAM* 1 (Jun 1910):back cover; ads in LF, *The Tuberculosis Situation in Pennsylvania in the Year 1909* (Philadelphia: Peter Reilly, n.d.); *The Dermady Cottage Sanatorium*, (1907), LFPM, vol. 86, no. 19; *Fern Cliff Sanatorium*, n.d., LFPM, vol. 116, no. 29; *The Orchards, White Haven, P.O., Luzerne County, Pa.*, n.d., LFPM, vol. 55, no. 32; and *Hillcrest Sanatorium for the Treatment of Pulmonary Tuberculosis, Hoyt, P.O., Montgomery Co., Pa.* (Mrs. Wilson's third sanatorium), n.d., LFPM, vol. 54, no. 10a.

17. *JOL* 3 (Apr 1906):119, 4 (Oct 1907):354 (for the two quotations), and *Radnor-Wayne Sanatorium*, 1905, 14.

18. *Radnor-Wayne Sanatorium for the Cure*; *Sunnyrest Sanatorium*, pamphlet 7750; C. R. Flick, *Dr. LF*, 88; and the Riordan photo album.

19. *Sunnyrest Sanatorium*, pamphlet 7750; ads for Dermady Sanatorium and Hill Crest Sanatorium, in LF, *Tuberculosis Situation*; and ad for Fern Cliff Sanatorium, *JOL* 3 (Apr 1906):119.

20. "Sanitarium and Sanatorium," *JOL* 2 (Feb 1905):13.

21. Tasks and judgments come from many examples in the LF papers.

22. *Sunnyrest Sanatorium*, pamphlet 722; Riordan interview and photo album; Nancy H. Kindley to LF, 22 Feb 1908; LF to Mother Walberg, 17 Dec 1913 (for the first quotation); LF to G. H. Sloan, 20 Jan 1911 (for the second quotation); and LF to M. J. Sweeney, 13 Mar 1911.

23. Mabel Morgan to LF, 16 Aug 1904, SS; ES to LF, 12 Mar 1905, 22 Oct 1904, both SS; Margaret G. O'Hara to LF, 23 May 1909, 25 Sep 1911; William Coniff to LF, 2 Dec 1907, SS; and J. V. Walsh to LF, 8 Jan 1908.

24. For charges, see citations in n. 16; ES to LF, 14 May 1914; sanatorium directories; and LF's frequent lists in his letters to patients. For other users, see *Sunnyrest Sanatorium*, pamphlet 7750; J. L. Hanley to LF, 25 Aug 1907, SS; Benj. Galland to LF, 19 Dec 1910; LF to J. M. Sheedy, 20 Feb 1909; and M. B. Carroll to LF, n.d. [filed 31 Dec 1907], SS.

25. For costs, see LF to Mrs. F. N. Robertson, 29 Apr 1911; LF to R. D. Caldwell, 20 Nov 1911; LF to C. R. Miller, 20 Jun 1910; and LF to L. A. Shipman, 26 Feb 1913. For physicians' fees, see LF to E. H. Craver, 7 Oct 1903; LF to J. B. Crone, 21 Dec 1903; LF to Isaac Morgan, 12 Jan 1909; and LF to C. R. Miller, 20 Jun 1910.

26. Frances A. Eastlake to LF, 2 Nov 1904, and Ella Hackenburg to LF, 28 Mar 1909. Eastlake decided instead to take "nervous" persons into her home.

27. U.S. Census, Springfield Township, 1910; Riordan interview and photo

album; and U.S. Census, East Side Borough and White Haven Borough, 1910. All "hospital" employees listed in East Side Borough came from four households, three of which were enumerated next to the Stockdale family. The fourth had eight boarders, four of them nurses. The Orchards had closed, and the White Haven Sanatorium, which had its own long list of staff, did not employ outside nurses.

28. U.S. Census, White Haven Borough, 1910, and the Bracken interview. In addition to the women who nursed in private families, census data from White Haven show only four other persons who might have worked in sanatoriums. One tuberculosis nurse boarded at McFadden's and one servant, one laborer, and one engineer worked in an "institution."

29. Clara C. Waugh to LF, 2 Feb 1906; ES to LF, 2 Jul 1906, SS, 11 Mar 1903; Helen McDevitt to LF, 29 Sep 1906, 23 May 1908; Walter F. Wood to LF, 24 Aug 1907; and Alex. Armstrong to LF, 27 Feb 1909.

30. Amy E. Potts to LF, 10 Apr 1906. See also Maddie Gaillard to LF, 8 Aug 1904, SS; ES to LF, 7 Apr 1905, 5 Apr 1906, both SS; and Mrs. J. D. Meise to LF, 22 Aug 1907, SS.

31. Daisy W. Laidley, 18 Apr 1905, SS; Richard Pollard to LF, 3 Jul 1905, SS; and ES to LF, 5 Apr 1906, SS. Frequent themes in the many complaints were poor food and lack of attention.

32. Riordan and Bracken interviews.

33. George E. Macklin to LF, 5 Nov 1904, SS, and Louis Woelfel to LF, 17 Dec 1904, SS.

34. Mary M. Wilson to LF, 23 Feb, SS, 5, 22 Mar 1905; LF to E. Luttgen, 9 Oct 1903; LF to Jas. Hancock, 14 Jun 1904; and LF to Mary M. Wilson, 8, 24 Mar 1905.

35. Mary M. Wilson to LF, 2 May, 7, 22 Jul 1905; Mrs. Kate B. Mervine to LF, n.d., [Jul 1905], SS; F. A. Griesmann to LF, 26 Jul 1905; Richard L. Field to LF, 19, 22, 26 July 1905, all SS; Mary M. Wilson to LF, 12 Sep 1905; and LF to Mary M. Wilson, 13 Sep 1905.

36. Record of the sheriff's sale, Chester County Court House, and LF to Katherine V. Henin, 25 Apr 1911. Potts returned to the Visiting Nurse Society of Philadelphia and took charge of its Main Line Branch (*ARVN* 24 [1910]:8, 15). For Wightman, see U.S. Census, Foster Twp., 1910.

37. *Clair Mont Sanatorium*, n.d., LFPM, vol. 111, no. 129; Jacobs, *Directory*, 61; LF to Agnes Heibel, 11 Aug 1910; LF to Joseph S. Neff, 16 Jul 1912; J. J. Best to LF, 19 Oct 1912; *White Haven, Pa., Brookhurst Sanitorium*, n.d., LFPM, vol. 116, no. 43; and LF to J. J. Best, 21 Oct 1912. Philadelphia's death rates for tuberculosis of the lungs had fallen from 265 per 100,000 people in 1890, to 210 in 1900, and to 194 in 1911.

38. J. J. Best to LF, 19 Oct 1912; records of property sales in the Carbon County Court House; and directories of the National Association through 1934. In 1912 Wightman bought Potts's share of the Orchards. The Orchards was reopened temporarily in 1914 by another White Haven graduate nurse (LF to C. R. Kitsmiller, 6 Jul 1914; *The Orchards*, n.d., LFPM, vol. 124, no. 174; and LF to Ella A. Trimble, 11 Jun 1914).

39. LF to F. N. Yeager, 7 Oct 1912, 12 Apr 1913, and LF to HP, 14 Jan 1914.

40. LF to Sr. Mary Louis, 1 Apr 1913; LF to P. H. Dale, 28 Feb 1913; LF to Samuel Griffith, 26 Mar 1913; Mary Mahony to LF, 31 Mar 1912, 18, 27 Feb 1913; and LF to Mary Mahony, 28 Feb, 14, 24 Mar 1913. Eagleville was the common name for the Philadelphia Jewish Sanatorium for Consumptives, Eagleville, Pa. For the furnishings, see LF to John A. Flick, 22 Apr 1914, and LF to Daniel D. Test, 3 Jul 1914. For many letters of announcement, see LFLP, 25 to 29 Apr 1913. For Flick's charges, see LF to B. Frank Hiestand, 21 Apr 1913; LF to I. G. Daly, 8 May 1913; and LF to Mary McLaughlin, 12 May 1913.

41. "Treatment sheets" and "Daily Records of Dinners," n.d. [filed 1, 31 May 1913], LFCU; LF to Richard Reeser, 24 Feb 1913; LF to H. Hurlburt Tomlin, 2, 15 Apr 1913; LF to B. Frank Hiestand, 21 Apr 1913; and LF to Mrs. Geo. Hiestand, 2 May 1913.

42. LF to Director Porter, 1 Apr 1913. See also LF to Supt. James Robinson, 14 Apr, 6 May 1913; LF to T. E. Mitten, 6 May 1913; LF to Director Porter, 26 Jun 1913; and Ella A. Shape to LF, 16 Sep 1913. Noise may have partly explained a move or expansion of Flick's sanatorium in Nov 1913 to 736 Pine Street, one house away from the corner (LF to Daisy W. Laidley, 3 Nov, 4 Dec 1913, and LF to J. C. Laidley, 7 Jan 1914).

43. Andrew R. Whitaker to LF, 31 Aug 1913; LF to H. Hurlburt Tomlin, 26 Jun 1913; and LF to Margaret G. O'Hara, 17, 29 Jul 1913.

44. Margaret G. O'Hara to LF, n.d. [Aug 1913]; LF to Margaret G. O'Hara, 15 Aug 1913; and LF to William J. Clark, 6 Aug 1914.

45. LF to Sr. Mary Louis, 14 Apr 1914. In letters to others, Flick consistently gave illness as his reason for closing his sanatorium.

46. Mary M. Gally to LF, 1 Jan 1903, and "A Growing Problem," *JOL* 4 (Apr 1907):100–101. See also Anna D. Pope to LF, 8 Jul 1904; Louise Sturtevant to LF, 17 Jul 1904; Charles H. Jackson to LF, 8 Feb 1906; Livingston Farrand to LF, 27 Mar 1909; James A. de Paul [?sp] to LF, 18 Mar 1910; Oscar E. Dooly to LF, 1 Feb 1915; W. K. McClure, "The Boycott of Consumptives," *Living Age* 251 (8 Dec 1906):624–29; and William G. Brown, "Some Confessions of a 'T. B.,'" *Atlantic Monthly* 113 (Jun 1914):747–54.

Chapter 11. Attention, Care, and Doctor's Orders: Tuberculosis Nursing

1. For background, see Susan M. Reverby, *Ordered to Care: The Dilemma of American Nursing, 1850–1945* (Cambridge: Cambridge University Press, 1987), 11–16, 40–59; Charles E. Rosenberg, *The Care of Strangers: The Rise of America's Hospital System* (New York: Basic Books, 1987), 212–36; Nancy Tomes, "'Little World of Our Own': The Pennsylvania Hospital Training School for Nurses, 1895–1907," *Journal of the History of Medicine and Allied Sciences* 33 (Oct 1978):507–30; and Patricia O'Brien, "'All a Woman's Life Can Bring': The Domestic Roots of Nursing in Philadelphia, 1830–1885," *Nursing Research* 36 (Jan/Feb 1987):12–17.

2. "Cured Consumptives Trained as Tuberculosis Nurses," *North American*, 11 Feb 1906, sec. 6. The nurses graduated late in 1905.

3. Ibid.

4. Joseph Walsh, "The Work of the Free Hospital for Poor Consumptives and White Haven Sanatorium Society," *ARFH* 17 (1915):3; LF, "Cured Patients as Tuberculosis Nurses," *JOL* 8 (Jan 1911):6; and Mary E. Lee to LF, 12 Jul 1904. The school at White Haven admitted two men and graduated one, not included in this summary. The experiment in training men, Flick noted, was "not satisfactory enough" to continue. Although the graduate was successful, there was "less demand" for men and "some difficulty training both sexes in the same class" (p. 7). Of the first fifty-four graduates from the White Haven training school, 37 percent came from Philadelphia, 33 percent from elsewhere in Pennsylvania, 26 percent from other states, and 2 percent each from Puerto Rico and Nova Scotia (*ARFH* 18 [1916]:32–33). Immigrants from Europe were notably absent. Surnames were predominantly English, Irish, Scottish, and German. I believe that all graduates were white. In 1910, 42.6 percent of the women in the nation's work force were unskilled (e.g., servants), 27.9 percent were semiskilled (e.g., garment-workers and factory operatives), and 13.9 percent held clerical or kindred jobs (Janet M. Hooks, *Women's Occupations through Seven Decades*, Women's Bureau Bulletin No. 218 [Washington, D.C.: U.S. Government Printing Office, 1947], 207).

5. Charles [J.] Hatfield, "Nursing in Tuberculosis," *JOL* 4 (Oct 1904):324; LF to GG, 2 Aug 1905; and Joseph Walsh, "The Methods of the Henry Phipps Institute for the Study, Treatment, and Prevention of Tuberculosis in Philadelphia," *Bulletin of the Johns Hopkins Hospital* 19 (Jun 1908):177.

6. ES to LF, 7 Jul 1904; Mary McNamee to LF, 20 Jun 1904; and Cha[rle]s J. Hatfield, H. R. M. Landis, and W. B. Stanton, "The Training School for Nurses of the Henry Phipps Institute," *RHPI* 5 (1908):443–44. The percentage who "lost courage" is based on thirty-two students, omitting four graduates from the previous year who were completing short terms of work. Another four pupils were dismissed because of incompetency or disobedience, and four broke down in health. The loss totaled 41 percent. For White Haven data, see names of pupil nurses, *ARFH* 10 (1908):75, 11 (1909):64, and frequent lists of graduates, *ARsFH*.

7. Anna G. Murphy to LF, 27 Sep 1904, 13 Nov 1905, and LF to Anna G. Murphy, 27 Sep 1904, 14 Nov 1905. See also "Nursing as an Employment for Young Women Who Have Had Tuberculosis," *FAM* 1 (Feb 1909):34–35; "Tuberculosis Nurses," *FAM* 1 (Apr 1910):12; and A. M. P., "A Plucky Nurse," *FAM* 1 (Jul 1910):12.

8. Rules for the Nurses of the Henry Phipps Training School, examinations in materia medica given to the first group of graduates, test scores of the early graduates, and Phipps Training School Examination, 11 May 1910, all in JW, vol. 2. White Haven's school was modeled on that at Phipps. For similar rules there, see JW, vol. 1.

9. LF, "Cured Patients," 6; Anna L. Morris, "White Haven Sanatorium Training School for Nurses," *ARFH* 15 (1913):9–10; Walsh, "Work of the FHPC," 4, 10; and Joseph Walsh, "The Advantage of Tuberculosis Nursing for Tuberculous Patients," *JOL* 20 (Nov 1923):408. Well over half of the graduates of general training schools went into private duty during this period (Reverby, *Ordered to Care*, 110).

10. Nurses' reports in LF papers; Hatfield, "Nursing in Tuberculosis," 322–23; and Charles J. Hatfield, "Training for Professional Nursing in Institutions for Tuberculous Patients," *TSICT*, vol. 3 (1908):409.

11. Hatfield, "Nursing in Tuberculosis," 322.

12. Paul H. Kretzschmar, "Dr. Dettweiler's Method of Treating Pulmonary Consumption," *New York Medical Journal* 47 (18 Feb 1888):178, and LF, "Home Treatment of Tuberculosis," *Therapeutic Gazette*, 3d ser., vol. 18 (15 Jun 1902): 369.

13. Hatfield, "Nursing in Tuberculosis," 322, and "Commencement at White Haven Sanatorium," *White Haven Journal*, 14 Jul 1911 (made available to me by Mrs. Charlotte Armstrong, Hazleton, Pa.).

14. Mrs. W. H. Thompson to LF, 29 Jan 1904, SS.

15. Chas. M. Levis to LF, 31 Jan 1905, SS.

16. Harriett E. Greene to LF, 8 Sep 1909.

17. Richard L. Field to LF, 28 Oct 1905, SS. See also idem, 19, 22 Jul 1905, both SS, and Mary M. Wilson to LF, 6 Jun 1905, SS.

18. LF to Mrs. Geo. Hiestand, 2 May 1913, and Elida W. [Mrs. Geo.] Hiestand to LF, 4 May 1913. Hiestand died at home on 31 Aug 1913.

19. E. G. Bobb to LF, 13 Jun, 8 Aug, 5 Sep 1911. Chester's older brother had died in 1907 at age twenty-two (U.S. Census, Blair County, 1910, and a gravestone in the Roaring Springs, Pa., cemetery). For Flick's medical priorities, see LF, "Tuberculosis As It Concerns the Physician," *Interstate Medical Journal* 18 (Feb 1911):197–98. For him, the highest medical function was prevention; cure was second. The alleviation of suffering, a poor third, was "a dangerous function" that had "trammeled the progress of scientific medicine and kept individual physicians, indeed the majority of all physicians, in the quagmire of mediocrity. The power to ease the sufferings of a fellow human being is so seductive that it constantly leads physicians to do things which, if fully analyzed and shown up in all their influences, would often reveal a broken thread of life which might have held out a while longer had that relief not been sought and given."

20. Anna M. Walsh to LF, 2 Oct 1911, and E. G. Bobb to LF, 6 Oct 1911.

21. LF to E. G. Bobb, 11 Oct 1911.

22. Ibid.; Anna M. Walsh to LF, 20 Nov 1911; and E. G. Bobb to LF, 3 Dec 1911.

23. Effie A. Boda to LF, 7 Jan 1914; Stella M. Brown to LF, 24 Jan 1913; and, for clothing and equipment for an out-of-town case, Katharine DeWitt, *Private Duty Nursing*, 2nd ed., enlarged (Philadelphia: J. B. Lippincott Co., 1917; reprint, New York: Garland Publishing, 1984), 58–64. See also Reverby, *Ordered to Care*, 95–105.

24. Anna L. Morris to LF, 4 Feb 1911, and Edith Metzler to LF, 4 Oct, 18 Nov 1911.

25. Hatfield, "Nursing in Tuberculosis," 322; Walsh, "Work of the FHPC," 3–4; and many letters that cite salaries in LF's papers. The monthly cost of maintaining a nurse at the Phipps Institute, including food, services, light, heat, and rent, was estimated at "a little over sixteen dollars" (LF to GG, 29 May 1905).

26. LF to Edith Metzler, 20 Nov 1911; Reverby, *Ordered to Care*, 102–5;

and, for training schools in sanatoriums, *JOL* 11 (Jan 1914):25, and Walsh, "Advantage of Tuberculosis Nursing," 407.

27. Nellie K. Smith to LF, 23 Jul 1908, and Mrs. P. White to LF, 5 Mar 1908. See also Joseph M. Pile to LF, 21 Aug 1895, SS; Maurice J. Babb to LF, 6 May 1904; Mrs. Wm. H. Lewin to LF, 29 Jul 1907; Edith Marchant to LF, n.d. [answered 28 Oct 1910]; M. Etta Pierce to LF, 7 Aug 1912; and Mrs. F. P. Atherton to LF, 28 Feb 1914;

28. M. B. Holzman to LF, 1 Jan 1908. See also W. S. Long to LF, 4 Nov 1905, SS, and Samuel Ginsburg to LF, 23 Dec 1908.

29. Walsh, "Work of the FHPC," 3–4 (3 for the quotation), and idem, "Advantage of Tuberculosis Nursing," 408. The weekly earnings of female production workers in twenty-five manufacturing industries in 1914 averaged $7.75 for a 50.1-hour week (*Historical Statistics of the United States, Colonial Times to 1970* [Washington, D.C.: U.S. Bureau of the Census, 1975], 172).

30. Walsh, "Work of the FHPC," 4, and Anna G. Murphy to LF, 15 Nov 1908.

31. Walsh, "Advantage of Tuberculosis Nursing," 408. Mortality rates reported for the graduates, calculated from the four sources cited in n. 9, ranged from 7 percent in 1913 to 21 percent in 1923.

32. U.S. Census, Northampton County, 1880, 1900; Employee Register (1883–1895), Guardians of the Poor, PCA; and Stephanie Stachniewicz and Jean K. Axelrod, *The Double Frill: The History of the Philadelphia General Hospital School of Nursing* (Philadelphia: George F. Stickley Co., 1978), 17–42, 218.

33. Student Record, Bureau of Charities, Philadelphia General Hospital, Training School for Nurses, 15 Nov 1894 to 7 Oct 1897, PCA; Reverby, *Ordered to Care*, 49–57; and Tomes, "'Little World of Our Own,'" 526–28.

34. David Riesman to LF, 3, 18 Jan, 21 Apr 1902; Jas-Hendrie Lloyd to LF, 27 Aug 1902; and ES to LF, 2, 3 Jan [1903].

35. ES to LF, 9 Feb 1903; LF to Mary Mahoney [sic], 24 Nov 1903; Mary Mahony (MM hereafter) to LF, 25 Nov 1903; LF to HP, 4 Apr 1904; MM to LF, 10 Apr, 16 May 1904; LF to GG, 4 Jun 1904; MM to LF, 15 Jul 1904, 17 Apr 1905, SS; LF to MM, 20 Jun 1905; and *Radnor-Wayne Sanatorium for the Cure of Tuberculosis*, (n.p., n.d.), LFPM, vol. 55, no. 28. Mahony took cases with other physicians and there are times unaccounted for.

36. MM to LF, 23 Apr, 9 May, 6 Jul, 5, 17 Nov 1908, 14 Jan 1909, n.d. [answered 30 Mar 1909], 6 Apr, 30 May, 20 Jun 1909, and LF to Philip Marvel, 5 Mar 1909.

37. LF to Chas. Stover, 16 Apr 1910; MM to LF, 28 Sep, 4 Dec 1910, 16 Jan, 1 Mar, 28 Sep 1911; LF to MM, 29 Sep 1910; and P. M. Sharples to LF, 16 Jul 1911.

38. MM to LF, 19 July, 1, 5 Aug, 2 Dec 1911.

39. MM to LF, 6, 11, 25 Dec 1911.

40. MM to LF, 31 Mar 1912, 18, 27 Feb, 17 Mar, 6 Aug 1913; LF to Anna G. Murphy, 19 Apr 1912; LF to MM, 14, 28 Feb, 24 Mar, 5, 15 Aug 1913; LF to H. [Hurlburt] Tomlin, 26 Jun 1913; and LF to Margaret G. O'Hara, 17, 29 Jul 1913.

41. MM to LF, 7 Sep, 25 Oct 1913, 9 Mar 1914; LF to MM, 10 Sep, 27, 30 Oct 1913, 30 Sep 1914; and Jane E. Mahony to LF, 8 Oct 1914.

42. LF to Philip Marvel, 5 Mar 1909; Martin F. Sloan, "Tuberculosis Nursing as a Profession," *JOL* 10 (Nov 1913):336; and gravestone of MM and five members of her family in the cemetery, St. Joseph's Church, Easton. Flick replied to a later inquiry: "Miss Mary Mahony broke down whilst nursing a case and never recovered. . . . I . . . tried to persuade her to go to the White Haven Sanatorium as those of us who were interested in her tried to save her but she declined. . . . I have every reason to believe that she is enjoying a well merited reward" (LF to Mrs. F. S. Forgeus, 24 Mar 1920).

Chapter 12. The Final Years of George E. Macklin

1. GG to LF, 28 Apr 1903; F. N. Hoffstot to GM, 29 Apr 1903, SS; and Geo. E. Macklin (GM hereafter) to LF, 30 Apr 1903, SS.

2. GM to LF, 13, 25 May 1903, both SS. Macklin tended to use many periods and capital letters in his writing. His secretary did not.

3. GM to LF, 25 May, 2 Jun 1903, both SS.

4. GM to LF, 2 Jun 1903, SS.

5. GM to LF, 7 Jul 1903, SS.

6. C. J. Hunt to LF, 7, 20 Jul 1903, both SS. Rales were abnormal sounds in Macklin's breathing.

7. GM to LF, 4 Aug 1903, SS.

8. GM to LF, 18, 21, 23, 29 Aug, 9, 26 Sep 1903, all SS.

9. GM to LF, 19 Oct, 25 Nov, 30 Dec 1903, all SS, and LF to GM, 31 Dec 1903.

10. GM to LF, 15 Jan 1904, SS, and LF to GM, 16 Jan 1904. An "effusion" refers to fluid in the pleural space, around the lung. The rationales for fly-blisters and other treatments changed with new medical ideas. According to Flick in 1909, microbial infection caused hyperemia (vascular congestion), which in turn caused pain. Toxins associated with infection could also cause pain, both by contributing to the hyperemia and by irritating nerve fibers. A fly-blister drew blood away from the diseased part, Flick believed, and thereby relieved pain. It also drew antitoxins to the surface and, when the blister so raised was allowed to absorb, it produced a reaction in the body and enhanced immunity. Depletion therapy, as by purging, eliminated toxins through the stools, while scrub baths with soap and hot water eliminated them through the skin. See LF, "The Therapeutics of Pain," *Monthly Cyclopaedia and Medical Bulletin* 2 (Aug 1909):456–60.

11. GM to LF, 2, 15 Feb, 21 May, 1 Jun 1904, all SS.

12. GM to LF, 21 Jun 1904, SS.

13. GM to LF, n.d. [filed 7 Aug 1904, but probably 2 or 3 Aug], SS.

14. LF to GG, 4 Aug 1904, and GM to LF, 7 Aug 1904.

15. GM to LF, 10, 16, 19 Aug 1904, all SS, and LF to GM, 9, 17 Aug 1904.

16. GM to LF, 19 Aug 1904, SS. In LFSB, vol. 1, 177, an undated clipping

shows a photo of Dr. B[oswell] P. Anderson and, below it, the title, "Whose Strong Refutations of Dr. Flick's Fallacies Regarding the Cure of Tuberculosis are Bringing Many Sufferers to the City of Sunshine."

17. LF to GM, 23, 27 Aug 1904.

18. GM to LF, 27 Aug 1904, SS.

19. LF to GM, 30 Aug 1904.

20. GM to LF, 30 Aug 1904, SS.

21. GM to LF, 3, 26, 28 Sep 1904, all SS, and LF to GM, 5, 13, 22 Sep, 14 Oct 1904.

22. GM to LF, 15, 17 Oct 1904, both SS, and LF to GM, 18 Oct 1904.

23. GM to LF, 5 Nov 1904, SS.

24. GM to LF, 5 Nov, 5, 14 Dec 1904, all SS, and LF to GM, 7 Nov, 6 Dec 1904. James J. Corbett was a champion heavyweight boxer, 1892–1897.

25. LF to GM, 15 Dec 1904, 9 Jan 1905, and GM to LF, 7, 9 Jan 1905, both SS.

26. GM to LF, 7, 14, 16 Feb 1905, SS, and the following from the Camden Archives and Museum: The Kirkwood Hotel Register, 9 Mar 1903–13 Apr 1905; Floor Plans of the Kirkwood; and W. S. Alexander and Jno. W. Corbett, *A Descriptive Sketch of Camden, S.C.* (Charleston, S.C.: Walker, Evans & Cogswell Co., Printers, 1888), 3–4. Macklin occupied Room 310; Charles Bacher, the room directly across the corridor to the rear of the building.

27. Charles Bacher to LF, 16 Feb 1905, SS. Dr. Corbett coauthored *A Descriptive Sketch of Camden* (n. 26).

28. LF to GM, 18 Feb 1905.

29. LF to GM, 20 Feb 1905.

30. Charles Bacher to LF, 19 Feb 1905, SS; Elizabeth Macklin to LF, 20 Feb 1905, SS; and LF to GM, 20 Feb 1905.

31. Jno. W. Corbett to LF, 21 Feb 1905, SS; LF to Jno. W. Corbett, 23 Feb 1905; and LF to Elizabeth Macklin, 23 Feb 1905. Bacher did not mention Corbett's use of calomel, to which the latter attributed a better assimilation of food. There was no unanimity of medical opinion as to the best treatment of hemorrhage. Flick himself had used opium and ergot, as he reported in 1898, but when they failed in one of his cases he switched to nitroglycerine. He reported three cases successfully treated. Constriction of the blood vessels by the older treatments simply increased the force in the blood vessels, he reasoned, thus increasing the risk of hemorrhage, whereas a reduction in this force was desired. Nitroglycerine and depletion of the body by purges—as by Epsom salts (sulphate of magnesia)—were helpful, he believed, because they reduced the force in the vessels. For the opinions of Flick and others who more or less agreed with him, see LF, "Nitroglycerine as a Hemostatic in Hemoptysis," *Philadelphia Medical Journal* 1 (19 Feb 1898):344; William Osler, *The Principles and Practice of Medicine* 5th ed. (New York: D. Appleton, 1903), 639–41; and Albert P. Francine, *Pulmonary Tuberculosis—Its Modern and Specialized Treatment* (Philadelphia: J. B. Lippincott, 1906), 121–59. For support of Corbett's treatment, see James Tyson, *The Practice of Medicine*, 3rd ed. (Philadelphia: P. Blakiston's Son, 1903), 274–75.

32. Elizabeth G. Macklin to LF, 26 Feb 1905, SS, and LF to Elizabeth Macklin, 1 Mar 1905.

33. GM to LF, 12 Mar 1905, SS.
34. GM to LF, 15 Mar 1905, SS.
35. LF to GM, 13, 17 Mar 1905.
36. GM to LF, 18 Mar 1905, SS.
37. Charles Bacher to LF, 18 Mar 1905, SS.
38. Ibid.
39. LF to Charles Bacher, 20 Mar 1905, and LF to GM, 20 Mar 1905.
40. Elizabeth Macklin to LF, 30 Mar 1905, SS, and LF to Elizabeth Macklin, 3 Apr 1905. A "private car" meant a private railroad car.
41. Charles L. Minor to LF, 8 Apr 1905, SS.
42. Elizabeth Macklin to LF, 6 Apr 1905, SS.
43. LF to Charles L. Minor, 10 Apr 1905; "George E. Macklin," *Pittsburg Post*, 27 Jun 1905; and William Shakespeare, *Measure for Measure*, act 3, sc. 1, lines 2–3, 11–13, quoted in James R. Leaming, "The Philosophy of Climatic Treatment of Chest Disease," *TACA* 4 (1887):30. Charles Bacher later worked at the Kensington Dispensary for the Treatment of Tuberculosis, Philadelphia. He died in the Home for Consumptives at Chestnut Hill in 1910.
44. John B. Huber, *Consumption, Its Relation to Man and His Civilization, Its Prevention and Cure* (Philadelphia: J. B. Lippincott, 1906), 114.

Chapter 13. Into the Homes, Minds, and Lives of the Poor: Visiting Nurses

1. Carroll Smith-Rosenberg, *Religion and the Rise of the American City Mission Movement 1812–1870* (Ithaca, N.Y.: Cornell University Press, 1971); Paul Boyer, *Urban Masses and Moral Order in America, 1812–1920* (Cambridge: Harvard University Press, 1978), 15, 18–19, 24, 38, 150–61; Allen Davis, *Spearheads for Reform: The Social Settlements and the Progressive Movement, 1890–1914* (New York: Oxford University Press, 1967); and Kathleen D. McCarthy, "Parallel Power Stuctures: Women and the Voluntary Sphere," and Anne F. Scott, "Women's Voluntary Associations: From Charity to Reform," both in *Lady Bountiful Revisited: Women, Philanthropy, and Power*, ed. Kathleen D. McCarthy (New Brunswick, N.J.: Rutgers University Press, 1990). For the antecedents and early history of public health nursing in the U.S., see Annie M. Brainard, *The Evolution of Public Health Nursing* (Philadelphia: W. B. Saunders, 1922), 180–261, and Karen A. Buhler-Wilkerson, "False Dawn: The Rise and Decline of Public Health Nursing, 1900–1930," (Ph.D diss., University of Pennsylvania, 1984), 1–30.
The transition in leadership from the ladies to the nurses marks the generational shift from bourgeois matron to the "new woman" identified by Smith-Rosenberg in *Disorderly Conduct: Visions of Gender in Victorian America* (New York: Alfred A. Knopf, 1985), 167–81. This new woman, born between the late 1850s and 1900, developed a career outside of the home, took part in public affairs, and was socially and economically autonomous.
2. Mabel Jacques, *District Nursing* (New York: Macmillan Co., 1911), 100–103; Ellen N. La Motte, *The Tuberculosis Nurse: Her Function and Her Qualifications* (New York: G. P. Putnam's Sons, 1915), 70–107; and Anna G. Murphy to LF, 7,

15 Jan [1913]. In the 1920s, when nurses from the city health department visited tuberculous patients at home, Flick opposed their seeing his private patients (LF to Wilmer Krusen, 29 Sep 1924; LF to A. A. Cairns, 13 Oct 1926; and LF to Ward Brinton, 18 Oct 1926).

3. Brainard, *Evolution*, 214–18 (216–17 for the quotations). Jenks was the daughter of John Henry Towne, a very successful Philadelphia industrialist (E. Digby Baltzell, *Philadelphia Gentlemen: The Making of a National Upper Class* [New York: Free Press, 1958; reprint Philadelphia: University of Pennsylvania Press, 1978)], 103–4, and "Towne, John Henry, 1818–1875," a clipping, UPA). She had paid for the first cottage at Trudeau's Adirondack Cottage Sanitarium (Edward L. Trudeau, *An Autobiography* (Philadelphia: Lea and Febiger, 1915), 170.

4. Brainard, *Evolution*, 218–19.

5. *ARVN* 28 (1914):16–17, and "Object of the Society," *ARVN* 9 (1895):4.

6. Statistical data calculated from the annual reports, and, for chronic complaints, *ARVN* 7 (1893):6, 8 (1894):6. The year ending early in 1888 was atypical: 9.5 percent of the cases had consumption. In early 1900, there were forty-nine cases of phthisis; in 1901, fifty-one.

7. LF, "The Contagiousness of Phthisis (Tubercular Pulmonitis)," *Transactions of the Medical Society of Pennsylvania* 20 (Jun 1888):173–77; William Osler, "The Home in Its Relation to the Tuberculosis Problem," *Medical News* 83 (12 Dec 1903):1105–6 (for the quotations), 1108–9; and LF, "House Infection of Tuberculosis," *Medical News* 84 (20 Feb 1904):345–50.

8. Adelaide Dutcher, "Where the Danger Lies in Tuberculosis. A Study of the Social and Domestic Relations of Tuberculous Out-Patients," *Philadelphia Medical Journal* 6 (1900):1031–32; Harvey Cushing, *The Life of Sir William Osler*, vol. 1 (Oxford: Clarendon Press, 1925), 536; and Brainard, *Evolution*, 273–75.

9. Ruth B. Sherman, "Baltimore's Work in Tuberculosis," *American Journal of Nursing* 1 (Jun 1901):626–29 (628 for the quotations).

10. R. Thelin, "The Report of the Visiting Nurse in Homes of Tuberculous Patients for Seven Weeks," *Johns Hopkins Nurses Alumnae Magazine* 3 (Mar 1904): 33–34; Brainard, *Evolution*, 275–78; and M. A. Nutting, "The Visiting Nurse for Tuberculosis," *Charities and the Commons* 16 (7 Apr 1906):51–55 (54 for the quotation).

Visiting (or district) nursing had strong roots in the ideas of Florence Nightingale. Nightingale had advised William Rathbone in his efforts to develop district nursing in Liverpool, England, and one of her papers, "Sick-Nursing and Health-Nursing," was read at the Chicago Exhibition in 1893. Although Nightingale opposed the germ theory, twentieth-century nurses easily grafted the specific precautions against tubercle bacilli onto the strong stock of her sanitary reform, with its emphasis on ventilation, cleanliness, and light. Along with rest and good nutrition, this constituted the regimen for tuberculosis.

11. L. W. Quintard, "Report of Head Nurse and Matron," *ARVN* 20 (1906): 8, and "Nurses Need Funds to Fight Tuberculosis," *North American*, 29 Jul 1906, a clipping, VN-CSHN.

12. Historical Record Book Class Admitted 1897 to 1909, Archives of the

Department of Nursing Service, Hospital of the University of Pennsylvania; lists of graduates in the annual reports of the Hospital of the University of Pennsylvania; Henry M. Fisher to LF, 25 Oct 1909; and U.S. Census, Jersey City, N.J., 1900, and Buffalo, N.Y., 1910. The Historical Record Book contains comments on Jacques through 30 Dec 1904. She had been demoted a year.

13. "Special Tuberculosis Work of the Visiting Nurse Society, Philadelphia, Pa.," LFPM, vol. 65, no. 57; Mabel Jacques, "The Visiting Nurse in Tuberculosis, Her Importance as an Educational Agent," *JOL* 6 (May 1909): 134–36; idem, "The Tuberculosis Nurse and Her Work," *Trained Nurse and Hospital Review* 47 (Nov, Dec 1911):284–85, 344–46, 48 (Jan 1912):19–20; "Nurses Need Funds to Fight Tuberculosis"; "A Good Angel to Poor Consumptives," *Philadelphia Press*, 7 Oct 1907; "Seek Assistance of State in War on Consumption," *Philadelphia Inquirer*, 18 Feb 1909 (source of the quotation); "Foes of Tuberculosis Sadly in Need of Funds," *North American*, 18 Jul 1909, sec. 1, pt. 2; and Margaret Lehmann, "Report of the Superintendent," *ARVN* 25 (1911):8–9.

Data were reported on the disposition of patients between 1 Aug 1907 and 28 Feb 1911. Of the 758 patients, 40 percent died, 29 percent were judged suitable for family care after instruction, and 20 percent were sent to hospitals or sanatoriums. The remaining 11 percent had various other outcomes. An additional 167 patients were still under care at the time of the reports. See *ARVN* 22 (1908):15, 23 (1909):11, 24 (1910):12, 25 (1911):11.

14. Jacques, "Visiting Nurse in Tb," 135–36; Mable [*sic*] Jacques, "Report of Special Nurse on Tuberculosis," *ARVN* 23 (1909):11–13; and L. W. Quintard, "Report of the Superintendent," *ARVN* 23 (1909):9.

15. Board Minutes, Visiting Nurse Society of Philadelphia, 7 Jun 1907, VN-CSHN; L. W. Quintard, "Report of the Superintendent," *ARVN* 22 (1908):6–7; Mable [*sic*] Jacques, "Report of Special Nurse on Tuberculosis," *ARVN* 22 (1908): 15–16; Jacques, "Visiting Nurse in Tb," 134–36; idem, "Report of Special Nurse," 1909, 12; idem, "District Nursing versus Friendly Visiting," *JOL* 7 (Jan 1910): 386; "St. Stephen's Has Its First Clinic," n.d., a clipping, VN-CSHN; and "Medical Men Reinforced by Churches and Other Institutions in Fight against Tuberculosis," *North American*, 23 Feb 1908, sec. 3. Work at the Church of the Crucifixion lasted a few months; the class at St. Stephen's, two years.

16. Joseph H. Pratt, "The Class Method of Treating Consumption in the Homes of the Poor," *TNA* 3 (1907):59–68; idem, "The Class Method in the Home Treatment of Tuberculosis, and What It Has Accomplished," *TACA* 27 (1911): 87–118; and idem, "Results Obtained by the Class Method of Home Treatment in Pulmonary Tuberculosis During a Period of Ten Years," *Boston Medical and Surgical Journal* 176 (4 Jan 1917):13–15.

Pratt initiated his work at the Emmanuel Church with the aid of its rector, the Rev. Elwood Worcester. Worcester had previously been the rector of St. Stephen's in Philadelphia, where neurologist S. Weir Mitchell was a friend and parishioner. Worcester later, with colleagues, developed a psychotherapeutic healing method that became known as the Emmanuel Movement; he traced his ideas to a conversation with Mitchell and to the success of Pratt's class. See John G. Greene, "The Emmanuel Movement, 1906–1929," *New England Quarterly* 7 (Sep 1934):494–532.

17. Jacques, "Tb Nurse and Her Work," 284–85, and idem, *District Nursing*,

32–37 (34–35 for the quotation). A "fasch" was a long piece of cotton fabric with which Italian mothers wrapped their babies when they put them in bed until they were three or four months old. The arms were placed straight against the body and the legs straight together (interviews in Philadelphia by Linda V. Walsh with Theresa Serater, 7 Oct 1988, and Maria Leone, 30 Aug 1988, personally reported to the author).

18. Philadelphia's Bureau of Health reported 3,157 deaths from tuberculosis of the lungs in 1907. By a contemporary rule of thumb, the death rate was tripled to estimate the number of active living cases.

19. Jacques, *District Nursing*, 94–99, and La Motte, *Tb Nurse*, 28–32.

20. Jacques, "Tb Nurse and Her Work," 285, 344.

21. Jacques, "Visiting Nurse in Tb," 134. Flies were commonly thought to carry tubercle bacilli and spread infection.

22. Ibid., 134–35.

23. Ibid., 135. Florence Nightingale considered old wallpaper and other areas where dirt and "animal matters" accumulated to be sources of disease: "Old papered walls of years' standing, dirty carpets, uncleansed furniture, are just as ready sources of impurity to the air as if there were a dung-heap in the basement." She recommended frequent lime-washing (whitewashing) of walls. See "Notes on Nursing: What It Is and What It Is Not" (1859) and "Nursing the Sick" (1882), both in Lucy Ridgely Seymer, comp., *Selected Writings of Florence Nightingale* (New York: Macmillan, 1954), 138, 338. Early-twentieth-century reformers believed that tubercle bacilli lurked in dust and dirt; although, unlike Nightingale, they used disinfectants, their approach to cleanliness was similar.

24. "Foes of Tb Sadly in Need of Funds." The Visiting Nurse Society, like Flick, was skillful at using the press to promote its cause. For Jacques on promotion, see her *District Nursing*, 111–16.

25. Names of tuberculosis nurses and numbers of tuberculous patients in the *ARsVN*; Record of Gifts to the Endowment Fund of the Visiting Nurse Society of Philadelphia, VN-CSHN; and "Obituary: William Furness Jenks, M.D.," *Boston Medical and Surgical Journal* 105 (24 Nov 1881):503–4.

26. "Special Tuberculosis Work;" Jacques, "Visiting Nurse in Tb," 136; and idem, *District Nursing*, 35–36 (for the quotation). For pay, see Quintard, "Report of Head Nurse," 9–10; Jacques, *District Nursing*, 61, 91–92; and Board Minutes, VNSP, 4 Mar 1910, 5 Apr 1912. If a nurse lived at 1340 Lombard Street (VNS headquarters as of 1893), she received board, lodging, and laundry but twenty-five dollars less. Although a visiting nurse's salary was less than could be earned in private duty, Jacques considered the steadiness of the work advantageous. In 1913, the state dispensaries paid nurses sixty to seventy dollars a month.

27. Jacques, *District Nursing*, 7–12, 14–16 (16 for the third quotation), 21, 42, 76–77 (76 for the first two quotations), 92 (for the fourth quotation), 109–12, 120–21.

28. Board Minutes, VNSP, 1 Nov 1908; Quintard, "Report of Superintendent," (1909):8; "A Most Interesting Section," attributed to the *Evening Star*, 28 Sep [1908], a clipping, VN-CSHN; *TSICT*, vol. 5 (1908):240–41, 307–8; and "Seek Assistance of State in War on Consumption," *Philadelphia Inquirer*, 18 Feb 1909.

29. "Pioneers in Public Health: Ellen N. La Motte," *Trained Nurse and Hospital Review* 81 (Sep 1928):312; Ellen N. La Motte, "Tuberculosis Work of the Instructive Visiting Nurse Association of Baltimore," *American Journal of Nursing* 6 (Dec 1905):141–47; idem, "The Present Attitude of the Tuberculosis Nurse towards Her Work," *Johns Hopkins Hospital Bulletin* 21 (Apr 1910):115–17; and Vern L. Bullough, Olga M. Church, and Alice P. Stein, *American Nursing: A Biographical Dictionary*, s.v. La Motte, Ellen Newbold, and s.v. Lent, Mary E.

30. Ellen N. La Motte, "The Unteachable Consumptive," *TSICT*, vol. 3 (1908):256–60 (257–58 for quotations). La Motte wrote extensively, and her *Tuberculosis Nurse* is the best single source on the subject.

31. Mary E. Lent, "The True Functions of the Tuberculosis Nurse," *TSICT*, vol. 3 (1908):576–80.

32. Mabel Jacques, "Saving the Home," *JOL* 6 (Nov 1909):323–24 (323 for the quotation).

33. Jacques, "District Nursing versus Friendly Visiting," 387, and, for work colonies, idem, "Home Occupations in Families of Consumptives and Possible Dangers to the Public," *TSICT*, vol. 3 (1908):568–69. Jacques's emphasis on the effects of happiness on mind and health almost certainly reflected ideas of the Emmanuel movement (see n. 16). Dr. Carl E. Grammer, the rector who succeeded Worcester at St. Stephen's, was apparently using Worcester's "mental therapeutics" in the tuberculosis class there ("St. Stephen's Has Its First Clinic").

34. Mabel Jacques, "Saving the Home," 323–24. Note the similarity of Jacques's example to Superintendent Durburow's in 1883 (pp. 47–48).

35. Ibid., 324. Lent's paper from the Congress was reprinted in *JOL* 6 (Sep 1909):265–69. At the editor's invitation, Lent had added photographs of the bad conditions that justified her position.

36. Henry Fisher to LF, 25 Oct 1909; *Annual Report of the Department of Health of Buffalo*, New York (1910):69; and *Annual Report of the District Nursing Association of Buffalo* 26 (1911):17, 23–24. Jacques published through Jan 1912, but I have found no later trace of her.

37. Margaret Lehmann, "Report on Metropolitan Work," *ARVN* 25 (1911): 12, and Lee K. Frankel, "Standards in Visiting Nurse Work," read at the meeting of the National Organization for Public Health Nursing, 22 Jun 1915, 8–10, LFPM, vol. 130, no. 46. See also Philip P. Jacobs, "Welfare Work of the Metropolitan Life Insurance Company," *Survey* 24 (13 Aug 1910):705–7; Louis I. Dublin, *A 40 Year Campaign against Tuberculosis* (New York: Metropolitan Life Insurance Co., 1952), 54–55; and Diane B. Hamilton, "The Metropolitan Life Insurance Company Visiting Nursing Service (1909–1953)," (Ph.D. diss., University of Virginia, 1987). An industrial life insurance policy was the cheapest variety sold and required weekly premiums.

38. Board Minutes, VNSP, 7 Jun 1912, 4 Oct 1912; Lee K. Frankel and Louis Dublin, "Visiting Nursing and Life Insurance. Statistical Summary of Eight Years of Public Health Nursing for Industrial Policyholders of the Metropolitan Life Insurance Company, New York," *Quarterly Publications of the American Statistical Association Journal* 16 (Jun 1918; reprint, New York: Metropolitan Life Insurance Co., n.d.), 102; Katharine Tucker, "Report of the Superintendent," *ARVN* (1917):9; and statistics, *ARVN*, 1911–1929.

39. "Tuberculosis Work in Philadelphia," *Monthly Bulletin of the Department of Public Health and Charities of Philadelphia* 4 (Jun 1919):85–86; *ARKD* 3 [1909]: 41; *Annual Report of the Presbyterian Hospital in Philadelphia* 39 (Jan 1910):103; *RPS* (1916):16–17, (1917):17–18, (1918):8, 13, (1921):18–28; sources in chap. 11, n. 9; Anna G. Murphy to LF, 7, 15 Jan [1913]; and lists of dispensary staff, *ARCH*, 1909 through 1912. The small proportion of graduates who entered this field was not unusual then.

40. Albert P. Francine's discussion of W. L. Dunn, "The Responsibility for Relapse of Tuberculous Patients after Discharge," *TNA* 6 (1910):181; Albert P. Francine, "Principles of Social Service Work and Their Application in Practice at the State Tuberculosis Dispensary, Philadelphia," *American Journal of Public Health* 3 (Jul 1913):695–96; idem, "The State Tuberculosis Dispensaries," *PMJ* 17 (Sep 1914):940; and William G. Turnbull, "The State Sanatoria for Tuberculosis," *PMJ* 17 (Sep 1914):943. For the nurses' role, see *ARCH* 3 (1908):453–54, 4 (1909): 336–39, 5 (1910):404–7, 7 (1912):840–41; B. Franklin Royer, "The Department of Health's Activity in Handling Tuberculosis in Pennsylvania," *PMJ* 16 (Feb 1913):387–88; and Francine, "Principles of Social Service Work," 688–96.

41. Jacques, "District Nursing versus Friendly Visiting," 387; Buhler-Wilkerson, "False Dawn," 85–93; and Francine, "Principles of Social Service Work," 689–90. As of 1909, nurses in the state dispensaries were also supervised by a chief visiting dispensary nurse (Alice M. O'Halloran) and her assistant, but their visits were infrequent.

42. Mabel Jacques, "Relief, and the Tuberculosis Family," *Trained Nurse and Hospital Review* 46 (May 1911):276–77 (277 for the quotations); Ellen N. La Motte, "Tuberculosis Work," 143; and Francine, "Principles of Social Service Work," 693. By 1913 Maryland, New Jersey, New York, Wisconsin, and Minnesota had legalized compulsory institutionalization for selected consumptives, and by 1922 thirty-four cities (Philadelphia not among them) had followed suit. See "Compulsory Segregation Law," *Survey* 28 (24 Aug 1912):667; David R. Lyman, "The Control of the Careless Consumptive," *ART* 2 (Mar 1918):37; "Tuberculosis: A Chapter of a Forthcoming Report of the Committee on Municipal Health Department Practice of the American Public Health Association," *ART* 6 (Dec 1922):962; and Michael E. Teller, *The Tuberculosis Movement: A Public Health Campaign in the Progressive Era* (New York: Greenwood Press, 1988), 93–94.

The not-poor, operationally defined by many health departments as those who had private physicians, were usually exempted from visits by nurses and medical inspectors from the health departments. Jacques's assessment of the power of money was correct. See, for example, Daniel M. Fox, "Social Policy and City Politics: Tuberculosis Reporting in New York City, 1889–1910," *BHM* 49 (Summer 1975):169–95.

Chapter 14. Persuasion, Choice, and Circumstance

1. Lists of officers and boards of directors, *RPS*.

2. Treasurer's reports, *RPS*; *RPS* (1911):12–13; Esther G. Price, *Pennsylvania Pioneers Against Tuberculosis* (New York: National Tuberculosis Association,

1952), 206–7; Leigh M. Hodges, *The People against Tuberculosis: The Story of the Christmas Seal* (New York: National Tuberculosis Association, 1942); and Richard H. Shryock, *National Tuberculosis Association, 1904–1954. A Study of the Voluntary Health Movement in the United States* (New York: National Tuberculosis Association, 1957; reprint, Arno Press, 1977), 127–34.

3. Price, *Pennsylvania Pioneers*, 63; Charles J. Hatfield, "Introduction," *RPS* (1908):4; and treasurer's reports, *RPS*.

4. "Four Hundred Sick for One Bed!" *FAM* 1 (Jan 1909):14–15, and *RPS* (1911):5–6, (1913):3–20, (1914):5–6, 63–64. Bed capacity for tuberculous patients at Philadelphia General Hospital was 174 in 1904, 300 in 1908, 411 in 1916, and 495 in 1919 (directories of the National Association). For persisting need, see *AMP*, vol. 3 (1908):30; *FAM* 1 (Feb 1909):17; *AMP* vol. 3 (1912):47; and "A Tuberculosis Program for Pennsylvania," *RPS* (1913):16–18.

5. *RPS* (1911):10–12 (11 for the quotation), (1912):10, (1915):14–15.

6. Howard S. Anders, "Address and Annual Report by the President," *RPS* (1903):9 (for the quotations), and "Consumption 'Cures,'" *FAM* 2 (Feb 1911): 11. See also "A 'Sure Cure,'" *FAM* 2 (Mar 1911):5–7, 10–12; "Patent Medicines and Their Effects," *FAM* 2 (Sep 1911):15–16; and *Nostrums and Quackery. Articles on the Nostrum Evil and Quackery Reprinted, with Additions and Modifications, from the Journal of the American Medical Association*, 2nd ed. (Chicago: American Medical Association Press, 1912), 76–182 for "consumptive cures."

7. From 1909 through 1916, when the lengthy *ARCH* ceased, each report included favorable clinical studies of "Dixon's fluid," often with testimonials from physician-employees of the state system. All reports were statistically flawed. Flick acknowledged that his diet of milk and eggs was based on empiricism, not on exact scientific data (LF to Irving Fisher, 24 Oct 1905).

8. *RPS*; tracts of the Society; and *FAM*, 1909–1911.

9. Howard S. Anders, "The President's Address," *RPS* (1905):8; M. S. C., "How the Schools Can Aid in the Prevention of Tuberculosis," *FAM* 1 (Mar 1909):8–11; "Fifteen Thousand Children to Learn How to Fight Tuberculosis," *FAM* 2 (Sep 1911):1; "What the School Children Have Learned about Tuberculosis," *FAM* 2 (Oct 1911):3–6 (3 for the quotation); and *RPS* (1911):7–8, (1912):12–13, (1913):22–23, (1917):3.

10. Shryock, *NTA*, 102; James M. Anders, et al., to Bishop Mackay-Smith, 3 Mar 1910, copy of a letter to be sent to bishops, etc., as heads of churches in Pennsylvania, LFPM, vol. 137, no. 1; Asa S. Wing to LF, 23 Oct 1912, LFPM, vol. 124, no. 21; "800 Sermons on Tuberculosis," *RPS* (1913):21–22; and *RPS* (1914):5, (1915):5–6.

11. *RPS* (1912):8, (1916):7. The Society reported yearly on its press activities. The *JOL*, which originated as *The Outdoor Life* at Saranac Lake in 1904, was adopted as the official organ of the National Association for the Study and Prevention of Tuberculosis in 1906 (Robert G. Paterson, "Periodicals Devoted to Tuberculosis in the United States of America," *ART* 53 [May 1946]:502). The *FAM* failed to compete successfully for subscribers ("Shall There Be a Fresh Air Magazine?" LFPM, vol. 111, no. 47, and *RPS* 20 [1912]:10).

12. "How the Red Cross Seals Were Sold," *FAM* 2 (Dec 1911):5–7; "Why

the Red Cross Seal?" *FAM* 2 (Nov 1911):10; S. Adolphus Knopf, *A History of the National Tuberculosis Association: The Anti-Tuberculosis Movement in the United States* (New York: National Tuberculosis Association, 1922), 55–66; and Shryock, *NTA*, 127–34. The American Red Cross sold the seals before the NTA did. The NTA participated, and then in 1920 took over.

13. "The Work of the Y.M.C.A. Against Tuberculosis," *FAM* 1 (Jan 1909): 34–36; John Meade, "Of Interest to Wage Earners. Participation of Trade Unionists in Crusade Against Tuberculosis," *FAM* 1 (Jan 1909):20–22; "Department of Social Work," *FAM* 1 (Jan 1909):36–40; "Preliminary Report to the Labor Unions of Philadelphia," *FAM* 1 (Feb 1909):23–27; "The Work of the Y.M.C.A.," *FAM* 1 (Mar 1909):23–24; "Labor Unions and Tuberculosis," *FAM* 2 (Aug 1911):8; *RPS* (1911):9–10, (1914):6, (1915):7, (1916):4–5; and Price, *Pennsylvania Pioneers*, 196–229. Baby Saving Shows were displays designed to teach healthful methods of infant care.

14. "The Public Drinking Cup," *PHB*, no. 4 (Oct 1909):8–9; "Little Dangers to Be Avoided in the Daily Fight against Tuberculosis," *PHB*, no. 7 (Jan 1910):1–5; "Tuberculosis Exhibit," *ARCH* 7 (1912):840; "The Pulpit and the Great White Plague. Tuberculosis Sunday,'" *ARCH* (1913):97; "Health Exhibits of the Department," *ARCH* 10 (1915):796–99; *ARCH* 11 (1916):814–18; and for Dixon's promotion of dispensaries, *ARCH* 3 (1908):16–20.

15. *The Outdoor Life* to LF, 14 Nov, 8 Dec 1904; *FAM* 1 (Feb 1909):36; P. R. McDevitt to LF, 2 Jan 1906; Anna Curtin to LF, 9 Jan 1906; Eunice McKenna to LF, 17 Jan 1906; Class of 1905, St. Francis H. S. C., to LF, 9 Jan 1906; K. C. Melhour to the Civic Club, 2 Jan 1906, LFCP; and Louise S. Hatfield to LF, 10, 20 Jan, 10 Feb 1906. Flick's book was published in seven editions between 1903 and 1914. See also Samuel H. Adams to LF, 7 May 1904; Samuel H. Adams, "Tuberculosis: The Real Race Suicide," *McClure's Magazine* 24 (Jan 1905):234–49; *RPS* (1916):7; "A New Four-Reel Motion-Picture on Tuberculosis," *Bulletin of the National Association for the Study and Prevention of Tuberculosis* 1 (Jun 1915):1, 3; and "Health Exhibits of the Department," *ARCH* 10 (1915):793–95.

16. Metropolitan Life Insurance Company of New York, *A War upon Consumption*, 1909; Philip P. Jacobs, "Welfare Work of the Metropolitan Life Insurance Company," *Survey* 24 (13 Aug 1910):705–7; and Louis I. Dublin, *A 40 Year Campaign against Tuberculosis* (New York: Metropolitan Life Insurance Company, 1952), 53–54.

17. For language cited in this and the next paragraph, "An Institution Being Established Every Other Day in the United States," *FAM* 1 (Jan 1909):23; "Tuberculosis Campaign's Great Progress," *FAM* 1 (Feb 1909):14–15; Editorial, *FAM* 1 (Feb 1909):16–17; LF, "The Twentieth-Century Crusade," *FAM* 1 (Jun 1910):3–4; and J. Byron Deacon, "What the Philadelphia Health Department Is Doing to Prevent Tuberculosis," *FAM* 2 (Feb 1911):2–4 (3 for the quotation).

18. David A. Stewart, "Heroes of Tuberculosis," *FAM* 2 (Oct 1911):10–12 (11 for the quotation), and "Scientific Giving," *FAM* 2 (Dec 1911):12–14 (13 for the quotation). See also *ARCH* 4 (1909):29–30; "What One Little Woman Has Accomplished," *FAM* 1 (Feb 1909):27–29; "A Patient's Story," *FAM* 2 (Apr 1911):1–3; and "How I Got Well," *FAM* 2 (Jun 1911):5–6. In "The Industrialist

as Hero: An Emerging Educational Theme in Nineteenth-Century America," *Educational Studies* 12 (Spring 1981):69–83, Anthony F. C. Wallace discusses the hero myth in establishing new social values.

19. George R. Brown, "True Heroism," *Spunk* 3 (Jun 1911):4–5.

20. W. S. Ramsey to LF, 14 Dec 1908, SS.

21. For the two quotations, see Mrs. A. Birnbryer to LF, 9 Apr 1908, and Amelie A. Turner to LF, 21 Aug 1907, SS.

22. "The Public Drinking Cup," 8–9; Hugh Moore, "The Poisoned Cup," *FAM* 1 (Sep 1910):7; "Little Dangers to Be Avoided," 1–5; "Warns of Germs in Books," *Public Ledger*, 29 May 1916; Clara Atherton to LF, 31 May 1906; and Jos. F. Hayward to Chas. H. Thomas, LFCP, 30 Jul 1901. Flick thought that the state had become too alarmist and cited the fact that patients' mail from Mont Alto was stamped "disinfected" ("Proceedings of the Joint Committee of the Senate and House of Representatives," *Pennsylvania Legislative Journal*, Appendix [1913]: 5697). Other people expressed their worries to Flick about contacts at work, in schoolrooms, gymnasiums, and rented housing, on city streets, in their own neighborhoods, and elsewhere.

23. Elmer E. McKee, "Pro and Con—Mostly Con," *Spunk* 6 (Sep 1914):16–17.

24. Mary Mahony to LF, 17 Apr 1905, SS; F. A. Rigby to LF, 15 Oct 1911; and James P. Hood to LF, 27 Dec 1910. Mrs. Levis, having tried both Sunnyrest and Fern Cliff, died at White Haven about seven weeks after Mahony's report.

25. C. W. Gerhart to LF, 2 Apr 1909, and Lilla N.[?sp] Davis to LF, 28 Aug 1909.

26. E. R. Bush to LF, 5 Apr 1903.

27. *RPS* (1911):9, and Mrs. D. P. Stackhouse to LF, 24 Oct 1908.

28. Elizabeth L. Martin to LF, 1 Oct 1904.

29. LF, "Prognosis in Tuberculosis," *Amercian Medicine* 11 (6 Jan 1906):15–16; LF, "Tuberculosis As It Concerns the Physician," *Interstate Medical Journal* 18 (Feb 1911):202, 204; LF to Mrs. Mary A. South, 23 Nov 1907; and LF to Rev. James M. Grant, 28 Feb 1913.

30. Joseph S. Neff, "Tenth Annual Report of the Department of Public Health and Charities," *AMP*, vol. 3 (1912):21–22, and "Report on Former Patients of the Dispensaries Visited or Traced during 1914," *ARCH* 9 (1914):733.

31. George Hiestand to LF, n.d. [filed 16 Feb 1909].

32. Elmer E. McKee, "A Warning," *Spunk* 8 (Dec 1916):25.

33. LF, "Home Treatment of Tuberculosis," *Therapeutic Gazette*, 3d ser., vol. 18 (15 Jun 1902):369. See also LF, "Communities without Health Departments in the Crusade against Tuberculosis," *NYPMJ* 79 (11 Jun 1904):1129–30; George W. Norris, "The Diagnosis of Incipient Pulmonary Tuberculosis," *Medical News* 85 (17 Sep 1904):545–46; Thomas H. A. Stites, "The Tuberculosis Dispensary System of the Pennsylvania Department of Health: A Sketch of Its Organization and Methods," *PMJ* 12 (Jun 1910):701; "Producers and Consumers," *PHB*, no. 18 (Dec 1910):4; and Albert P. Francine, "The State Tuberculosis Dispensaries," *PMJ* 17 (Sep 1914):940–41. In discussing Stites's paper, "Tuberculosis Dispensary System," 711–12, William B. Stanton cited another reason why general

practitioners referred far-advanced patients to sanatoriums as if they had early tb. "In many cases he realizes that the patient is not a suitable one, but so much pressure is brought to bear by the family and friends and by patients who have been improved at sanatoriums that the physician has not the moral courage to refuse to send them."

34. Figures are calculated from tuberculosis beds in hospitals and sanatoriums listed in the directories of the National Association. Philadelphia and Pittsburgh had the only approved municipal facilities through 1911. In 1919, the White Haven Sanatorium had 250 beds (the largest number reported in the voluntary/private sector), and the Home for Consumptives at Chestnut Hill had 110 beds. Additional governmental expenditures included the care of consumptives in almshouses, insane asylums, and prisons, and state appropriations to voluntary institutions.

35. This principle, not understood in Flick's period, may be illustrated by a life-line marked with four points:

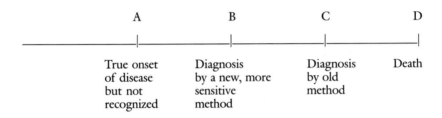

A	B	C	D
True onset of disease but not recognized	Diagnosis by a new, more sensitive method	Diagnosis by old method	Death

The apparent duration of life with a disease detected by an older, less sensitive method lies along the line from C to D. A new, more sensitive diagnostic method increases this duration to BD, thus increasing apparent survival by the interval BC. The patient dies, however, at the unchanged point D.

36. Symptoms of early tuberculosis were subtle, Flick asserted, and physicians should search for a history of occasional cough, loss of appetite, morning malaise, afternoon headaches, "occasionally a hypersensitiveness of the entire nervous system" or "alternative vivacity and depression." Physical signs could also be slight: a small rise in temperature "possibly reaching 99 or sometimes 100; a pulse above the normal and pupils dilated, perhaps one or both." On chest examination, the physician might find "slight bronchovesicular breathing," some increase in tactile fremitus and vocal resonance, slight bronchophony, and, usually, impaired resonance over the lesion. These signs, "more apt to be found over the back," could also be heard above or over the clavicle (LF, "Diagnosis and Treatment of Early Cases of Tuberculosis," *Interstate Medical Journal* 16 (Jul 1909):479.

In retrospect, none of these data are clear evidence of active tuberculosis. The symptoms have many possible explanations, and on physical examination the chest signs of inactive (healed) tuberculosis may be identical to those of active disease. Except for impaired resonance, these chest signs may even be found in normal persons. Large pupils and slightly elevated temperatures are not necessarily abnormal. A patient with all of these manifestations might, of course, have tuberculosis, and the odds in favor of that would have been much higher in Flick's day than now, especially among patients referred to a chest specialist. For recognition of overdiagnosis, see H. R. M. Landis, "The Tuberculosis Dispensary and Home Treatment," *Illinois Medical Journal* 20 (Dec 1911):648, and idem, "A Study of the Ultimate Results in the Dispensary Treatment of Tuberculosis," *TNA* 8 (1912):388–89.

Studies elsewhere documented erroneous diagnoses in sanatoriums. Of 1,400 patients sent to the Cook County Hospital for Consumptives in Illinois, presumably with advanced tuberculosis, 8.5 percent were found clinically nontuberculous (C. M. Wood, "Necessity of Examination of the Sputum in the Diagnosis of Pulmonary Tuberculosis," *JAMA* 35 [20 Oct 1900]:1019–20). Of 198 autopsies performed at the Boston Consumptives Hospital, 11.5 percent showed no active tuberculous lesions (J. Earle Ash, "The Pathology of the Mistaken Diagnoses in a Hospital for Advanced Tuberculosis," *JAMA* 64 [2 Jan 1915]:11–15). Overdependency on clinical evaluation without bacteriological study explains some of these errors, but physicians had a dilemma: active tuberculosis could exist with or without demonstrable tubercle bacilli.

37. Cecilia R. Flick, *Dr. Lawrence F. Flick As I Knew Him* (Philadelphia: Dorrance, 1956), 83, and Ella M. E. Flick, *Beloved Crusader: Lawrence F. Flick, Physician* (Philadelphia: Dorrance, 1944), 385 (for the quotation). In 1916, the Philadelphia General Hospital treated 2,371 patients in its tuberculosis department, but the roentgen ray laboratory, which examined only 312 chest, heart, and lung cases in the entire hospital, reported 107 cases of pulmonary tuberculosis. Most patients in the tuberculosis department, therefore, did not have chest x-rays.

38. Livingston Farrand, "A Comprehensive Program for the Prevention of Tuberculosis, *TSICT*, vol. 3 (1908):237 (see also 239); Lawrason Brown, "The Ultimate Results of Sanatorium Treatment," *TSICT*, vol. 1, pt. 2 (1908):927–39; Herbert M. King, "A Preliminary Study of the Value of Sanatorium Treatment," *TNA* 8 (1912):82–112; Albert P. Francine's discussion of W. L. Dunn, "The Responsibility for Relapse of Tuberculous Patients After Discharge," *TNA* 6 (1910):181; Homer Folks, "Address of the President. Some Adverse Factors of the Past Year," *TNA* 9 (1913):17–22; and Thomas J. Mays, "Effect of Present Prevention on the Spread of Consumption," *Medical Record* 82 (30 Nov 1912):977–80 (979 for the quotations). Farrand ranked hospitals for advanced and hopeless cases, unlike sanatoriums for curable patients, very high.

Chapter 15. Waiting Lists and Empty Beds

1. National Association for the Study and Prevention of Tuberculosis, comp., *A Tuberculosis Directory* (New York: National Association for the Study and Prevention of Tuberculosis, 1916); *Report of the Auditor General of Pennsylvania* (1915):647; and W. G. Turnbull, "County Tuberculosis Needs," *LP* 4 (Apr 1926):4.

2. Fred C. Johnson, "Pennsylvania State Sanatorium for Tuberculosis No. 1,

Mont Alto," *ARCH* 11 (1916):885, and Wm. G. Turnbull, "Pennsylvania State Sanatorium for Tuberculosis No. 2, Cresson," *ARCH* 11 (1916):915.

3. Franklin Royer, "The Public Aspect of Tuberculosis," *Public Health Journal* 12 (May 1921):213–14. Royer was speaking generally here.

4. *Report of the Auditor General* (1916):599, (1920):1064, and *Pennsylvania Department of Health Yearbook 1929*, 154–55. Expenditures and admissions fell before appropriations did, suggesting a departmental, not a legislative, decision. Appropriations for the tb program first diminished in 1919; those for the health department, in 1923 (*Smull's Legislative Handbook and Manual of Pennsylvania*). By 1921, the health department was devoting only 42 percent of its budget to tuberculosis. By 1923, admissions had decreased 34 percent from their peak in 1916. The *ARCH* ceased after 1916, and in the summer of 1916 the *PHB* deteriorated into repetitive "Little Talks on Health and Hygiene." Epidemics of poliomyelitis and typhoid fever occurred in 1916; influenza, in 1918. Martin had also been Director of Health and Charities in Philadelphia between 1903 and 1905. For fiscal issues, see "$90,000,000 Set as Sproul's Limit," *Public Ledger*, 27 Jan 1921; "Economy in State Offices Demanded," *Public Ledger*, 4 Jun 1921; "Pinchot Demands $130,000,000 Cut in State Budget," *Public Ledger*, 18 Dec 1922; "Four Years of Pennsylvania's Department of Health," *LP* 1 (Jan 1923):1; and *Biennial Report of the Auditor General of Pennsylvania* (1925):196, (1931):20;

5. Karl Schaffle, "The Functions of the Tuberculosis Dispensary," Wm. G. Turnbull, "Tubercle Bacillus Infection," and J. D. McLean, "The Department's Future Tuberculosis Campaign," all in *PHB*, no. 104 (Feb 1920):105–6, 111–14, 118–19 respectively; Edward Martin to LF, 20 Feb 1920; W. G. Turnbull to Mr. DeWees, 23 Sep 1920, copy, LFCU; and A. P. Francine, "State Tuberculosis Clinics," *LP* 1 (Jan 1923):16. Mont Alto's hospital reopened in Nov 1923 for tuberculous veterans whose care was paid for by the federal government. The federal contract lapsed in 1923, and in 1924 the building reopened for children (Charles H. Miner, "Opening Address at the Mont Alto Camp of Instruction," *LP* 2 (Jul–Aug 1924):5.

6. A. P. Francine, "The State Tuberculosis Work, What Is Being Done, and Future Plans," *PMJ* 24 (Mar 1921):412–13; idem, "Local Responsibility for Community Welfare with Special Reference to Tuberculosis," *PMJ* 25 (Apr 1922): 469–72 (including discussion); idem, "Suggestions Concerning County Tuberculosis Sanatoria in Pennsylvania," *PMJ* 25 (Aug 1922):789–93; *RPS* (1921):4 (for the quotation); and "State Department of Health, Harrisburg, Pa.," *PMJ* 25 (Dec 1921):202.

7. Francine, "Local Responsibility," 470–71 (470 for the first quotation); idem, "State Tuberculosis Work," 411–12 (for the second quotation); McLean, "Department's Future Campaign," 117; and Edgar T. Shields, "Tuberculosis Clinics Section," *LP* 3 (Mar–May 1925):7.

8. Ward Brinton, "The Tuberculosis Question in Philadelphia," *MBDH* 8 (Dec 1923):8–18 (17 for the quotation).

9. *The Report of the Citizens' Committee on the Finances of Pennsylvania to Hon. Gifford Pinchot*, Part 3 (1923), 170–71; *Biennial Report, Pennsylvania Department of Health* (1930):96, 101, 107–9; E. C. Allison, "Sanatoria Training Schools," *Spunk*

17 (Feb 1926):19; Henry A. Gorman, "The Aim of the Sanatorium Training School," *Spunk* 18 (Nov 1926):17–18; *Yearbook 1929*, 153; T. H. A. Stites, "Cresson," *Pennsylvania's Health* 10 (Jan–Feb 1932):71; "Patient Nurses Training Class," *Spunk* 23 (Mar 1932):48; and Fannie A. Daugherty, "Nursing History in State Sanatorium of South Mountain, Pennsylvania," *Spunk* 29 (Jun 1937):36–41.

10. Arnold C. Klebs, "The Frequency of Tuberculosis," in *Tuberculosis* (New York: D. Appleton, 1909), 105–16; C. von Pirquet, "The Frequency of Tuberculosis in Childhood," *TSICT*, vol. 2 (1908):559–61; Lawrason Brown, "The Specificity, Danger, and Accuracy of the Tuberculin Tests," *American Journal of the Medical Sciences*, n.s., 142 (Oct 1911):469–76; and H. R. M. Landis, "The Tuberculosis Crusade, *PMJ* 17 (Nov 1913):103–4. For the children's movement, see S. Josephine Baker, *Fighting for Life* (New York: Macmillan, 1939); Lela B. Costin, *Two Sisters for Social Justice: A Biography of Grace and Edith Abbott* (Urbana: University of Illinois Press, 1983); and Alisa C. Klaus, "Women's Organizations and the Infant Health Movement in France and the United States, 1890–1920," in *Lady Bountiful Revisited: Women, Philanthropy, and Power*, ed. Kathleen D. McCarthy (New Brunswick, N.J.: Rutgers University Press, 1990).

11. "Will Organize School Children as Health Crusaders," *Spunk* 8 (Dec 1916):40–41; *RPS* (1917):17, (1918):12, (1919):23, 34, 38, (1920):5–6, (1921):5–8; Richard H. Shryock, *National Tuberculosis Association, 1904–1954: A Study of the Voluntary Health Movement* (New York: National Tuberculosis Association, 1957; reprint, Arno Press, 1977), 170–73; Sarah D. Wyckoff, "Nutrition Classes for Children," *PMJ* 25 (Feb 1922):320–29; and Walter S. Cornell, "Medical Inspection of the Public Schools of Philadelphia," *MBDH* 10 (Sep 1925):108–11, 116–18.

12. William N. Bradley, "Tuberculosis in Children," *PMJ* 24 (Feb 1921): 285–87; Cornell, "Medical Inspection," 113; John D. Donnelly, "Malnutrition as a Pretuberculous State in Children," *PMJ* 25 (Feb 1922):317–20; and *ARKD* 26 (1931):23.

13. "Phipps Institute Outdoor School," *FAM* 2 (Sep 1911):3–6; *RPS* (May 1913):64; "County Society Reports," *PMJ* 19 (Mar 1916):474; Walter S. Cornell to LF, 30 Nov 1915; and Walter S. Cornell, "Modern Application of School Medical Inspection," *MBDH* 5 (Feb 1920):21. For open-air schools elsewhere, see Isabel F. Hyams and James J. Minot, "Boston's Outdoor School," *JOL* 6 (Jul 1909):187–93; Leonard P. Ayres, "Open-Air Schools," *TNA* 7 (1911):77–83; and H. W. Hetherington, "Open-Air Schools for the Treatment of Tuberculous Children," *ART* 20 (Oct 1929):511–31.

14. Alfred F. Hess, "The Tuberculosis Preventorium," *Survey* 30 (30 Aug 1913):666–68 (667 for the quotation), and idem, "The Significance of Tuberculosis in Infants and Children, with Measures for Their Protection," *JAMA* 72 (11 Jan 1919):83–88. For a personal account, see Eileen Simpson, *Orphans: Real and Imaginary* (New York: Weidenfeld and Nicolson, 1987), 47–61.

15. "Fifth Anniversary of the Woman's Auxiliaries," *ARKD* 5 (1911):46–47; "Sister Maria Roeck," *ARKD* 34 (1939):13; J. Willoughby Irwin, "Report of Medical Director and Physician In Chief," *ARKD* 3 (1909):39; idem, "Report of Medical Director and Physician in Chief," *ARKD* 4 (1910):15–16; Ida W. Hutzel,

"Annual Report of the Board of Managers," *ARKD* 5 (1911):11; A. S. W., "Our Farm," *ARKD* 5 (1911):87–88; and Sr. Maria Roeck, "Report of Sister-in-Charge," *ARKD* 8 (1914):13.

16. "Hamburg Highlights," *Spunk* 14 (Sep 1922):44 (for the quotation); W. L. Latimer, "The Children's Hospital," *Spunk* 16 (Nov 1924):20; William G. Turnbull, "Tuberculosis Sanatoria," *LP* 3 (Mar–May 1925):25–27; "The Health Camp for Children," *LP* 3 (Oct 1925):24; and *Yearbook 1929*, 156, 163–64. Of 191 children reported in 1928, River Crest had only one definite and two suspicious cases of tuberculosis. Eighty-one children (42 percent) had had contact with definite cases (*ARKD* 22 [1928]:27).

17. Harry W. Goos, "Report of Children's Clinic," *ARKD* 7 (1913):41; Cornell, "Medical Inspection," 106–10, 117–18; Latimer, "Children's Hospital," 20; A. J. Bohl, "Testing for Tuberculosis," *Pennsylvania's Health* 8 (Sep–Oct 1930): 20–21; W. G. Turnbull, "Helio Therapy at Cresson," *LP* 1 (Jan 1923):23 (for the quotation); idem, "Practical Heliotherapy," *Atlantic Medical Journal* 27 (Dec 1923):132–34; idem, "Heliotherapy," *LP* 4 (Nov–Dec 1926):6–7; and notes and photographs in *Spunk*. At the Kensington Dispensary, defects were corrected through the children's clinic, not at River Crest. Auguste Rollier, a Swiss physician, had popularized heliotherapy for tb of the skin, bones, and joints (Paul de Kruif, *Men Against Death* [New York: Harcourt, Brace, 1932], 300–316).

18. Annette S. Woll, "A Word from 'River Crest,'" *ARKD* 13 (1919):32; "Creating an Immunity," *Spunk* 17 (Aug 1925):26; and Theodore B. Appel to Hon. John S. Fisher, Governor of Pennsylvania, 5 Sep 1928, Pennsylvania State Archives, RG 11, Records of Department of Health, folder 1. Walter Ziegler, who as a (nontuberculous) boy was sent to the Children's Hospital at Mont Alto, gained forty pounds and was grateful for his stay (interview with author, South Mountain, Pa., 21 Apr 1986).

19. *RPS*, and directories of the National Association.

20. M. L. Faust, "Sources of Revenue of the States with a Special Study of the Revenue Sources of Pennsylvania," *Annals of the American Academy of Political and Social Science* 95 (May 1921):113–22; *RPS* (1926):4; *RPS* (1927):3; W. G. Turnbull, "County Tuberculosis Needs," *LP* 4 (Apr 1926):4; J. C. Reifsnyder, "County Tuberculosis Sanatoria," *LP* 5 (Jan–Feb 1927):5; and Schaffle, "Functions of the Tb Dispensary," with discussion, 106–8 (for the quotations).

21. Turnbull, "County Tb Needs," 4–7 (6 for the quotation), and idem, "Philadelphia's Use of State Sanatoria," *MBDH* 13 (Apr 1928):11–12.

22. Turnbull, "County Tb Needs," 6–7.

23. Theodore B. Appel, "Health and the Depression," *Pennsylvania's Health* 11 (Jul–Aug 1933):10–11, and directories of the National Association.

24. Numbers of deaths (tb of all forms) from the U.S. Bureau of the Census, *Mortality Statistics*; beds in hospitals and sanatoriums from directories of the National Association; and, for NTA recommendations, Shryock, *NTA*, 154. Death rates were more reliable than case rates.

25. LF papers; *ARsFH*; and Mary G. Marren to LF, 26 Jul 1926.

26. H. M. Neale to LF, 24 Mar 1915; LF to H. M. Neale, 27 Mar 1915; LF to Anna L. Morris, 13 Sep 1916; Isadore Kaufman to LF, 4 Oct 1916; LF to Mary

G. Marren, 4 Oct 1926; *Weekly Roster and Medical Digest* 22 (16 Oct 1926):6; and mortality rates and durations of stay from *ARsFH*. According to "Hospital Management," 3 Dec 1932, a clipping, LFSB, vol. 4, the White Haven Sanatorium paid its medical staff during the year honoraria totaling fourteen thousand dollars.

27. Anna L. Morris to LF, 24 May 1920; Mary G. Marren to LF, 19 Feb 1921; lists of guarantors, *ARFH*, 1923–1935; "Tb Drop Hits White Haven" [1926], a clipping, LFSB, vol.4; and Alex. Armstrong to LF, 7 Jul 1926. Between 1923 and 1931, White Haven also took tuberculous veterans and was paid by the U.S. government.

28. For the public and voluntary functions of general hospitals, see Rosemary Stevens, *In Sickness and in Wealth: American Hospitals in the Twentieth Century* (New York: Basic Books, 1989).

29. Charles H. Miner to LF, 10 Dec 1931, and LF to Anna L. Morris, 12 Dec 1931.

30. *Wilkes-Barre Record*, 19 Oct 1917; Edward M. Keck, interview with author, Allentown, Pa., 8 Jul 1983; gravestone of Margaret G. O'Hara, Holy Cross Cemetery, Yeadon, Pa.; Kathryn Riordan, interview with author, Gwynedd, Pa., 6 Jan 1981; and A. J. Cohen to LF, 28 May 1931.

31. Anna L. Morris to Joseph Walsh, 15 Dec 1931, LFCU.

32. Joseph Walsh to LF, 16 Dec 1931; LF to Anna L. Morris, 16 Dec 1931; and Anna L. Morris to LF, 17 Dec 1931. Flick's letters stop for several months after this episode, but there is no evidence that the farming-out plan was ever effected.

33. LF to Anna L. Morris, 28 Jan 1920, 9, 16 Feb 1933, and Anna L. Morris to LF, 14 Feb 1933.

34. LF to Jas. J. Walsh, 28 Oct 1925; LF to Jacob Billikopf, 16 Mar 1927 (for the quotations); "After Thirty-Eight Years," *ARFH* 35 (1933):4; Charlotte B. Parish to White Haven Sanatorium Association, 2 Jun 1934, LFCU; Charlotte B. Parish to LF, 7 Jun 1934; LF to Charlotte B. Parish, 8 Jun 1934; "Report of the Board of Directors," *ARFH* 38 (1936):7; and, for diagnoses, *ARsFH*. Diagnoses included heart and mental disorders, but most were of chest diseases, particularly anthracosilicosis, a condition common among local miners.

35. Joseph Walsh to the Members of the Visiting Staff, White Haven Sanatorium, 22 Jun 1934, LFCU.

36. For preventoriums, LF to Alex H. Davisson, 27 Dec 1935, and LF to Harold L. Ickes, 20 Apr 1935 (for the quotation). For hospitals, James M. Anders, "Some Practical Aspects of the Subject of Additional Hospitals for Tuberculosis Patients in Philadelphia," *MBDH* (Aug 1930):15–22; LF to J. J. Sullivan, 17 Apr 1931, 10 Jun 1931; A. J. Cohen to LF, 28 May 1931; LF to A. J. Cohen, 1 Jun 1931; LF to Harry Mackey, 7 Dec 1931; Harvey D. Brown to [Jacob] Billikopf, 17 Dec 1931, LFCU; LF to Jacob Billikopf, 23 Dec 1931; and LF to John Beardsley, 16 Nov 1932.

37. Dorothy E. Wiesner, "The Care of Tuberculosis Patients in General Hospitals in Philadelphia," *ART* 33, suppl. (Jan 1936):109–37.

38. Wiesner, "Care of Tb," 117–18; J. W. Cutler, "Ambulatory Pneumothorax and Public Health," *Medical Journal and Record* 137 (19 Apr 1933):326–30; and idem, "The Increasing Importance of Pneumothorax Therapy in Pulmonary Tuberculosis," *JAMA* 106 (18 Apr 1936):1366–73.

39. G. L. Leslie, "Collapse Measures for Pulmonary Tuberculosis," *Spunk* 26 (Jul 1934):24.

40. "Symposium on Thoracic Surgery," *PMJ* 32 (Sep 1929):855–66; John B. Flick and John H. Gibbon, "The Application of Thoracoplasty to the Treatment of Pulmonary Tuberculosis," *PMJ* 39 (Jul 1936):768–71; and Moses Behrend, "Surgery of the Tuberculous Lung," *MBDH* (Nov–Dec 1935):3–9.

41. Behrend, "Surgery," 3; "Supplementary Medical Report," *ARFH* 39 (1937):9; and Frank A. Craig, "Address of the President," *ARFH* 40 (1938):3, 5. Pneumothorax was used at White Haven long before this change in facilities (Alexander Armstrong, "Present Status of Therapeutic Pneumothorax in Pulmonary Tuberculosis," *PMJ* 23 [Mar 1920]:317, and Frank A. Craig, *The Story of the White Haven Sanatorium* [n.p., n.d.], 43–44).

42. "Modern Weapons and Education in State-wide Fight on Tuberculosis," *RPS* (1936):7; "Steps Toward Meeting Shortage of Tuberculosis Hospital Beds in State," *Spunk* 29 (May 1937):14; Edith MacBride Dexter, "Our Major Problem," *Pennsylvania's Health* 14 (Jul 1937):1–9; "Official State Tuberculosis Program Outlined," *PMJ* 41 (May 1938):736–37; Commonwealth of Pennsylvania, *New, Reestablished, and Reorganized Services of the Department of Health, January 15, 1935– March 1, 1938*, (n.p., n.d.), 18–19, 23–24; *Pennsylvania Department of Health: Story in Pictures of Four Years of Progressive Achievement* (n.p., n.d.), (for the quotations); and Mary Henderson, "Review of Hamburg," *Spunk* 31 (Apr 1939):59.

Chapter 16. "P.S. I . . . Am Colored"

1. Robert D. Freeman to LF, 18 Nov 1906.

2. W. E. B. Du Bois, *The Philadelphia Negro: A Social Study* (1899; reprint, New York: Schocken Books, 1967), 108–9. For background, see also Vincent P. Franklin, *The Education of Black Philadelphia: The Social and Educational History of a Minority Community, 1900–1950* (Philadelphia: University of Pennsylvania Press, 1979); Allen B. Ballard, *One More Day's Journey: The Making of Black Philadelphia* (Philadelphia: ISHI Publications, 1987); Theodore Hershberg, ed., *Philadelphia: Work, Space, Family, and Group Experience in the Nineteenth Century* (Oxford: Oxford University Press, 1981); and Roger Lane, *Roots of Violence in Black Philadelphia, 1860–1900* (Cambridge, Mass.: Harvard University Press, 1986).

3. Du Bois, *Philadelphia Negro*, 90–92.

4. Ibid., 113–14; "No. 743, An Act," *Laws of the General Assembly of Pennsylvania, Session of 1913*, 1223; N[athan] F. Mossell, "The Modern Hospital Largely Educational," *JNMA* 8 (Jul–Sep 1916):133–34; B. C. H. Harvey, "Provision for Training Colored Medical Students," *JNMA* 22 (Oct–Dec 1930):186–89; Herbert M. Morais, *The History of the Negro in Medicine*, International Library of Negro Life and History (New York: Publishers Co., 1967–1968); David McBride, *Integrating the City of Medicine: Blacks in Philadelphia Health Care, 1910–1965* (Philadelphia: Temple University Press, 1989), 85–107; and Vanessa N. Gamble, "The Negro Hospital Renaissance: The Black Hospital Movement, 1920–1940" (Ph.D. diss., University of Pennsylvania, 1987).

5. Virginia M. Alexander, "The Social, Economic and Health Problems of

North Philadelphia Negroes and Their Relation to a Proposed Interracial Public Health Demonstration Center," typescript, 1935, 86–121 (121 for the quotation), Papers of Virginia M. Alexander, UPA.

6. Hospital Library and Service Bureau, "Report on Informal Study of the Educational Facilities for Colored Nurses and Their Use in Hospital, Visiting and Public Health Nursing," in *Black Women in the Nursing Profession: A Documentary History*, ed. Darlene C. Hine (New York: Garland Publishing, 1985), 46, 49; Mossell, "Modern Hospital," 134; and Negro History Files, Record Group 41, Records of the WPA Pennsylvania Historical Survey, Pennsylvania State Archives.

7. Morais, *History*, 39–70, 74–88; Todd L. Savitt, "Lincoln University Medical Department—A Forgotten 19th-Century Black Medical School," *Journal of the History of Medicine and Allied Sciences* 40 (Jan 1985):42–65; Gamble, "Negro Hospital Renaissance"; "Some Events in the History of the Frederick Douglass Memorial Hospital and Training School," *ARFD* 10–11 (1905–1906):60–68; "The Douglass Hospital," *Crisis* 3 (Jan 1912):118–20; Alfred Gordon, "Frederick Douglass Memorial Hospital and Training School," in *Philadelphia—World's Medical Centre* [Philadelphia, ca. 1930], 58–60; Elliott M. Rudwick, "A Brief History of Mercy-Douglass Hospital in Philadelphia," *Journal of Negro Education* 20 (Winter 1951):50–66; and Russell F. Minton, "The History of Mercy-Douglass Hospital," *JNMA* 43 (May 1951):153–59. Frederick Douglass—ex-slave, abolitionist, orator, and human rights leader—died early in 1895.

8. Population figures from U.S. Census Reports, tabulated in Franklin, *Education*, 8, and Du Bois, *Philadelphia Negro*, 75–76. The white population grew 23.6 percent in this decade. See also W. E. B. Du Bois, *The Souls of Black Folk*, (1903; reprint, New York: New American Library, 1969); and Frederick L. Hoffman, "The Decline in the Tuberculosis Death-Rate, 1871–1912," *TNA* 9 (1913):128–29. Tb death rates during slavery, poorly documented, may well have been lower (Vanessa N. Gamble, "Introduction," *Germs Have No Color Line: Blacks and American Medicine, 1900–1940* [New York: Garland Publishing, 1989]).

9. Du Bois, *Philadelphia Negro*, 113–14, 162 (114 for the quotation); *ARFD* 2 (1987):12; Elsie Witchen, *Tuberculosis and the Negro in Pittsburgh: A Report of the Negro Health Survey* (Tuberculosis League of Pittsburgh, 1934), 53; Wilbert C. Jordan, "Voodoo Medicine," in *Textbook of Black-Related Diseases*, ed. Richard A. Williams (New York: McGraw-Hill Book Co., 1975), 715–38; Loudell F. Snow, "Sorcerers, Saints and Charlatans: Black Folk Healers in Urban America," *Culture, Medicine and Psychiatry* 2 (Mar 1978):69–106; and Hans A. Baer, "Toward a Systematic Typology of Folk Healers," *Phylon* 43 (Winter 1982):327–43.

10. Alexander, "Social Problems," 60–65, 69, 121 (61, 62, 121 for quotations).

11. Murray P. Horwood, "A Tuberculosis Survey of Philadelphia," *American Journal of Public Health* 14 (Jan 1924):32; Du Bois, *Philadelphia Negro*, 160–61 (160 for the quotation); Gamble, "Introduction"; and Marion M. Torchia, "Tuberculosis among American Negroes: Medical Research on a Racial Disease, 1830–1950," *Journal of the History of Medicine and Allied Sciences* 32 (Jul 1977):252–79. For conjecture about other groups, see Lilian Brandt, "Consumption in the United States. Part 3. Race," *Charities* 9 (6 Dec 1902):570–75, and John B. Huber,

Consumption: Its Relation to Man and His Civilization, Its Prevention and Cure (Philadelphia: J. B. Lippincott, 1906), 100–107.

12. Livingston Farrand to LF, 31 Aug 1905; LF to Mary M. Wilson, 8 Sep 1905; Mary M. Wilson to LF, 11 Sep 1905; and LF to Livingston Farrand, 11, 12 Sep 1905.

13. National Tuberculosis Association, comp. *A Directory of Sanatoria, Hospitals, Day Camps and Preventoria* (New York: National Tuberculosis Association, 1923), 99–105, and Henry M. Minton, "The Proper Disposition of the Tuberculosis Case," *JNMA* 16 (Apr–Jun 1924):143. According to national directories, 1923 to 1938, Pennsylvania tb institutions admitting blacks increased from 41 to 72 percent. The latter figure includes Mercy and Douglass, both termed "colored," not the usual "Negroes admitted."

14. ES to LF, 2 Nov 1901.

15. *RHPI* 1 (1904):12 (for the quotation). See also *RHPI* 2 (1905):13–14, 3 (1906):16–17; T. S. Burwell, "Pulmonary Tuberculosis: Some Observations from a Study of Three Hundred Cases," *JNMA* 15 (Jan–Mar 1923):45, and Minton "Proper Disposition," 142–43.

16. Harold E. Farmer, interview with author, Wayne, Pa., 2 Jul 1985. Dr. Farmer graduated from the University of Pennsylvania Medical School in 1932 and worked at the Phipps Institute between 1935 and 1937. Deficiency in intestinal lactase has been reported in up to 80 or 90 percent of black adults in the U.S. (Norman Kretchmer, "Lactose and Lactase," *Scientific American* 227 [Oct 1972]: 70–78, and Norton J. Greenberger and Kurt J. Isselbacher, "Disorders of Absorption," in *Harrison's Principles of Internal Medicine* 11th ed., ed. Eugene Braunwald et al. [New York: McGraw-Hill, 1987], 1274).

17. *Spunk* 11 (Sep 1919):12.

18. Alex. Armstrong to LF, 11, 23 May 1910, and F. A. Rigby to LF, 15 Oct 1911.

19. LF to Alex. Armstrong, 12, 24 May 1910, and LF to Francis B. Bracken, 7 Dec 1914.

20. LF to Anna L. Morris, 1 Dec 1914, including a copy of the patients' first protest and LF's response, and "Committee for patients" to M. S. Kemmerer, 4 Dec 1914, LFCU.

21. LF to Anna L. Morris, 1–2, 4, 19 Dec 1914; LF to Francis B. Bracken, 9 Dec 1914; LF to M. S. Kemmerer, 2 Jan 1915; LF to Frank A. Craig, 23 Dec 1914; Frank A. Craig to LF, 21 Jan 1915; and Application Blank for White Haven Sanatorium, LFPM, vol. 137, no. 115. The medical administration committee refused to accept the resignation, and Flick continued as medical director until 1917, when Joseph Walsh replaced him.

22. Mabel Jacques, "The Visiting Nurse in Tuberculosis: Her Importance as an Educational Agent," *JOL* 6 (May 1909):136–37.

23. W. G. Turnbull, "Philadelphia's Use of State Hospitals and Sanatoria," *MBDH* 13 (Apr 1928):12–13. See also Witchen, *Tuberculosis and the Negro*, 45–46.

24. C[harles] J. H[atfield], "Henry Robert Murray Landis, 1872–1937," *ART* 37 (Jan 1938):100–103 (102 for the quotation); D. J. McCarthy, "Memoir of

Henry Robert Murray Landis, M.D.," *TSCP* 4th ser., vol. 6 (1938–1939):254–55; and Harold E. Farmer, "The Education of Henry Robert Murray Landis, 1872–1937," *Bryn Mawr Hospital Bulletin* 6 (Summer 1984):37–41.

25. *The Whittier Centre* [Nov 1, 1913]:1, 3, and *The Whittier Centre* (1914): 5. See also August Meier, *Negro Thought in America, 1880–1915: Racial Ideologies in the Age of Booker T. Washington* (Ann Arbor: University of Michigan Press, 1963).

26. *The Whittier Centre* (1914):4–5; H. R. M. Landis, "Colored Physicians and Colored Nurses for Colored Patients," *TNA* 12 (1916):378; and Harvey D. Brown, "Tuberculosis Work Among Negroes in Philadelphia," *ART* 36 (Dec 1937):788–89.

27. Mrs. E[lizabeth] W. Tyler, "Summary of Work, Feb 1st to Oct 1st, 1914," *The Whittier Centre* (1914):5–6. For Tyler, see Anna B. Coles, "The Howard University School of Nursing in Historical Perspective," *JNMA* 61 (Mar 1969); reprint, Hine, *Black Women*, 31; and Mary E. Carnegie, *The Path We Tread: Blacks in Nursing, 1854–1984* (Philadelphia: J. B. Lippincott Co., 1986), 148–49.

28. Tyler, "Summary of Work," 6–7, 9, and Landis, "Colored Physicians and Colored Nurses," 378.

29. H. R. M. Landis, "The Clinic for Negroes at the Henry Phipps Institute," *TNA* 17 (1921):431; idem, "The Tuberculosis Problem and the Negro," *Virginia Medical Monthly* 49 (Jan 1923):565; and *RPS* (1915):10.

30. W. Montague Cobb, "Henry McKee Minton, 1870–1946," *JNMA* 47 (Jul 1955):285–86, and Landis, "Clinic for Negroes," 430–31.

31. *RPS* (1915):11, (1916):11; and Board Minutes, Visiting Nurse Society of Philadelphia, VN-CSHN, 2 Jun, 6 Oct 1916. In 1913, Jefferson Hospital had taken over the old Phipps building for a chest department.

32. Brown, "Tuberculosis Work," 791–98; "The Philadelphia Health Council and Tuberculosis Committee," in *Philadelphia—World's Medical Centre*, 48–50; and *Twenty Years of Tuberculosis Work by the Philadelphia Health Council and Tuberculosis Committee*, (n.p. [ca. 1939]), 5–7, 14. For the clinics of the Negro Bureau, see *RsPS*; *The Story of the Whittier Centre*, (1924):14–15; Haven Emerson, Sol Pincus, and Anna C. Phillips, *Philadelphia Hospital and Health Survey* (Philadelphia: Philadelphia Hospital and Health Survey Committee, 1930), 219; and Philadelphia Health Council and Tuberculosis Committee, *Philadelphia Association of Tuberculosis Clinics: Statistical Summary of Clinics in 1932*. Inadequate funds closed Clinic No. 4 in 1933 and Clinic No. 3 by 1935 (Brown, "Tuberculosis Work," 793, and Fannie Eshleman, "The Negro Nurse in a Tuberculosis Program," *Public Health Nurse* 27 [Jul 1935]:378).

33. Landis, "Colored Physicians and Colored Nurses," 377–78; idem, "Clinic for Negroes," 433; idem, "Tb Problem and the Negro," 1923, 563–66; and idem, "Tuberculosis and the Negro," *Annals of the American Academy of Political and Social Science* 140 (Nov 1928):86–89.

34. Landis, "Tb Problem and the Negro," 1923, 561–63; "Negro Migration Problem," [edit.], *Public Ledger*, 29 May 1923, 10; Sadie T. Mossell, "The Standard of Living Among One Hundred Negro Migrant Families in Philadelphia," *Annals of the American Academy of Social and Political Science* 98 (Nov 1921):173–78; Pennsylvania Department of Welfare, *Negro Survey of Pennsylvania* (Harrisburg, Pa.,

1927), 89–90; and for background, C. Vann Woodward, *The Strange Career of Jim Crow*, 3rd rev. ed. (New York: Oxford University Press, 1974).

35. Henry M. Minton, "Negro Physicians and Public Health Work in Pennsylvania," *Opportunity: A Journey of Negro Life* 2 (Mar 1924):74; Meier, *Negro Thought in America*, 270–78; E. Franklin Frazier, "Human, All Too Human: The Negro's Vested Interest in Segregation," in *E. Franklin Frazier on Race Relations*, ed. G. Franklin Edwards (Chicago: University of Chicago Press, 1968), 283–91; and Franklin, *Education*. The idea that black nurses and physicians were uniquely qualified and more capable than whites in understanding and influencing black patients was repeatedly emphasized by Landis and was echoed by Fannie Eshleman in her "Negro Nurse in a Tb Program," 378. See also Pa. Dept. Welfare, *Negro Survey*, 90, 95.

36. For Minton as superintendent, see *Bi-Annual Report of the Mercy Hospital and School for Nurses* (1919–1921):6. At least three medical interns and twenty graduate nurses from Mercy took positions at the Phipps Institute between 1923 and 1934 (*RsHPI*; *Reports of the Mercy Hospital and School of Nursing*; and data attributed to Fannie Eshleman, Negro History Files, WPA).

37. *Report, Mercy Hospital* (1923–1924):25, (1924–1926):28–29; Fannie Eshleman, "Tuberculosis Training for Colored Student Nurses," *Public Health Nurse* 15 (Jun 1923):301–3; and idem, "Negro Nurse in a Tb Program," 375–78. In 1935, Eshleman noted that twenty-two of the seventy-seven graduates who had had this training found positions in public health.

38. Esmond R. Long, "Report of the Henry Phipps Institute," *RHPI* 27 (1936–1937):20, and, for Eshleman's observations, Julius L. Wilson, "The History of the Henry Phipps Institute of Philadelphia," typescript, 50, CPP.

39. Long, "Report," 9, 15, 31, and Eugene L. Opie, "The Peripatetic Education of a Pathologist," *Medical Clinics of North America* (Jul 1957):943.

40. Brown, "Tuberculosis Work," 791–94.

41. H. R. M. Landis, "Tb Problem and the Negro," 1926, 378. In 1935, Eshleman still quoted this opinion ("Negro Nurse in a Tb Program," 376).

42. John S. Haller, Jr., *Outcasts from Evolution: Scientific Attitudes of Racial Inferiority, 1859–1900* (Urbana: University of Illinois Press, 1971); George M. Fredrickson, *The Black Image in the White Mind: The Debate on Afro-American Character and Destiny, 1817–1914* (New York: Harper and Row, 1971); Mark Aldrich, "Progressive Economists and Scientific Racism: Walter Willcox and Black Americans, 1895–1910," *Phylon* 40 (Spring 1979):1–14; Carol M. Taylor, "W. E. B. Du Bois's Challenge to Scientific Racism," *Journal of Black Studies* 11 (Jun 1981):449–60; Carter G. Woodson, *The Negro Professional Man and the Community* (Association for the Study of Negro Life and History, 1934; reprint, New York: Negro Universities Press, 1969), 95–96, 143–47; Darlene C. Hine, "The Ethel Johns Report: Black Women in the Nursing Profession, 1925," *Journal of Negro History* 67 (Fall 1982):212–28; and Ethel Johns, "A Study of the Present Status of the Negro Woman in Nursing," 1925, Rockefeller Archives Center.

43. LF to Gifford Pinchot, 3 Mar 1933.

44. LF to Frederick M. Kirby, 29 Nov, 5, 16 Dec 5 1932, and LF to J. S. Caldwell, 1 Dec 1932.

45. Nathan F. Mossell, "Autobiography," typescript, Papers of Nathan F. Mossell, UPT 50 M913, Box 1, folder 1, UPA; W. Montague Cobb, "Nathan Francis Mossell, M.D., 1856–1946," *JNMA* 46 (Mar 1954):118–30; J. H. Gray, "Biographical Sketch of Nathan F. Mossell, M.D.," *ARFD* 25 (1920):18–25; Horace M. Bond, *Education for Freedom: A History of Lincoln University, Pennsylvania* (Lincoln University, Pa.: Lincoln University, 1976), 338–41, 346–50; and Gamble, "Negro Hospital Renaissance," 15–18.

46. "Some Events," 62–68; Du Bois, *Philadelphia Negro*, 230; and *ARPB* 1904–1914.

47. Rudwick, "Brief History," 50–52; and Gamble, "Negro Hospital Renaissance," 19–34.

48. Cobb, "Mossell," 124–25; "Row over Hospital Funds," newspaper clipping, 14 Mar 1917, TUPA; "Appropriation Committee Hears Douglass Case," *Philadelphia Tribune*, 17 Mar 1917; "Douglass Hospital Board of Managers Show Clear Record," *Philadelphia Tribune*, 24 Mar 1917; "Insists upon the Removal of Hospital Chief," *Philadelphia Tribune*, 21 Apr 1917; "Chamber of Commerce Withdrew Endorsement from Douglass Hospital before Controversy," *Philadelphia Tribune*, 5 May 1917; "Douglass Hospital Gets $24000 with String Attached," *Philadelphia Tribune*, 19 May 1917; "Dr. N. F. Mossell Tendered a Large Reception," *Philadelphia Tribune*, 16 Jun 1917; "Doctor Mossell Makes an Explicit Criticism of the Actions of the State Board of Charities," *Philadelphia Tribune*, 22 Feb 1919; "State Aid Refused Douglass Hospital," *Public Ledger*, 20 Feb 1919; "State Board Aims to Oust Mossell," *Public Ledger*, 12 Jul 1919; "Douglass Hospital Loses $22,000 by Board's Choice," *Philadelphia Inquirer*, 1919, LFSB, vol. 4; and "Chronology, 1917–1920," *ARFD* (1920):111–12. The Charities Bureau endorsed organizations as worthy of contributions; the Welfare Federation, which succeeded it, raised funds for its member organizations.

49. Johns, "Study," Exhibit E, 8–10; Gray, "Biographical Sketch"; and Patrick O'Connell, "Abstract of Address," *ARFD* (1920):27–28.

50. Gordon, "FDMH and TS," 60; *ARFD* 2 (1897):35; and "State Board Aims to Oust Mossell." See also Mossell, Autobiographical Writings, Papers of Nathan F. Mossell, folder 2; idem, "Modern Hospital," 133–34, idem, "Report of Medical Director and Superintendent," *ARFD* 25 (1920):35–37; idem, "An Address on Hospital Efficiency," *ARFD* 18–20 (1916):13–15; idem, an untitled statement, LFCU, 25 Apr 1933; and N[athan] F. Mossell to the Board of Managers of the FDMH, 11 Jan 1935, LFCU.

51. Johns, "Study," Exhibit E, 8–9. Johns found Minton to be "a cultured gentleman" and "by far the most outstanding negro physician in the public health field" ("Study," 35, and Exhibit E, 3).

52. According to Emerson, *Philadelphia Hospital and Health Survey*, 579, 695–96, 709, occupancy rates at Douglass between 1924 and 1928 ranged from 27 to 37 percent of capacity, the lowest recorded in Philadelphia hospitals. State appropriations varied between $6,322 and $8,550. Occupancy rates at Mercy during this period ranged from 60 to 72 percent. For conditions at Douglass and the state requests, see Mrs. I. Albert Liveright to Charles A. Lewis, 1 Jun 1933, attached to Gifford Pinchot to LF, 2 Jun 1933.

53. Memo, Betty Read to [Charles] Israel, 29 Sep [1932], *Bulletin* file, TUPA; LF to Seth A. Brumm, 20 Jan 1933; and LF to Lawrence Farrell, 28 Jan 1933. According to the 1938 directory of the National Tuberculosis Association, Mercy Hospital opened a small tuberculosis ward in 1933.

54. LF to Fred. M. Kirby, 25 Jan 1933 (for first quotation); LF to Lessing J. Rosenwald, 11 Feb 1933 (for second quotation); LF to Richard J. Beamish, 17 Feb 1933 (for third quotation), 22 Feb 1933; LF to Michael M. Davis, 23 Feb 1933; LF to Gifford Pinchot, 3 Mar 1933 (for fourth quotation); Seth A. Brumm to LF, 19 Jan 1933; Michael M. Davis to LF, 27 Feb 1933, and LF to Fred. M. Kirby, 4 Mar 1933 (for fifth quotation).

55. LF to Fred. M. Kirby, 4 Mar 1933; LF to Richard J. Beamish, 14 Mar 1933; and LF to N. F. Mossell, 23, 27 Mar 1933.

56. LF to C. H. Garlick, 30 Mar 1933; LF to Gifford Pinchot, 29 May 1933; "Dr. Flick Appeals for Hospital Aid," *Philadelphia Inquirer*, 4 Jun 1933, sec. 1; LF to the Board of Directors of the Free Hospital for Poor Consumptives and White Haven Sanatorium Association, 7 Jun 1933; "Dr. Flick Obtains $1,000 for Douglass," *Philadelphia Record*, 10 Jun 1933; LF to Wm. H. Heard, 12 Jun 1933; LF to Fred. M. Kirby, 12 Jun 1933; "Belated State Funds Will Save Douglass," *Philadelphia Tribune*, 8 Feb 1934.

57. "Unveil Flick Plaque," *Evening Bulletin*, 30 Apr 1937, a clipping, TUPA; LF to William C. Duncan, 24 Mar 1934; LF to Harry A. Mackey, 28 Apr 1936; LF to N. F. Mossell, 28 Apr 1937; Papers of Sadie T. Mossell Alexander, UPT 50, A374, STMA 77, folders 57, 58; and *ARsFH*.

58. Gray, "Biographical Sketch," 24 (for the quotation); Bond, *Education for Freedom*, 350; N. F. Mossell, untitled statement, LFCU; Mossell, Autobiographical Writings; "Mossell Forced off Board of Douglass Hospital When State Denies Appropriation," *Philadelphia Tribune*, 22 Jun 1933, 3; Franklin, *Education*, 67–68; and Meier, *Negro Thought in America*.

59. For the politics of Mercy-Douglass, see for starters the clippings on the hospitals, TUPA. The hospitals had the support of competing factions within the Republican party, members of which helped to raise funds. In 1919, Mercy Hospital, following the advice of the Chamber of Commerce and the State Board of Public Charities, moved out of the central city, which was crowded with white hospitals, to southwest Philadelphia. Douglass remained in the highly competitive environment.

60. *The Whittier Centre* [Nov 1, 1913], 3.

Chapter 17. The Decline of Tuberculosis

1. Flick had his paper, *The Crusade Against Tuberculosis in Philadelphia*, published privately in 1932, and made three hundred copies available at the Society's meeting (LF to Francis A. Faught, 12 Nov 1932). Page numbers are from that version. The paper was also published in the Society's *Weekly Roster and Medical Digest* 28 (26 Nov 1932):17–30. Flick could only estimate the numbers of Philadelphians isolated. He tried to persuade institutions to cull their statistical data

for Philadelphians. When they did not, he made estimates. The numbers were inaccurate, as Flick acknowledged.

2. "Health Seal Sale Funds Misspent, Dr. Flick Asserts," *Public Ledger*, 24 Nov 1932, and "Physicians Differ on Seal-Sale Row," *Public Ledger*, 25 Nov 1932. See also "Flick Criticism of Seal Fund Use Assailed, Upheld," *Philadelphia Inquirer*, 25 Nov 1932. Flick made another attack on the Pennsylvania Society and the Philadelphia Health Council in *The Pennsylvania Society for the Prevention of Tuberculosis* (n.p., 1935).

3. Annual rates of death from tuberculosis of the lungs and from all forms of tuberculosis were reported by the city's health department. The names of both the department and the reports vary, and periodic minor revisions and other changes affected the figures. Errors in estimating the city's population between the decennial counts of the federal census caused some erratic fluctuations in these rates, and diagnostic uncertainties persisted throughout the period.

4. J. Willoughby Irwin, "A Statistical Study of Tuberculosis in Philadelphia for the Time of Official Registration, 1861 to 1903, Inclusive," *RPI* (1904):89–118. Irwin's figures generally agree with the health department's. His "tuberculosis" (90–93) included consumption of the lungs (by far the biggest subgroup), hemorrhage of the lungs, lupus (tuberculosis of the skin), scrofula (tuberculosis of the lymph nodes of the neck), ulceration of the lungs, hectic fever, and consumption of the bowels, larynx, liver, stomach, kidney, and bladder. For diagnoses in "probably" and "possibly tuberculosis," see pp. 94–97, 100–103.

5. LF, *Crusade*, 9, and, for an earlier update of Irwin's study, LF, "The Progress in the Tuberculosis Campaign in Pennsylvania up to 1911," *International Clinics*, 21st ser., vol. 2 (1911):89–113. Around 1904, when the health department changed its nomenclature, the rates for diagnoses that Flick included in his "probably tuberculosis" plummeted dramatically. There was no reciprocal rise in the rates of death from tuberculosis of the lungs. Rates of tuberculosis in all forms did rise for a few years, but only moderately.

6. LF, *Crusade*, 10, and H. R. M. Landis, "The Tuberculosis Crusade," *PMJ* 17 (Nov 1913):103.

7. E. M. E. Flick, *Beloved Crusader: Lawrence F. Flick, Physician* (Philadelphia: Dorrance, 1944), 7 (for the quotation).

8. For a way to understand this process, see Mary Douglas, *How Institutions Think* (Syracuse, N.Y.: Syracuse University Press, 1986).

9. Frederick L. Hoffman, "The Decline in the Tuberculous Death-Rate, 1871–1912," *TNA* 9 (1913):101–37; Thomas McKeown and R. G. Record, "Reasons for the Decline of Mortality in England and Wales during the Nineteenth Century," *Population Studies* 16 (Nov 1962):104, 108–9; and Simon Szreter, "The Importance of Social Intervention in Britain's Mortality Decline c. 1850–1914: A Re-interpretation of the Role of Public Health," *Social History of Medicine* 1 (April 1988):1–37. According to Hoffman (116–17), the rates of death per 100,000 from pulmonary tuberculosis in fifty American cities dropped from 318 in the decade 1872–81 to 186 in 1902–11. Rates for Massachusetts, Rhode Island, and Connecticut combined fell over this period from 291 to 146.

10. Mary Dempsey, ed., "Statistical Data," *ART* 46 (Oct 1942):452.

11. LF to Irvin P. Knipe, 24 Mar 1927.

12. William Osler's textbook, *The Principles and Practice of Medicine* (New York: D. Appleton), first mentioned the diagnostic use of x-rays in tuberculosis in its 8th edition, which was revised by Thomas McCrae of Jefferson Medical College in 1912. X-ray examination, although acknowledged to be of great value when used skillfully, could not prove the cause or the activity of lung disease. "More than any others," the author cautioned, "radiographers need the salutary lessons of the dead house to correct their visionary interpretations of shadows." A somewhat softened admonition persisted in the text through at least 1938.

For a sampling of results, see J. A. Rutledge and John B. Crouch, "The Ultimate Results in 1,654 Cases of Tuberculosis Treated at the Modern Woodmen of America Sanatorium," *ART* 2 (Feb 1919):755–63; H. E. Hilleboe, "The Comparative Mortality of Patients Discharged from Tuberculosis Sanatoria," *ART* 34 (Dec 1936):713–24; idem, "Post-Sanatorium Tuberculosis Survival Rates in Minnesota," *Public Health Reports* 56 (23 Apr 1941):895–907; Stefan Grzybowski and Donald A. Enarson, "The Fate of Cases of Pulmonary Tuberculosis under Various Treatment Programmes," *Bulletin of the International Union Against Tuberculosis* 53 (Jun 1978):70–75; and K. Styblo, "State of the Art. I. Epidemiology of Tuberculosis," *Bulletin of the International Union Against Tuberculosis* 53 (Sep 1978):145, 147. Within the minimal, moderatedly-advanced, and far-advanced groups, patients with demonstrable bacilli in their sputum had much worse outlooks than those without them. Those without bacilli included unknown numbers of people with inactive tuberculosis or nontuberculous diseases. Changing classifications of the stage of disease complicate comparisons over time. Compared to physical examination, x-ray studies identified more patients and detected a greater extent of disease.

For diagnostic error, see chap. 14, n. 36; also Thomas McCrae and Elmer H. Funk, "The Diagnosis of Chronic Pulmonary Tuberculosis," *JAMA* 73 (19 Jul 1919):161–65; B. Stivelman, "Conditions Commonly Mistaken for Pulmonary Tuberculosis: Report of a Study of 1700 Consecutive Cases," *ART* 4 (Jan 1921): 856–65; and Carolyn K. Wells, et al., "Diagnostic Criteria and Technology as Sources for Changing Incidences of Pulmonary Diseases," *American Journal of Medicine* 88 (Feb 1990):117–22.

13. For evaluation of bed rest with chemotherapy, see Nicholas D. D'Esopo, "Clinical Trials in Pulmonary Tuberculosis," *American Review of Respiratory Disease* 125 (Mar 1982, pt. 2):87–88.

14. A study by Norman G. Hawkins, Robert Davies, and Thomas H. Holmes, "Evidence of Psychosocial Factors in the Development of Tuberculosis," *American Review of Tuberculosis and Pulmonary Diseases* 75 (May 1957):768–80, is frequently cited, but its research design is flawed. Most important, the dependent variable, tuberculosis, almost certainly contributed to the measured independent variable, a "life-organizational stress situation."

15. Theodore B. Sachs, "Artificial Pneumothorax in the Treatment of Pulmonary Tuberculosis: Results Obtained by Twenty-four American Observers," *JAMA* 65 (27 Nov 1915):1861–66; Joseph Walsh, "Artificial Pneumothorax with Necropsy," *ART* 9 (Jun 1924):337–45; Max Pinner, *Pulmonary Tuberculosis in the Adult: Its Fundamental Aspects* (Springfield, Ill.: Charles C. Thomas, 1945), 481–

82; and John D. Boice, Jr., and Richard R. Monson, "Breast Cancer in Women After Repeated Fluoroscopic Examinations of the Chest," *Journal of the National Cancer Institute* 59 (Sep 1977):823–32. Pneumothorax also had strong advocates until effective chemotherapy was established.

16. Robert F. Martin, *National Income in the United States, 1799–1938* (New York: National Industrial Conference Board, 1939; reprint, Arno Press, 1976), 4–17.

17. John S. Chapman and Margaret D. Dyerly, "Social and Other Factors in Intrafamilial Transmission of Tuberculosis," *American Review of Respiratory Diseases* 90 (Jul 1964):48–60, and Gretchen A. Condran and Rose A. Cheney, "Mortality Trends in Philadelphia: Age- and Cause-Specific Death Rates 1870–1930," *Demography* 19 (Feb 1982):118–19.

18. Edith M. Lincoln, "Epidemics of Tuberculosis," *Advances in Tuberculosis Research* 14 (1965):57–201; V. N. Houk, et al., "The Epidemiology of Tuberculosis Infection in a Closed Environment," *Archives of Environmental Health* 16 (Jan 1968):26–35; George D. Hanzel, "Tuberculosis Control in the United States Navy: 1875–1966," *Archives of Environmental Health* 16 (Jan 1968):7–21; William W. Stead, "Undetected Tuberculosis in Prison: Source of Infection for Community at Large," *JAMA* 240 (1 Dec 1978):2544–47; Charles B. Mosher, "Unusually Aggressive Transmission of Tuberculosis in a Factory," *Journal of Occupational Medicine* 29 (Jan 1987):29–31; William W. Stead, et al., "Tuberculosis as an Endemic and Nosocomial Infection among the Elderly in Nursing Homes," *New England Journal of Medicine* 312 (6 Jun 1985):1483–87; E. Nardell, et al., "Exogenous Reinfection with Tuberculosis in a Shelter for the Homeless," *New England Journal of Medicine* 315 (18 Dec 1986):1570–75; and David J. Rothman, *The Discovery of the Asylum: Social Order and Disorder in the New Republic* (Boston: Little, Brown, 1971.) At the Philadelphia Hospital in 1875, for example, physicians attributed one-third of the deaths on the medical wards and one-fifth of the deaths in the Insane Department to phthisis of the lungs; in the city's House of Correction, this fraction reached almost one-tenth (*AMP* [1875]:659–60, 664–71, 1258–59).

19. C. R. Vernon Gibbs, *Passenger Liners of the Western Ocean*, 2nd ed. (New York: John de Graff, 1957); Maldwyn A. Jones, *Destination America* (New York: Holt, Rinehart and Winston, 1976), 24–44; Philip Taylor, *The Distant Magnet: European Immigration to the U.S.A.* (New York: Harper and Row, 1971), 131–41; and Kerby A. Miller, *Emigrants and Exiles: Ireland and the Irish Exodus to North America* (New York: Oxford University Press, 1985), 252–63.

20. Gibbs, *Passenger Liners* (29–30, 125, 157, 180 for passage times), and Jones, *Destination America*, 40.

21. Morrill Wyman, *A Practical Treatise on Ventilation* (Cambridge, [Mass.]: Metcalf and Co., 1846); John H. Griscom, *The Uses and Abuses of Air*, 3rd ed. (New York: Redfield, 1854); David Boswell Reid, *Ventilation in American Dwellings* (New York: Wiley and Halsted, 1866); H[arriet] B[eecher] Stowe, "The Chimney-Corner for 1866. VII. Bodily Religion: A Sermon on Good Health," *Atlantic Monthly* 18 (Jul 1866):85–93; Lewis W. Leeds, *A Treatise on Ventilation: Comprising Seven Lectures Before the Franklin Institute, Philadelphia, 1866–68* (New York: John Wiley and Son, 1871); John S. Billings, *The Principles of Ventilation and*

Heating and Their Application, 2nd ed. (New York: Sanitary Engineer, 1884); Charles E. Rosenberg, *The Care of Strangers: The Rise of America's Hospital System* (New York: Basic Books, 1987), 122–41; and Nancy Tomes, "The Private Side of Public Health: Sanitary Science, Domestic Hygiene, and the Germ Theory, 1870–1900," *BHM* 64 (Winter 1990):509–39.

22. The Hagley Museum and Library, Greenville, Delaware, has a rich collection of trade catalogs, pamphlets, and books on heating and ventilation, e.g., S. A. Harrison, *Hints on Warming and Ventilation of Public and Private Buuildings* [1852]; *Peters and Johnson's Warming and Ventilation Apparatus, As Applied to Churches, Public Buildings, Halls, Factories, Stores, School-Houses, and Private Dwellings* (Boston, 1853); Henry A. Gouge, *New System of Ventilating Which Has Been Tested under the Patronage of Many Distinguished Persons* (New York, 1866); Morris, Tasker and Co., *Tasker's Patent Self-regulating Hot Water Furnace Adapted to Warm Private Residences, Hospitals, Churches, Halls of Justice, Conservatories, School and Green Houses* (Philadelphia, 1868); and *Ventilation and Warming of Buildings, upon the Principles As Designed and Patented by Isaac D. Smead* (Toledo, Ohio: Isaac D. Smead and Co., 1889). Neither the trade publications nor the reformers are good sources with which to assess actual ventilation. The trade typically judged as inadequate all devices except the splendid ones they were currently selling. Reformers continued to be dissatisfied.

23. George T. Palmer, "What Fifty Years Have Done for Ventilation," in *A Half Century of Public Health*, ed. Mazÿck P. Ravenel (New York: American Public Health Association, 1921), 342–44; C.-E. A. Winslow, *Fresh Air and Ventilation* (New York: E. P. Dutton, 1926), 90–91; *Illustrated Catalogue of B. F. Sturtevant's Pressure Blowers and Exhaust Fans* (Boston, 1873); C. S. Onderdonk, *The Blackman's Wheel* (Philadelphia, 1880); George M. Kober, "History of Industrial Hygiene and Its Effects on Public Health," in Ravenel, *Half Century*, 375; and J. Lynn Barnard, *Factory Legislation in Pennsylvania: Its History and Administration* (Philadelphia: University of Pennsylvania, 1907), 59.

24. Leeds, *Treatise*, 70, 167–68; Susan Strasser, *Never Done: A History of American Housework* (New York: Pantheon Books, 1982), 53–54; and Ruth S. Cowan, *More Work for Mother: The Ironies of Household Technology from the Open Hearth to the Microwave* (New York: Basic Books), 53–61, 96–97.

25. Condran and Cheney, "Mortality Trends," 115–16; Richard O. Cummings, *The American and His Food: A History of Food Habits in the United States* (Chicago: University of Chicago Press, 1940), 53–90; Daniel J. Boorstin, *The Americans: The Democratic Experience* (New York: Vintage Books, 1974), 313–30; Cowan, *More Work for Mother*, 20–22, 71–73; Strasser, *Never Done*, 11–31; Robert W. Fogel, "Nutrition and the Decline in Mortality Since 1700: Some Preliminary Findings," *Studies in Income and Wealth* 51 (1986):465; and Grace Wyshak and Rose E. Frisch, "Evidence for a Secular Trend in Age of Menarche," *New England Journal of Medicine* 306 (29 Apr 1982):1033–35. As Fogel notes (446), height reflects nutritional intake minus the claims against it, e.g., physical activity and infections. Thus, rising height [and earlier menstruation] may be due to rising food intake, decreased physical exertion, or decreased infections of various kinds. Their meaning is therefore arguable.

26. For a classic review of these factors, see Rene and Jean Dubos, *The White Plague: Tuberculosis, Man, and Society* (Boston: Little, Brown, 1952). As the quality of milk improved, bovine tuberculosis (which mainly caused nonpulmonary disease in children) undoubtedly decreased during the twentieth century. Because bovine tuberculosis seldom produced lung disease in adults, this improvement does not explain the falling rates of death from tuberculosis of the lungs.

27. E. R. N. Grigg, "The Arcana of Tuberculosis," *American Review of Tuberculosis and Pulmonary Diseases* 78 (Aug, Sep, Oct 1958):151–72, 426–53, 583–603; George W. Comstock, "Tuberculosis in Twins: A Re-Analysis of the Prophit Survey," *American Review of Respiratory Disease* 117 (Apr 1978):621–24; and, for the critic, Guy P. Youmans, *Tuberculosis* (Philadelphia: W. B. Saunders, 1979), 362–63.

28. Death rates from 1905 through 1915 come from *AMP* (1930):384–85; those from 1920 through 1935, from *AMP* (1938):450. Inadequate enumeration of the black population made the rates for blacks especially faulty and volatile. For national figures, see Anthony M. Lowell, "Tuberculosis Morbidity and Mortality and Its Control," in *Tuberculosis* (Cambridge, Mass.: Harvard University Press, 1969), 69–70.

Chapter 18. Conclusions and Epilogue

1. For two other campaigns, see James T. Patterson, *The Dread Disease: Cancer and Modern American Culture* (Cambridge: Harvard University Press, 1987), and Allan M. Brandt, *No Magic Bullet: A Social History of Venereal Disease in the United States Since 1880*, expanded ed. (New York: Oxford University Press, 1987).

2. Lewis Thomas, *The Lives of a Cell: Notes of a Biology Watcher* (New York: Viking Press, 1974), 31–36.

3. Ella M. E. Flick, *Dr. Lawrence F. Flick, 1856–1938* (n.p.: White Haven Sanatorium Association, 1940), 47, and LF to Robert L. Pitfield, 11 Nov 1936.

4. LF to Sr. Mary Louis, 16 Nov 1937, and LF to Mr. and Mrs. C. F. Snowden, 2 May 1935.

5. LF to Mrs. Bessie Karr, 18 Jun 1938, and "Lawrence F. Flick, Jr., Dies," *Bulletin of the Pennsylvania Tuberculosis Society* 26 (Nov–Dec 1945):11. The autopsy report is at the Pennsylvania Hospital.

6. Horace M. Bond, *Education for Freedom: A History of Lincoln University, Pennsylvania* (Lincoln University, Pa.: Lincoln University, 1976), 350, 551; W. Montague Cobb, "Nathan Francis Mossell, M.D., 1856–1946," *JNMA* 46 (Mar 1954):122; and "In Penn Procession," *Philadelphia Tribune*, 26 Sep 1940.

7. Elliott M. Rudwick, "A Brief History of Mercy-Douglass Hospital in Philadelphia," *Journal of Negro Education* 20 (Winter 1951), 54–66; "Mercy-Douglass—A Victim of Integration," *Philadelphia Inquirer*, 29 Jul 1973, sec. B; and "Neighbors Seek Voice on Future of Mercy-Douglass Site," *Philadelphia Inquirer*, 9 Dec 1982, sec. B.

8. *Pennsylvania Manual* (1939):95, (1961–1962):813, (1965–1966):822,

and Julius H. Comroe, Jr., "Pay Dirt: The Story of Streptomycin," *American Review of Respiratory Disease* 117 (Apr, May 1978):773–81, 957–68.

9. The intended state sanatorium in western Pennsylvania (Butler) first opened in 1942 as a U.S. Army hospital. In 1946, it became a Veterans Administration hospital.

10. Frank A. Craig, *The Story of the White Haven Sanatorium* (n.p., n.d.), 7, 23–24.

Bibliography of Selected Secondary Sources

Ackerknecht, Erwin H. *A Short History of Medicine*. 1955. Revised printing. New York: Ronald Press, 1968.

Aldrich, Mark. "Progressive Economists and Scientific Racism: Walter Willcox and Black Americans, 1895–1910." *Phylon* 40 (Spring 1979):1–14.

Baker, S. Josephine. *Fighting for Life*. New York: Macmillan, 1939.

Ballard, Allen B. *One More Day's Journey: The Making of Black Philadelphia*. Philadelphia: ISHI Publications, 1987.

Baur, John E. "The Health Seeker in the Westward Movement, 1830–1900." *Mississippi Valley Historical Review* 46 (Jun 1959):91–110.

Bordley, James III, and A. McGehee Harvey. *Two Centuries of American Medicine, 1776–1976*. Philadelphia: W. B. Saunders, 1976.

Boyer, Paul. *Urban Masses and Moral Order in America, 1820–1920*. Cambridge, Mass.: Harvard University Press, 1978.

Brainard, Annie M. *The Evolution of Public Health Nursing*. Philadelphia: W. B. Saunders, 1922.

Brieger, Gert H. "The Use and Abuse of Medical Charities in Late Nineteenth Century America." *American Journal of Public Health* 67 (Mar 1977):264–67.

Bryder, Linda. *Below the Magic Mountain: A Social History of Tuberculosis in Twentieth-Century Britain*. Oxford: Clarendon Press, 1988.

Buhler-Wilkerson, Karen A. "False Dawn: The Rise and Decline of Public Health Nursing, 1900–1930." Ph.D diss., University of Pennsylvania, 1984.

Burt, Nathaniel, and Wallace E. Davies. "The Iron Age 1876–1905." In *Philadelphia: A 300-Year History*. Edited by Russell F. Weigley. New York: W. W. Norton, 1982.

Carnegie, Mary E. *The Path We Tread: Blacks in Nursing, 1854–1984*. Philadelphia: J. B. Lippincott Co., 1986.

Cayleff, Susan E. *Wash and Be Healed: The Water-Cure Movement and Women's Health*. Philadelphia: Temple University Press, 1987.

Clement, Priscilla F. "The Response to Need, Welfare and Poverty in Philadelphia, 1800 to 1850." Ph.D. diss., University of Pennsylvania, 1977.

Cobb, W. Montague. "Nathan Francis Mossell, M.D., 1856–1946." *Journal of the National Medical Association* 46 (Mar 1954):118–30.

Cobb, W. Montague. "Henry McKee Minton, 1870–1946." *Journal of the National Medical Association* 47 (Jul 1955):285–86.

Corner, George W. *A History of the Rockefeller Institute, 1901–1953: Origins and Growth*. New York: Rockefeller Institute Press, 1964.

Corner, George W. *Two Centuries of Medicine: A History of the School of Medicine, University of Pennsylvania*. Philadelphia: J. B. Lippincott, 1965.

Corper, H. J. "The Centenary of the Birth of Hermann Brehmer." *Colorado Medicine* 24 (Jan 1927):16–19.

Costin, Lela B. *Two Sisters for Social Justice: A Biography of Grace and Edith Abbott.* Urbana: University of Illinois Press, 1983.

Craig, Frank A. *Early Days at Phipps.* Henry Phipps Institute for the Study and Prevention of Tuberculosis, University of Pennsylvania, 1952.

Craig, Frank A. *The Story of the White Haven Sanatorium.* N.p., n.d.

Dain, Norman. *Concepts of Insanity in the United States, 1789–1865.* New Brunswick, N.J.: Rutgers University Press, 1964.

Davis, Allen. *Spearheads for Reform: The Social Settlements and the Progressive Movement, 1890–1914.* New York: Oxford University Press, 1967.

Donegan, Jane B. *"Hydropathic Highway to Health": Women and Water-Cure in Antebellum America.* New York: Greenwood Press, 1986.

Douglas, Mary. *How Institutions Think.* Syracuse, N.Y.: Syracuse University Press, 1986.

Dubos, Rene, and Jean Dubos. *The White Plague: Tuberculosis, Man and Society.* Boston: Little, Brown, 1952.

Fellman, Anita Clair, and Michael Fellman. *Making Sense of Self: Medical Advice Literature in Late Nineteenth-Century America.* Philadelphia: University of Pennsylvania Press, 1981.

Flick, Ella M. E. *Dr. Lawrence F. Flick, 1856–1938.* White Haven Sanatorium Association, 1940.

Flick, Ella M. E. *Beloved Crusader: Lawrence F. Flick, Physician.* Philadelphia: Dorrance, 1944.

Flick, Cecilia R. *Dr. Lawrence F. Flick—As I Knew Him* Philadelphia: Dorrance, 1956.

Fox, Daniel M. "Social Policy and City Politics: Tuberculosis Reporting in New York, 1889–1900." *Bulletin of the History of Medicine* 49 (Summer 1975):169–95.

Franklin, Vincent P. *The Education of Black Philadelphia: The Social and Educational History of a Minority Community, 1900–1950.* Philadelphia: University of Pennsylvania Press, 1979.

Frazier, E. Franklin. "Human, All Too Human: The Negro's Vested Interest in Segregation." In *E. Franklin Frazier on Race Relations.* Edited by G. Franklin Edwards. Chicago: University of Chicago Press, 1968.

Fredrickson, George M. *The Black Image in the White Mind: The Debate on Afro-American Character and Destiny, 1817–1914.* New York: Harper and Row, 1971.

Funnell, Charles E. *By The Beautiful Sea: The Rise and High Times of That Great American Resort, Atlantic City.* New York: Alfred A. Knopf, 1975.

Gamble, Vanessa N. "The Negro Hospital Renaissance: The Black Hospital Movement, 1920–1940." Ph.D. diss., University of Pennsylvania, 1987.

Gamble, Vanessa N. Introduction to *Germs Have No Color Line: Blacks and American Medicine, 1900–1940.* New York: Garland Publishing, 1989.

Glassberg, Eudice. "Philadelphians in Need: Client Experiences with Two Philadelphia Benevolent Societies, 1830–1880." Doctor of Social Work diss., University of Pennsylvania, 1979.

Golab, Caroline. "The Immigrant and the City: Poles, Italians, and Jews in Philadelphia, 1870–1920." In *The Peoples of Philadelphia: A History of Ethnic Groups and Lower-Class Life, 1790–1940*. Edited by Allen F. Davis and Mark H. Haller. Philadelphia: Temple University Press, 1973.

Greene, John G. "The Emmanuel Movement, 1906–1929." *New England Quarterly* 7 (Sep 1934):494–532.

Grob, Gerald N. *Mental Institutions in America: Social Policy to 1875*. New York: The Free Press, 1973.

Haller, John S., Jr. *Outcasts from Evolution: Scientific Attitudes of Racial Inferiority, 1859–1900*. Urbana: University of Illinois Press, 1971.

Hamilton, Diane B. "The Metropolitan Life Insurance Company Visiting Nursing Service (1909–1953)." Ph.D. diss., University of Virginia, 1987.

Hendrick, Burton J. *The Life of Andrew Carnegie*. Garden City, N. Y.: Doubleday, Doran, 1932 (q.v. for Henry Phipps also).

Henry, Frederick P., ed. *Founders' Week Memorial Volume*. Philadelphia: City of Philadelphia, 1909.

Hershberg, Theodore, ed. *Philadelphia: Work, Space, Family, and Group Experience in the Nineteenth Century*. Oxford: Oxford University Press, 1981.

Hine, Darlene C. "The Ethel Johns Report: Black Women in the Nursing Profession, 1925." *Journal of Negro History* 67 (Fall 1982):212–28.

Ingalls, Theodore H. "Three Men in Tandem." *Harvard Medical Alumni Bulletin* 37 (Fall 1962):14–21.

Jones, Billy M. *Health Seekers in the Southwest, 1817–1900*. Norman: University of Oklahoma Press, 1967.

Kalisch, Philip A., and Beatrice J. Kalisch. *The Advance of American Nursing*. 2d ed. Boston: Little, Brown, 1986.

Katz, Michael B. *In the Shadow of the Poorhouse: A Social History of Welfare in America*. New York: Basic Books, 1986.

Kinghorn, Hugh M. "Brehmer and Dettweiler: A Review of Their Methods of Treatment of Pulmonary Tuberculosis," *American Review of Tuberculosis* 5 (Feb 1922):950–72.

Klaus, Alisa C. "Women's Organizations and the Infant Health Movement in France and the United States, 1890–1920." In *Lady Bountiful Revisited: Women, Philanthropy, and Power*. Edited by Kathleen D. McCarthy. New Brunswick, N.J.: Rutgers University Press, 1990.

Knopf, S. A[dolphus]. "Hermann Brehmer and the Semi-Centennial Celebration of Brehmer's Sanatorium for the Treatment of Consumptives; The First Institution of Its Kind (July 2, 1854–July 2, 1904)." *New York Medical Journal and Philadelphia Medical Journal* 80 (2 Jul 1904):3–6.

Knopf, S. Adolphus. *A History of the National Tuberculosis Association: The Anti-Tuberculosis Movement in the United States*. New York: National Tuberculosis Association, 1922.

Knopf, S. Adolphus. "Peter Dettweiler (1837–1937): Initiator and Promulgator of the Rest Cure in Pulmonary Tuberculosis, the One Hundredth Anniversary of His Birth." *Medical Record* 147 (18 May 1938):464–67.

Lane, Roger. *Roots of Violence in Black Philadelphia, 1860–1900*. Cambridge, Mass.: Harvard University Press, 1986.

Long, Esmond R. "Weak Lungs on the Santa Fé Trail." *Bulletin of the History of Medicine* 8 (Jul 1940):1040–54.

Ludmerer, Kenneth M. *Learning to Heal: The Development of American Medical Education.* New York: Basic Books, 1985.

McBride, David. *Integrating the City of Medicine: Blacks in Philadelphia Health Care, 1910–1965.* Philadelphia: Temple University Press, 1989.

McCarthy, Kathleen D. "Parallel Power Stuctures: Women and the Voluntary Sphere." In *Lady Bountiful Revisited: Women, Philanthropy, and Power.* Edited by Kathleen D. McCarthy. New Brunswick, N.J.: Rutgers University Press, 1990.

McFarland, Joseph. "The Beginning of Bacteriology in Philadelphia." *Bulletin of the Institute of the History of Medicine* 5 (Feb 1937):149–198.

McKeown, Thomas, and R. G. Record. "Reasons for the Decline of Mortality in England and Wales During the Nineteenth Century." *Population Studies: A Journal of Demography* 16 (Nov 1962):94–122.

Meier, August. *Negro Thought in America, 1880–1915: Racial Ideologies in the Age of Booker T. Washington.* Ann Arbor: University of Michigan Press, 1963.

Minton, Russell F. "The History of Mercy-Douglass Hospital," *JNMA* 43 (May 1951):153–59.

Morais, Herbert M. *The History of the Negro in Medicine.* International Library of Negro Life and History. New York: Publishers Co., 1967–1968.

Morman, Edward T. "Scientific Medicine Comes to Philadelphia: Public Health Transformed, 1854–1899." Ph.D. diss., University of Pennsylvania, 1986.

O'Brien, Patricia. "'All a Woman's Life Can Bring': The Domestic Roots of Nursing in Philadelphia, 1830–1885." *Nursing Research* 36 (Jan/Feb 1987):12–17.

O'Hara, Leo J. *An Emerging Profession: Philadelphia Doctors 1860–1900.* New York: Garland Publishing, 1989.

Price, Esther G. *Pennsylvania Pioneers Against Tuberculosis.* New York: National Tuberculosis Association, 1952.

Rauch, Julia B. "Unfriendly Visitors: The Emergence of Scientific Philanthropy in Philadelphia, 1878–1880." Ph.D. diss., Bryn Mawr College, 1974.

Reniers, Perceval. *The Springs of Virginia: Life, Love, and Death at the Waters.* Chapel Hill: University of North Carolina Press, 1941.

Reverby, Susan M. *Ordered to Care: The Dilemma of American Nursing, 1850–1945.* Cambridge: Cambridge University Press, 1987.

Risse, Guenter B., Ronald L. Numbers, and Judith W. Leavitt, eds. *Medicine Without Doctors: Home Health Care in American History.* New York: Science History Publications/USA, 1977.

Rogers, Frank B. "The Rise and Decline of the Altitude Therapy of Tuberculosis." *Bulletin of the History of Medicine* 43 (Jan–Feb 1969):1–16.

Rosen, George. "The Impact of the Hospital on the Physician, the Patient and the Community." *Hospital Administration* 9 (Fall 1964):15–33.

Rosen, George. *Preventive Medicine in the United States, 1900–1975, Trends and Interpretations.* New York: Prodist, 1977.

Rosenberg, Charles E. "The Therapeutic Revolution: Medicine, Meaning, and Social Change in Nineteenth-Century America." *Perspectives in Biology and Medicine* 20 (Summer 1977):485–506.

Rosenberg, Charles E. "From Almshouse to Hospital: The Shaping of Philadelphia General Hospital." *Milbank Memorial Fund Quarterly/Health and Society* 60 (Winter 1982):108–54.

Rosenberg, Charles E. *The Care of Strangers: The Rise of America's Hospital System.* New York: Basic Books, 1987.

Rothstein, William G. *American Physicians in the Nineteenth Century: From Sects to Science.* Baltimore: Johns Hopkins University Press, 1972.

Rothstein, William G. *American Medical Schools and the Practice of Medicine: A History.* New York: Oxford University Press, 1987.

Rudwick, Elliott M. "A Brief History of Mercy-Douglass Hospital in Philadelphia," *Journal of Negro Education* 20 (Winter 1951):50–66.

Savitt, Todd L. "Lincoln University Medical Department—A Forgotten 19th Century Black Medical School." *Journal of the History of Medicine and Allied Sciences* 40 (Jan 1985):42–65.

Scott, Anne F. "Women's Voluntary Associations: From Charity to Reform." In *Lady Bountiful Revisited: Women, Philanthropy, and Power.* Edited by Kathleen D. McCarthy. New Brunswick, N.J.: Rutgers University Press, 1990.

"Short Life Story of Dr. Lawrence F. Flick and Brief Account of His Work in Tuberculosis." In *The Strittmatter Award, 1933, to Dr. Lawrence F. Flick.* Philadelphia: Philadelphia Medical Society, n.d.

Shryock, Richard H. *American Medical Research, Past and Present.* New York: Commonwealth Fund, 1947.

Shryock, Richard H. *The Development of Modern Medicine: An Interpretation of the Social and Scientific Factors Involved.* New York: Alfred A. Knopf, 1947.

Shryock, Richard H. *National Tuberculosis Association, 1904–1954: A Study of the Voluntary Health Movement in the United States.* New York: National Tuberculosis Association, 1957. Reprint, Arno Press, 1977.

Sigerist, Henry E. "American Spas in Historical Perspective." *Bulletin of the History of Medicine* 11 (Feb 1942):133–47.

Smith-Rosenberg, Carroll. *Religion and the Rise of the American City Mission Movement 1812–1870.* Ithaca, N.Y.: Cornell University Press, 1971.

Smith-Rosenberg, Carroll. *Disorderly Conduct: Visions of Gender in Victorian America.* New York: Alfred A. Knopf, 1985.

Stachniewicz, Stephanie A., and Jean K. Axelrod. *The Double Frill: The History of the Philadelphia General Hospital School of Nursing.* Philadelphia: George F. Stickley, 1978.

Stephens, Irby. "Asheville: The Tuberculosis Era." *North Carolina Medical Journal* 46 (Sep 1985):455–63.

Stephenson, Mary V. *The First Fifty Years of the Training School for Nurses of the Hospital of the University of Pennsylvania.* Philadelphia: J. B. Lippincott, 1940.

Stevens, Rosemary. "Sweet Charity: State Aid to Hospitals in Pennsylvania, 1870–1910." *Bulletin of the History of Medicine* 58 (Fall, Winter 1984):287–314, 474–95.

Stevens, Rosemary. *In Sickness and in Wealth: American Hospitals in the Twentieth Century.* New York: Basic Books, 1989.

Szreter, Simon. "The Importance of Social Intervention in Britain's Mortality Decline c. 1850–1914: A Re-interpretation of the Role of Public Health." *Social History of Medicine* 1 (April 1988):1–37.

Taylor, Carol M. "W. E. B. Du Bois's Challenge to Scientific Racism." *Journal of Black Studies* 11 (Jun 1981):449–60.

Teller, Michael E. *The Tuberculosis Movement: A Public Health Campaign in the Progressive Era*. New York: Greenwood Press, 1988.

Tomes, Nancy. *A Generous Confidence: Thomas Story Kirkbride and the Art of Asylum-Keeping, 1840–1883*. Cambridge: Cambridge University Press, 1984.

Tomes, Nancy. "'Little World of Our Own': The Pennsylvania Hospital Training School for Nurses, 1895–1907." *Journal of the History of Medicine and Allied Sciences* 33 (Oct 1978):507–30.

Torchia, Marion M. "Tuberculosis Among American Negroes: Medical Research on a Racial Disease, 1830–1950." *Journal of the History of Medicine and Allied Sciences* 32 (Jul 1977):252–79.

Trudeau, Edward L. *An Autobiography*. Philadelphia: Lea and Febiger, 1916.

Weiss, Harry B., and Howard R. Kemble. *The Great American Water-Cure Craze: A History of Hydropathy in the United States*. Trenton, N.J.: Past Times Press, 1967.

West, Roberta M. *History of Nursing in Pennsylvania*. Pennsylvania State Nurses' Association, n.d.

Whorton, James C. *Crusaders for Fitness: The History of American Health Reformers*. Princeton, N.J.: Princeton University Press, 1982.

Woodward, C. Vann. *The Strange Career of Jim Crow*. 3rd rev. ed. New York: Oxford University Press, 1974.

Index

University of Pennsylvania Press
Studies in Health, Illness, and Caregiving in America
Joan E. Lynaugh, General Editor

Barbara Bates. *Bargaining for Life: A Social History of Tuberculosis, 1876–1938*. 1992.
Janet Golden and Charles Rosenberg. *Pictures of Health: A Photographic History of Health Care in Philadelphia*. 1991.
Anne Hudson Jones. *Images of Nurses: Perspectives from History, Art, and Literature*. 1987.
June S. Lowenberg. *Caring and Responsibility: The Crossroads Between Holistic Practice and Traditional Medicine*. 1989.
Elizabeth Norman. *Women at War: The Story of Fifty Military Nurses Who Served in Vietnam*. 1990.
Elizabeth Brown Pryor. *Clara Barton, Professional Angel*. 1987.
Zane Robinson Wolf. *Nurses' Work, The Sacred and The Profane*. 1988.

This book has been set in Linotron Galliard. Galliard was designed for Mergenthaler in 1978 by Matthew Carter. Galliard retains many of the features of a sixteenth century typeface cut by Robert Granjon but has some modifications that give it a more contemporary look.

Printed on acid-free paper.